Pre- and Postsynaptic Receptors

MODERN PHARMACOLOGY-TOXICOLOGY
A Series of Monographs and Textbooks

COORDINATING EDITOR
William F. Bousquet
School of Pharmacy and Pharmacal Sciences
Purdue University
West Lafayette, Indiana

ASSOCIATE EDITOR
Roger F. Palmer
University of Miami
School of Medicine
Miami, Florida

Volume 1 A Guide to Molecular Pharmacology-Toxicology, Parts I and II
Edited by R. M. Featherstone

Volume 2 Psychopharmacological Treatment: Theory and Practice
Edited by Herman C. B. Denber

Volume 3 Pre- and Postsynaptic Receptors
Edited by Earl Usdin and William E. Bunney, Jr.

Additional Volumes in Preparation

Pre- and Postsynaptic Receptors

*Proceedings of a study group held at the
Thirteenth Annual Meeting of the
American College of Neuropsychopharmacology,
San Juan, Puerto Rico*

Editors

EARL USDIN
*Psychopharmacology Research Branch
National Institute of Mental Health
Rockville, Maryland*

WILLIAM E. BUNNEY, Jr.
*Adult Psychiatry Branch
National Institute of Mental Health
Bethesda, Maryland*

MARCEL DEKKER, INC. New York

COPYRIGHT © 1975 by MARCEL DEKKER, INC. ALL RIGHTS RESERVED

Neither this book nor any part may be reproduced or transmitted in any form or by any means, electronic or mechanical, including photocopying, microfilming, and recording, or by any information storage and retrieval system, without permission in writing from the publisher.

MARCEL DEKKER, INC.

270 Madison Avenue, New York, New York 10016

LIBRARY OF CONGRESS CATALOG CARD NUMBER: 75-4238

ISBN: 0-8247-6312-2

Current printing (last digit):
10 9 8 7 6 5 4 3 2 1

PRINTED IN THE UNITED STATES OF AMERICA

Preface

Each year the pressure of progress in psychopharmacology forces the program committee of the American College of Neuropsychopharmacology (ACNP) to prune carefully among the many proposed study groups. For the meeting of December 10-13, 1974 in San Juan, there were two proposed study groups (Bunney and Bloom; Usdin and Lovenberg) which had a common theme: pre- and postsynaptic receptors. The ACNP Council decided to combine these into one workshop. The interest in this combined workshop was attested by the fact that it had to be relocated to the largest available convention room to accommodate the large audience. Large size of audience is, of course, a mixed blessing: it indicates interest, but it also tends to inhibit interchange between speakers and the audience. It is hoped that such interchange has not been too badly stifled; the reader must reach his decision on the basis of the summaries of discussion at the end of each paper.

The papers covered the current state-of-the-art (and beyond) of both technique and theory. We are deeply appreciative that the authors were willing to discuss in San Juan and publish here many of their exciting unpublished results; we are also appreciative of the efforts of authors who have prepared succinct summaries of the present thinking in several sub-fields of receptor research.

Although it was not possible to have all of the leaders in the field present their work in a small workshop, we feel that we have good representation not only of American scientists, but also of their Swedish and English colleagues. We should like to thank the College and Marcel Dekker, Inc. for their financial (and other) support.

The helpful assistance of the ACNP Secretary-Treasurer, Dr. Alberto DiMascio, and his secretary, Ms. Lorraine Josof, is most gratefully acknowledged, as well as the long and loyal help in transcribing tapes, etc. of my secretaries, Ms. Dorothy Eisel and Mr. Michael Sprague.

Earl Usdin

This book was edited by Drs. Usdin and Bunney in their private capacities. No official support or endorsement by the NIMH is intended or should be inferred.

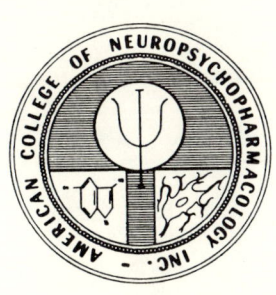

OFFICERS FOR 1974
AMERICAN COLLEGE OF NEUROPSYCHOPHARMACOLOGY

Leo E. Hollister, M.D., *President*
Philip R. A. May, M.D., *President-Elect*
Morris A. Lipton, Ph.D., M.D., *Secretary-Treasurer*
Jonathan O. Cole, M.D., *Assistant Secretary-Treasurer*
J. Richard Wittenborn, Ph.D., *Past-President*

Contents

INTRODUCTORY REMARKS

William E. Bunney, Jr.   1

DOPAMINE NEURONS: ROLE OF IMPULSE FLOW AND PRESYNAPTIC RECEPTORS IN THE REGULATION OF TYROSINE HYDROXYLASE

P.H. Roth, J.R. Walters, L.C. Murrin, and V.H. Morgenroth,III   5

    Introduction   5
    Effects of increased impulse flow in tyrosine hydroxylase   7
    Effects of inhibition of impulse flow on tyrosine hydroxylase   20
    Presynaptic receptor modulation of the activation of tyrosine hydroxylase produced by increased impulse flow   28
    Presynaptic receptor modulation of the activation of tyrosine hydroxylase produced by inhibition of impulse flow   32
    Summary   39
    Acknowledgments   41
    References   41

    Discussion   46

RECEPTOR-MEDIATED CONTROL OF DOPAMINE METABOLISM

A. Carlsson   49

    Introduction   49
    Complexity of receptor-mediated feedback control   49
    Possible implications of presynaptic receptors (or "Autoreceptors")   51
    Functional significance of receptor-mediated feedback control of transmitter synthesis   56
    Concluding remarks   57
    References   61

    Discussion   63

PHYSIOLOGICAL ASSESSMENT OF PRE- AND POSTSYNAPTIC RECEPTORS

F. E. Bloom   67

    Introduction   67
    Presynaptic receptors   68

Reflections of the long-loop feedbacks in neuronal
    discharge rates   72
Descriptive levels of analysis   77
Conclusions   79
References   82

Discussion   86

EVIDENCE FOR DRUG ACTIONS ON BOTH PRE- AND POSTSYNAPTIC CAT-
ECHOLAMINE RECEPTORS IN THE CNS

B.S. Bunney and G.K. Aghajanian   89

Introduction   89
Biochemical studies in CNS   91
Physiological studies in CNS   97
Summary and conclusions   108
Acknowledgments   112
References   113

Discussion   120

DOPAMINE-SENSITIVE ADENYLATE CYCLASE AND PROTEIN PHOSPHOR-
YLATION IN THE RAT CAUDATE NUCLEUS

Bruce K. Krueger, Javier Forn and Paul Greengard   123

Introduction   123
Regulation of adenylate cyclase activity in cell-free
    systems   125
Regulation of cyclic AMP levels in slices   134
Regulation of endogenous protein phosphorylation   138
Concluding remarks   141
References   144

Discussion   146

MECHANISMS OF RECEPTOR MEDIATED REGULATION OF CATECHOLAMINE
SYNTHESIS IN BRAIN

Walter Lovenberg and Eleanor A. Bruckwick   149

Introduction   149
In vivo synthetic rates and synthetic capacity   150
Mechanism and kinetic properties of brain tyrosine
    hydroxylase   151
Cofactor levels   153
Effect of dopamine agonists and antagonists on dopamine
    turnover   155
Receptor mediated feedback inhibition   156

CONTENTS

Neurotransmitter sensitive adenylate cyclases	157
Effects of neuroleptics on the kinetic properties of tyrosine hydroxylase	157
Attempts to define molecular events that occur during the transformation of tyrosine hydroxylase	158
Concluding remarks	164
References	166
Discussion	168

BEHAVIORAL SEQUELAE OF DOPAMINERGIC DEGENERATION: POSTSYNAPTIC SUPERSENSITIVITY?
Ian Creese and Susan D. Iver — 171

References	185
Discussion	188

BIOCHEMICAL IDENTIFICATION OF THE POSTSYNAPTIC SEROTONIN RECEPTOR IN MAMMALIAN BRAIN
Solomon H. Snyder and James P. Bennett, Jr. — 191

Subcellular localization	193
Regional Distribution of receptor binding and the effect of raphe lesions	193
Binding of LSD *in vivo* competes with endogenous serotonin	197
Saturation of LSD binding	197
Relative affinity of drugs and neurotransmitters for LSD and serotonin binding sites	200
A model for conformational alterations of the post-synaptic serotonin receptor	201
References	204
Discussion	205

STRUCTURE-ACTIVITY RELATIONSHIPS FOR AGONIST AND ANTAGONIST DRUGS AT PRE- AND POSTSYNAPTIC DOPAMINE RECEPTOR SITES IN RAT BRAIN
L.L. Iversen, A.S. Horn and R.J. Miller — 207

Introduction	207
Actions of agonists on cyclic AMP formation	208
Neuroleptic drugs as antagonists of dopamine-sensitive cyclic AMP formation in striatal homogenates	214
Effects of neuroleptic drugs on other transmitter and hormone receptors	226
Presynaptic actions of dopaminergic drugs	230
Effects of intracerebral injection of cholera toxin	233
References	235
Discussion	241

CRITERIA FOR AND PITFALLS IN THE IDENTIFICATION OF RECEPTORS

P. Cuatrecasas   245

    Introduction   245
    Problems and Pitfalls in the Study of Hormone Receptors   246
    Acknowledgment   262
    References   262

    Discussion   263

PINEAL BETA-ADRENERGIC RECEPTOR: REGULATION OF SENSITIVITY

Jorge A. Romero and Julius Axelrod   265

    Introduction   265
    Control of N-Acetyltransferase activity   268
    Receptor super- and subsenitivity   269
    References   280

    Discussion   282

STRATEGIES FOR THE SYSTEMATIC STUDY OF NEUROTRANSMITTER RECEPTOR FUNCTION IN MAN

William E. Bunney, Jr. and Dennis A. Murphy   283

    Introduction   283
    Pharmacological strategies   288
    Strategies utilizing lesions   303
    Strategies utilizing tissue models   304
    Possible neuronal receptor site sensitvity changes in bipolar manic-depressive illness   307
    Summary   308
    References   309

    Discussion   312

INDEX   313

Authors and Active Participants

Martin W. Adler
Department of Pharmacology, Temple University School of Medicine, Philadelphia, PA 19140

G. K. Aghajanian
Department of Psychiatry, Yale University School of Medicine, New Haven, CT 06520

Julius Axelrod
National Institute of Mental Health, Bethesda, MD 20014

James P. Bennett
Department of Pharmacology and Experimental Therapeutics, Johns Hopkins University School of Medicine, Baltimore, MD 21205

F. E. Bloom
National Institute of Mental Health, St. Elizabeth's Hospital, Washington, D. C. 20032

Eleanor A. Bruckwick
National Heart and Lung Institute, Bethesda, MD 20014

B. S. Bunney
Department of Psychiatry, Yale University School of Medicine, New Haven, CT 06508

William E. Bunney, Jr.
National Institute of Mental Health, Bethesda, MD 20014

Larry L. Butcher
Department of Psychology, University of California, Los Angeles, CA 90024

A. Carlsson
Department of Pharmacology, University of Göteborg, S-400 33 Göteborg 33, Sweden

William G. Clark
Veterans Administration Hospital, Sepulveda, CA 91343

Erminio Costa
National Institute of Mental Health, St. Elizabeth's Hospital, Washington, D. C. 20032

Ian Creese
Department of Pharmacology and Experimental Therapeutics, Johns Hopkins University School of Medicine, Baltimore, MD 21205

Pedro Cuatrecasas
Department of Medicine, Johns Hopkins University School of Medicine, Baltimore, MD 21205

John M. Davis
Illinois State Psychiatric Institute, Chicago, IL 60612

Guy M. Everett
Department of Pharmacology, University of California School of Medicine, San Francisco, CA 94122

Javier Forn
Department of Pharmacology, Yale University School of Medicine, New Haven, CT 06510

Kjell Fuxe
Department of Histology, Karolinska Institutet, S-104 01 Stockholm 60, Sweden

Silvio Garattini
Istituto de Ricerche Farmacol. 'Mario Negri', 20157 Milan, Italy

Gian L. Gessa
Istituto di Farmacologia, University of Cagliari, 09100 Cagliari, Italy

Paul Greengard
Department of Pharmacology, Yale University School of Medicine, New Haven, CT 06510

Sidney M. Hess
Department of Biochemical Pharmacology, Squibb Institute for Medical Research, Princeton, NJ 08540

A. S. Horn
Department of Pharmacology, Univeristy of Cambridge, Cambridge CB2 2QD, England

Oleh Hornykiewicz
Department of Psychopharmacology, Clarke Institute of Psychiatry, Toronto 2B, Ont., Canada

L. L. Iversen
Department of Pharmacology, University of Cambridge, Cambridge CB2 2QD, England

AUTHORS AND PARTICIPANTS

Bruce K. Krueger
Department of Pharmacology, Yale University School of Medicine, New Haven, CT 06510

Phil J. Langlais
Veterans Administration Hospital, Brockton, MA 02401

Louis Lemberger
Lilly Laboratories for Clinical Research, Marion Country General Hospital, Indianapolis, IN 46202

Walter Lovenberg
National Heart and Lung Institute, Bethesda, MD 20014

Lewis R. Mandel
Merck Sharp and Dohme Research Laboratories, Rahway, NJ 07065

Herbert Y. Meltzer
Department of Psychiatry, University of Chicago, Chicago, IL 60637

R. J. Miller
Department of Pharmacology, Michigan State University, East Lansing, MI 48823

Kenneth E. Moore
Department of Pharmacology, Michigan State University, East Lansing, MI 48823

V. H. Morgenroth, III
Department of Psychiatry, Yale University School of Medicine, New Haven, CT 06510

Dennis L. Murphy
National Institute of Mental Health, Bethesda, MD 20014

L. C. Murrin
Department of Psychiatry, Yale University School of Medicine, New Haven, CT 06520

Jorge A. Romero
National Institute of Mental Health, Bethesda, MD 20014

R. H. Roth
Department of Psychiatry, Yale University School of Medicine, New Haven, CT 06510

Saul Schanberg
Department of Pharmacology and Neurology, Duke University Medical Center, Durham, NC 27710

Robert C. Smith
Department of Psychiatry, University of Chicago, Chicago, IL 60637

Solomon H. Snyder
Department of Pharmacology and Experimental Therapeutics, Johns Hopkins University School of Medicine, Baltimore, MD 21205

Sydney Spector
Department of Pharmacology, Roche Institute of Molecular Biology Nutley, NJ 07110

Earl Usdin
National Institute of Mental Health, Rockville, MD 20852

J. R. Walters
Department of Psychiatry, Yale University School of Medicine, New Haven CT 06510

Norman Weiner
Department of Pharmacology, University of Colorado Medical Center, Denver, CO 80220

Chairmen of the Meeting were: *William E. Bunney, Jr. and Earl Usdin.*

Chairmen of the Sessions were: *F. E. Bloom and Walter Lovenberg.*

ABBREVIATIONS

ACTH = adrenocorticotrophin

AMPT = α-methyl-p-tyrosine

ATP = adenosine triphosphate

BH_4 = tetrahydrobiopterin

cAMP = cyclic adenosine monophosphate

CNS = central nervous system

DA = dopamine

$DMPH_4$ = 6, 7-dimethyl-5, 6, 7, 8-tetrahydropterin

DOPA = dihydroxyphenylalanine

DOPS = dihydroxyphenylserine

E = epinephrine

EGF = epidermal growth factor

EGTA = ethylene glycol bis (β-aminoethyl ether tetracetic acid

ET 495 = trivastal

FSH = follicle stimulating hormone

GABA = γ-aminobutyric acid

GHB = γ-hydroxybutyric acid

GBL = γ-butyrolactone

HIOMT = hydroxyindole-O-methyltransferase

5-HT = 5-hydroxytryptamine = serotonin

Hz = herz

i. p. s. p. = inhibitory postsynaptic potentials

LH = luteinizing hormone

LSD = lysergic acid diethylamide

MFB = median forebrain bundle

nA = nanoamperes

NA = noradrenaline = norepinephrine

NAS = N-acetylserotonin

NAT = N-acetyltransferase

NE = norephrine

NGF = nerve growth factor

n. m. r. = nuclear magnetic resonance

PGE_1 = prostaglandin E_1

RNA = ribonucleic acid

S. E. = standard error

S. E. M. = standard error of the mean

TRH = thyroid releasing hormone

TSH = thyroid stimulating hormone

VIP = vasoactive intestinal polypeptide

Pre- and Postsynaptic Receptors

INTRODUCTORY REMARKS

William E. Bunney, Jr.

A great deal of basic research has recently contributed to our increased understanding of the pre- and post-synaptic neuronal receptor. This book reviews recent research in this area. This work is specifically relevant to psychopharmacology since many of the behaviorally active pharmacological agents alter neurotransmitter receptor site function. Thus the eventual evaluation of neurotransmitter receptor site function in man may be of particular importance in: 1) understanding the modes of action and side effects of many acutely and chronically administered psychoactive agents and 2) it is possible that changes in neuronal receptor site function may be secondarily or even primarily involved in psychopathological processes, in neurological diseases, and perhaps in other metabolic illnesses in man. Disease processes may be reflected in altered or unstable receptor site sensitivity, both in chronic illnesses and in phases of recurrent illnesses. Many neuroleptic drugs which are specifically effective in schizophrenia block postsynaptic dopamine receptors, thus altering the ability of neurotransmitters to bind to these receptors. It has been suggested that this action of the neuroleptics may be involved in their therapeutic effect in schizophrenia.

Fig. 1 reviews some of the characteristics of neuronal receptors. A ligand binds to a receptor, forming a receptor-ligand complex which then leads to a metabolic response. There must be a recognition of the ligand molecule by the receptor. The reaction with the ligand involves a reversibility of the binding process, a high affinity for the receptor, and saturation of receptor sites; usually stereospecificity exists for the ligand.

Figure 2 schematically represents a neuronal receptor. Neurotransmitters released from the presynaptic terminals react with the pre- and/or post-synaptic receptor sites. The process of response at the post-synaptic receptors involves adenyl cyclase, ATP, protein kinase and other intermediate steps which ultimately lead to an active physiological process such as an action potential.

It has further been hypothesized, as will be discussed, that there are feedback loops from the post- to the pre-synaptic neuron.

Receptor + Ligand = Receptor Ligand Complex → Metabolic Response

1) Recognition of Ligand Molecule

2) Reaction with Ligand
   a) Reversibility of Binding Process
   b) Affinity for Receptor Must be High
   c) Receptor Sites Can Be Saturated
   d) Stereospecificity

Fig. 1. Receptor Characteristics

INTRODUCTORY REMARKS

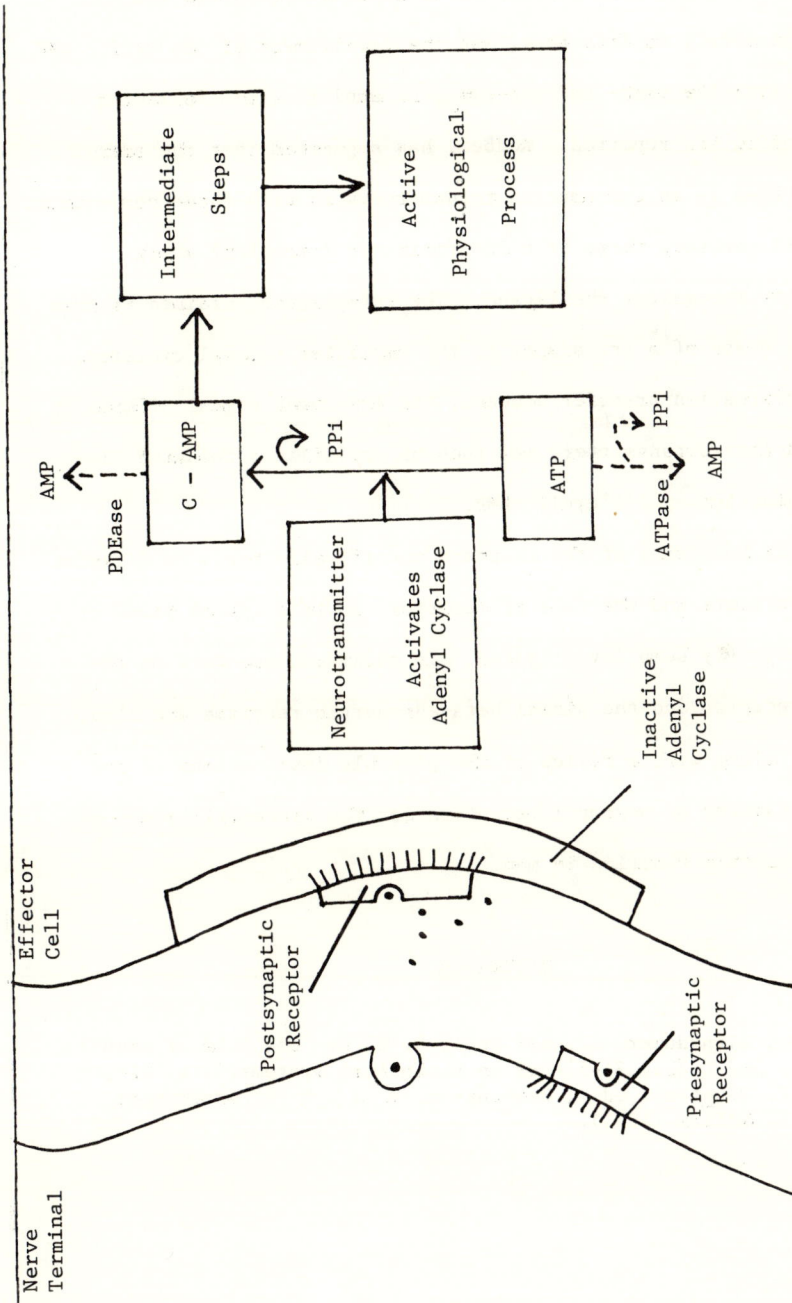

Fig. 2. SCHEMA FOR NEURONAL RECEPTOR. AMP = adenosine monophosphate, ATP = adenosine triphosphate, ATPase = adenosine triphosphatase, C - AMP = cyclic adenosine 3',5'-monophosphate, PDEase = phosphodiesterase, PP_i = pyrophosphate

The roles of the pre- and post-synaptic neuronal receptors are reviewed in detail in this book, and the involvement of the cyclic AMP system in both the post- and pre-synaptic amplification following ligand binding are reported. Rodbell has suggested that the adenyl cyclase system is an information transfer system with three components. At the cell surface, there is a discriminator (receptor) which specifically recognizes the ligand. The information obtained is then coupled by means of a transducer to the amplifier (adenyl cyclase). In this information transfer process, the low level signal offered by the ligand (neurotransmitter) may then be amplified a thousand times by the production of 3'5'cyclic-AMP.

In this book many of the chapters specifically focus on dopamine neurotransmitters and the role of receptors in this system since it has most recently been investigated. In addition, new work on the morphine receptor and the pineal beta-adrenergic receptor are also presented, along with a review of the possible implications of the new understanding of neuronal receptors for the systematic study of neuronal receptor function in man.

REFERENCE

Rodbell, M., Birnbaumer, I., and Pohl, S. L. in "The Role of Adenyl Cyclase and Cyclic 3'-5'-AMP in Biological Systems.", p. 51-, Rall, T. W. et al.,eds., Washington, D. C., U. S. Government Printing Office (1971).

DOPAMINE NEURONS: ROLE OF IMPULSE FLOW AND PRE-SYNAPTIC
RECEPTORS IN THE REGULATION OF TYROSINE HYDROXYLASE

R. H. Roth, J. R. Walters, L. C. Murrin and V. H. Morgenroth, III

Departments of Psychiatry and Pharmacology
Yale University School of Medicine
New Haven, Connecticut   06510

INTRODUCTION

Much evidence has accumulated in recent years to suggest that short term changes in transmitter synthesis are controlled by alterations in nerve impulse flow (Aghajanian et al., 1972; Roth et al., 1973; Weiner, 1970). In the case of the catecholaminergic neurons it has been postulated that the rate limiting biosynthetic enzyme, tyrosine hydroxylase, is regulated by end product inhibition. According to this model during periods of increased impulse flow when more transmitter is utilized synthesis should be accelerated, and during periods of quiescence or a reduction in impulse flow transmitter synthesis should be slowed as a result of a decreased utilization and a consequent buildup of the transmitter. This model is consistent with results obtained in both peripheral (Alousi and Weiner, 1966; Roth et al., 1966, 1967; Sedvall, 1969) and central (Arbuthnott et al., 1970; Korf et al., 1973a,b; Roth et al., 1974a) noradrenergic neurons where increases and decreases in neuronal activity appear to be well correlated with increases or decreases in norepinephrine metabolism and turnover. An increase in neuronal activity results in an acceleration of norepinephrine synthesis and turnover and a decrease or block in impulse flow leads to a reduction in synthesis and turnover.

Recent studies have demonstrated that central dopaminergic neurons behave in a fashion very similar to both peripheral and central noradrenergic neurons in their response to increases in impulse flow but paradoxically increase synthesis in response to a cessation of impulse flow (Roth et al., 1973, 1974b; Walters et al., 1973; Walters and Roth, 1974). The observed increase in synthesis in both cases appears to occur as a result of an increase in tyrosine hydroxylase activity. This unexpected observation in dopaminergic neurons of an increase in transmitter biosynthesis during periods of quiescence prompted our laboratory to investigate in more detail the alterations in tyrosine hydroxylase which occur in various central and peripheral catecholamine neurons during periods of altered impulse flow. It was found that electrical stimulation of both peripheral and central noradrenergic neurons and central dopaminergic neurons results in a kinetic activation of the tyrosine hydroxylase isolated from the tissue containing the terminals of the stimulated neurons (Murrin et al., 1974; Morgenroth et al., 1974; Roth et al., 1974a). This kinetic activation of tyrosine hydroxylase observed during enhanced neuronal activity appears to be mediated in both noradrenergic and dopaminergic neurons by an increased affinity of the enzyme for substrate tyrosine and pterin cofactors and by a decreased affinity of the enzyme for the natural endproduct inhibitor (i.e. norepinephrine or dopamine). No apparent change is observed in the V_{max} for either substrate or cofactor. Qualitatively similar alterations in the kinetic properties of striatal tyrosine hydroxylase are observed when impulse flow is blocked in the nigro-neostriatal dopamine pathway (Morgenroth et al., 1975; Roth et al., 1974b). However, it soon became clear that these changes produced by a cessation of impulse flow differed both quantitatively and mechanistically from the changes produced by increases in impulse flow in this pathway.

The following paper is an attempt to summarize our recent observations concerning the possible mechanisms by which alterations in impulse flow produce changes in the activity of neostriatal tyrosine hydroxylase. The role presynaptic receptors may play in modulating these changes will also be discussed. In this review consideration will only be given to the short term, minute to minute regulation of tyrosine hydroxylase which does not involve induction of new enzyme protein.

Effects of increased impulse flow on tyrosine hydroxylase

For the majority of studies mentioned in this review we chose a well defined central dopaminergic system, the nigro-neostriatal system. These neurons have their cell bodies localized primarily in the zona compacta of the substantia nigra and project mainly to the neostriatum and the central portions of the amygdaloid nucleus (Dahlström and Fuxe, 1965; Ungerstedt, 1971). Numerous studies have already demonstrated that drugs which increase impulse flow in this nigro-neostriatal pathway, such as the antipsychotic drugs, all cause a marked increase in the synthesis and turnover of dopamine in the neostriatum (Nybäck and Sedvall, 1968; Andén et al., 1971). However, until recently, it remained unclear whether or not the observed increase in synthesis was directly related to the degree of increased impulse flow.

In order to investigate directly whether a controlled alteration of impulse flow in the nigro-neostriatal pathway results in a predictable alteration in dopamine biosynthesis in the striatum we initially examined the effects of electrical stimulation of this pathway on the incorporation of labeled tyrosine into dopamine. In these experiments unilateral stimulation of the nigro-neostriatal neurons produced a significant increase in the formation of labeled dopamine from exogenous tyrosine, which was dependent upon impulse flow. A maximal increase (> 100%) in the accumulation of labeled dopamine occurred at a frequency of 15 Hz in experiments in which constant stimulation was applied for 20 minutes. Stimulation at varying frequencies of 5 to 30 Hz produced no significant alteration in the endogenous levels of dopamine in the neostriatum and the specific activity of tyrosine remained unchanged or slightly decreased when the stimulated side was compared to the contralateral side (Murrin and Roth, 1973).

In order to determine whether this increase in dopamine formation observed during neuronal stimulation was a result of an increase in tyrosine hydroxylase activity, we made use of a technique developed by Carlsson and coworkers (Carlsson et al., 1972) in which the short term accumulation of DOPA is measured following inhibition of DOPA decarboxylase and is used as an index of in vivo tyrosine hydroxylase activity. Employing this technique we observed that the accumulation of DOPA was linear for periods up to approximately one hour after administration of seryl-trihydroxybenzyl-hydrazine (RO-4-4602) in a dose (800 mg/kg) which completely blocked DOPA decarboxylase in the neostriatum (Walters and Roth, 1974). Stimulation of the nigro-neostriatal pathway for varying periods of time at frequencies of 5-30 Hz resulted in a stimulus dependent increase in DOPA accumulation (Murrin and Roth, unpublished data). Continuous stimulation for a period of 20 minutes at 15 Hz resulted in greater than a 100% increase in accumulation of DOPA in the neostriatum on the stimulated side when compared to the contralateral unstimulated neostriatum (Fig. 1). A further increase in DOPA accumulation was observed when the duration of the period of stimulation was increased from 20 to 30 minutes. Chloral hydrate administration, which is known to increase impulse flow in central dopaminergic neurons (Bunney et al., 1973), also caused a significant increase in the accumulation of DOPA in the neostriatum when compared to results obtained in unanesthetized rats.

Even more interesting was the observation that the apparent increase in tyrosine hydroxylase activity induced by electrical stimulation persisted following the termination of the stimulation

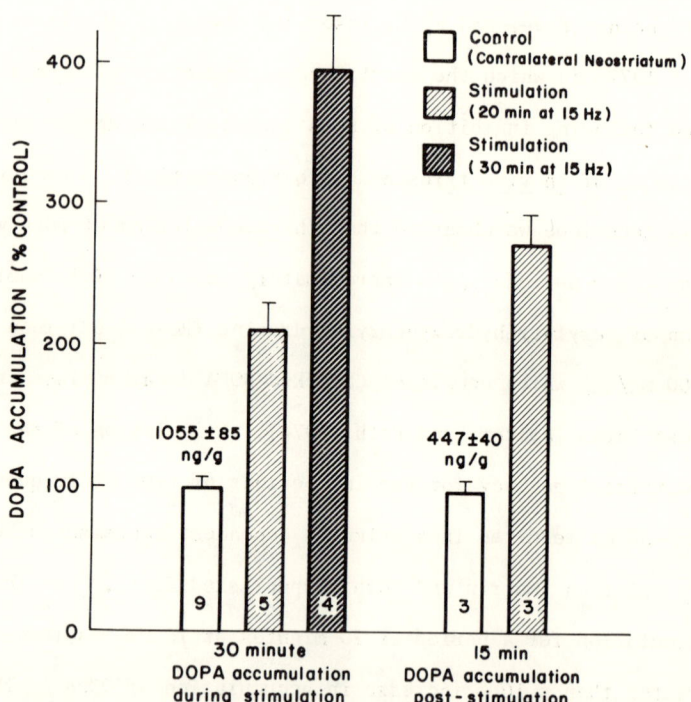

FIGURE 1. Accumulation of DOPA in the neostriatum during and following electrical stimulation of the nigro-neostriatal pathway. Rats were anesthetized with chloral hydrate (400 mg/kg) 15 minutes prior to beginning the stimulation period. DOPA was isolated and measured fluorometrically essentially by the technique of Kehr et al. (1972) as modified by Walters and Roth (1974). DOPA accumulation is expressed in terms of percent of the contralateral control neostriatum. Values are mean ± the S.E.M.

period. In experiments in which the accumulation of DOPA in the neostriatum was followed for 15 minutes after the termination of the stimulation we observed nearly a 180% increase in the DOPA levels in the neostriatum on the stimulated side when compared to the unstimulated contralateral side (Fig. 1). This observation indicates that the increase in tyrosine hydroxylase activity persists for a measurable amount of time following the a technique developed by Carlsson and coworkers (Carlsson et al., 1972) in which the short term accumulation of DOPA is measured following inhibition of DOPA decarboxylase and is used as an index of in vivo tyrosine hydroxylase activity. Employing this technique we observed that the accumulation of DOPA was linear for periods up to approximately one hour after administration of seryl-trihydroxybenzyl-hydrazine (RO-4-4602) in a dose (800 mg/kg) which completely blocked DOPA decarboxylase in the neostriatum (Walters and Roth, 1974). Stimulation of the nigro-neostriatal pathway for varying periods of time at frequencies of 5-30 Hz resulted in a stimulus dependent increase in DOPA accumulation (Murrin and Roth, unpublished data). Continuous stimulation for a period of 20 minutes at 15 Hz resulted in greater than a 100% increase in accumulation of DOPA in the neostriatum on the stimulated side when compared to the contralateral unstimulated neostriatum (Fig. 1). A further increase in DOPA accumulation was observed when the duration of the period of stimulation was increased from 20 to 30 minutes. Chloral hydrate administration, which is known to increase impulse flow in central dopaminergic neurons (Bunney et al., 1973), also caused a significant increase in the accumulation of DOPA in the neostriatum when compared to results obtained in unanesthetized rats.

Even more interesting was the observation that the apparent increase in tyrosine hydroxylase activity induced by electrical stimulation persisted following the termination of the stimulation

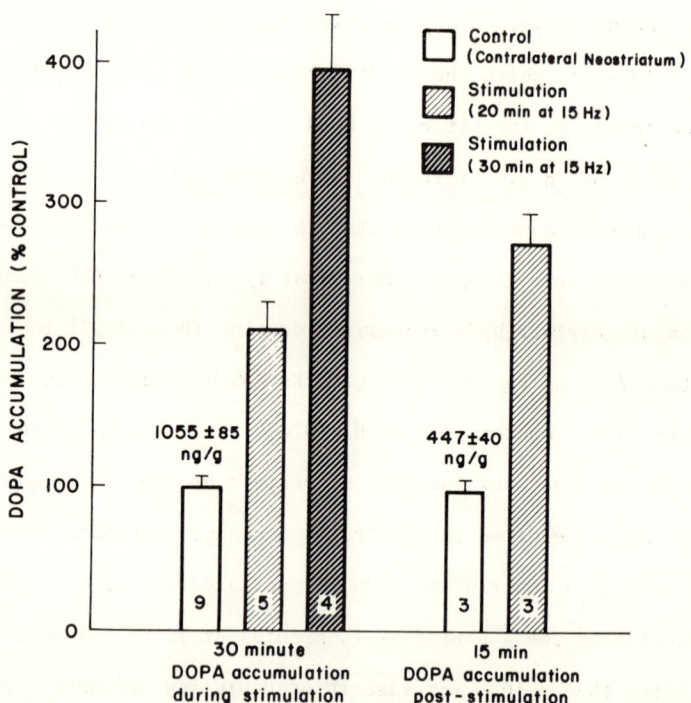

FIGURE 1. Accumulation of DOPA in the neostriatum during and following electrical stimulation of the nigro-neostriatal pathway. Rats were anesthetized with chloral hydrate (400 mg/kg) 15 minutes prior to beginning the stimulation period. DOPA was isolated and measured fluorometrically essentially by the technique of Kehr et al. (1972) as modified by Walters and Roth (1974). DOPA accumulation is expressed in terms of percent of the contralateral control neostriatum. Values are mean ± the S.E.M.

period. In experiments in which the accumulation of DOPA in the neostriatum was followed for 15 minutes after the termination of the stimulation we observed nearly a 180% increase in the DOPA levels in the neostriatum on the stimulated side when compared to the unstimulated contralateral side (Fig. 1). This observation indicates that the increase in tyrosine hydroxylase activity persists for a measurable amount of time following the termination of stimulation and thus we attempted to test whether this activation of tyrosine hydroxylase could be measured in homogenates of the neostriatum obtained from rats in which the nigro-neostriatal pathway was stimulated electrically. Success of such an experiment seemed likely since in previous experiments we had demonstrated that the post-stimulation increase in the activity of tyrosine hydroxylase, isolated from the vas deferens as well as the hippocampus, withstands the procedures of freezing, thawing and homogenization which are necessary to isolate the enzyme from the tissue (Morgenroth et al., 1974a; Roth et al., 1974a). In these experiments tyrosine hydroxylase activity was measured in the 100,000 x g supernatants obtained from the neostriatum by a modification of the methods of Shiman et al. (1971) and Coyle (1972) as described in detail by Morgenroth et al. (1974, 1975a) in the presence of subsaturating concentrations of tyrosine (10 μM) and pterin cofactor (100 μM).

Preliminary experiments demonstrated that stimulation of the nigro-neostriatal pathway for 20 minutes at 15 Hz produced a significant increase (> 50%) in the activity of tyrosine hydroxylase isolated from the neostriatum on the stimulated side when compared to the contralateral unstimulated side. Further studies indicated that it took about 10 minutes of continuous stimulation at 15 Hz to obtain a maximal activation of striatal tyrosine hydroxylase (Fig. 2). Furthermore, this activation persisted for about 15 minutes following the cessation of the stimulation (Fig. 3).

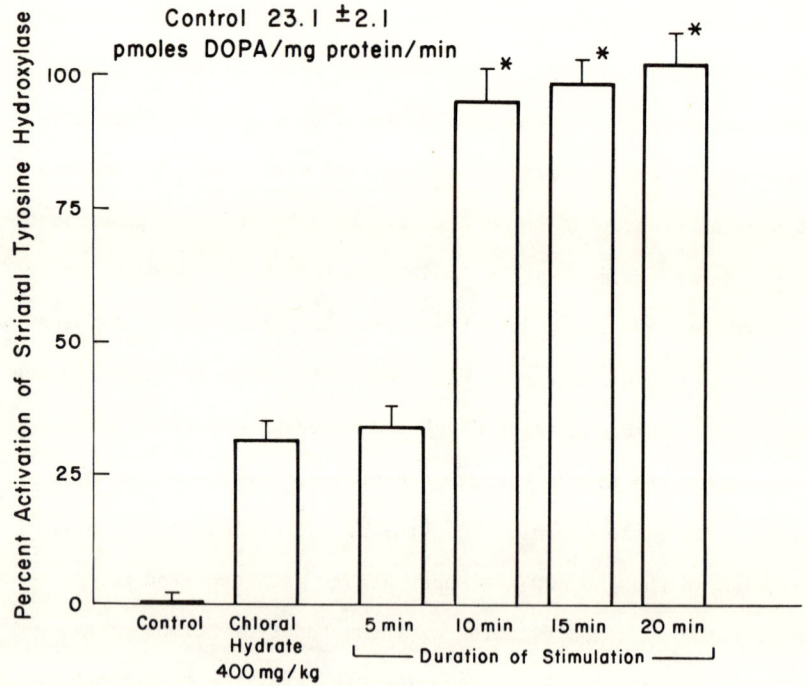

FIGURE 2. Time course for the activation of neostriatal tyrosine hydroxylase following electrical stimulation. The nigro-neostriatal pathway was stimulated at 15 Hz for the indicated periods of time and the tyrosine hydroxylase activity measured in the 100,000 x g supernatant of the neostriatum by a modification of the method of Shiman et al. (1971) as described by Morgenroth et al. (1974). Results are expressed as percent activation of tyrosine hydroxylase as compared to tyrosine hydroxylase isolated from the neostriatum of untreated control rats. Values are the means determined from 4 separate experiments. Vertical bars depict the S.E.M. * Indicates that the mean is significantly different from chloral hydrate treated rats, $P < 0.01$.

In an attempt to further understand this activation process we analyzed the effects of electrical stimulation of the nigro-neostriatal pathway on the kinetic properties of tyrosine hydroxylase isolated from the neostriatum. In these studies we focused our attention on determining the alterations in affinity

REGULATION OF TYROSINE HYDROXYLASE

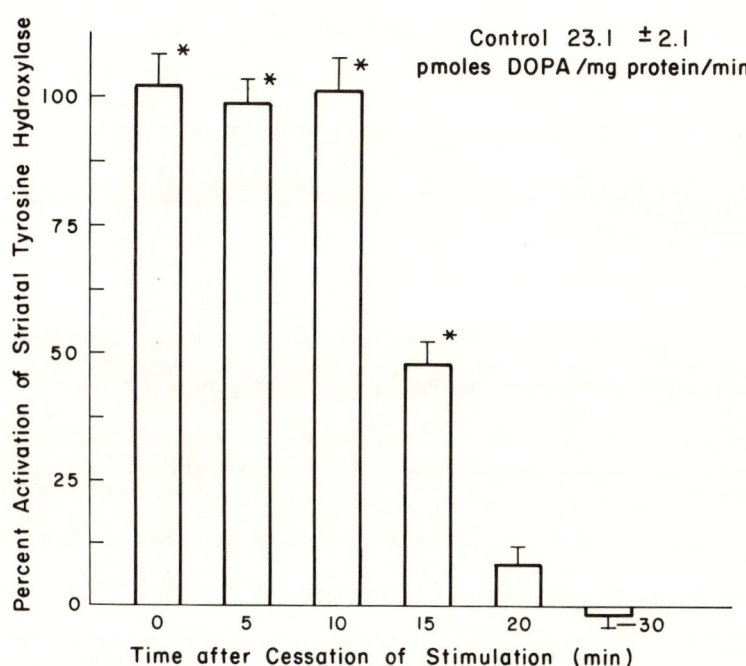

FIGURE 3. Time course for the decay of the post-stimulation activation of neostriatal tyrosine hydroxylase. The nigro-neostriatal pathway was stimulated for 20 min at 15 Hz and the rats killed at various time intervals following termination of the stimulation period. Results are expressed in terms of the decrease in activation of the enzyme isolated from the neostriatum on the stimulated side assuming that maximal activation of tyrosine hydroxylase occurs following stimulation of the nigro-neostriatal pathway for 20 minutes at 15 Hz. The activity of the maximally activated enzyme equals 48.4 $\pm$ 2.9 pmoles of DOPA/mg/protein/min or 209 $\pm$ 13% of tyrosine hydroxylase activity obtained from neostriatum of unanesthetized control rats. * Indicates that the mean is significantly different from value obtained from control striatum, $P < 0.01$.

of tyrosine hydroxylase for substrate, pterin cofactor and endogenous inhibitor, dopamine. In experiments in which the artificial pterin cofactor 6,7-dimethyl-5,6,7,8-tetrahydropterin ($DMPH_4$) was employed, electrical stimulation of the nigro-neostriatal pathway caused significant changes in the kinetic properties of the tyrosine hydroxylase isolated from the striatum on the stimulated side. Stimulation caused nearly a 2 1/2 or 3 fold decrease in the K_m of the enzyme for tyrosine when compared to the K_m of the enzyme isolated from the striatum of rats treated with chloral hydrate or untreated controls, respectively (Murrin et al., 1974). Additional experiments indicated that similar alterations in the K_m for tyrosine are obtained under assay conditions in which tetrahydrobiopterin (BH_4), the presumed natural cofactor, is employed as a cofactor. In no instance was a change in V_{max} for tyrosine observed. Electrical stimulation of the nigro-neostriatal pathway also caused about a 5 fold change in the affinity of neostriatal tyrosine hydroxylase for the pterin cofactor, BH_4, when compared to the enzyme isolated from the unstimulated side (Table 1).

In addition to altering the affinity of tyrosine hydroxylase for both substrate and pterin cofactor, electrical stimulation caused an apparent change in the affinity of the enzyme for the natural endproduct inhibitor, dopamine. This is reflected by a 5-fold increase in the K_i for dopamine of the tyrosine hydroxylase isolated from the neostriatum on the stimulated side.

Changes in the kinetic properties of striatal tyrosine hydroxylase similar to those found following electrical stimulation are observed when adenosine 3',5'-monophosphate (cAMP) (10 to 100 µM) is added to high speed supernatants prepared from the neostriatum (Harris et al., 1974, 1975; Table 1).

Under both experimental conditions tyrosine hydroxylase appears to have an increased affinity for substrate and pterin cofactor and a decreased affinity for dopamine. It is of interest in this regard that addition of cAMP to the tyrosine hydroxylase isolated from the neostriatum on the stimulated side produces no further activation of neostriatal tyrosine hydroxylase (Table 1). Also, the activation produced by electrical stimulation or by addition of cAMP to the high speed supernatant is not reversed following chromatography on Sephadex G-25. These findings are suggestive that the activation of tyrosine hydroxylase produced by these two conditions may occur by a similar mechanism.

Since it is known that during neuronal depolarization there is a significant increase in the accumulation of endogenous cAMP (Kakiuchi et al., 1969; Shimizu et al., 1970) it seems likely that this event could be responsible for mediating the observed activation of tyrosine hydroxylase produced during electrical stimulation of the nigro-neostriatal pathway. Although it was conceivable that cAMP might itself be an allosteric activator of tyrosine hydroxylase, in view of the delayed onset of action observed in both instances and the fact that, after a 10 min pre-incubation period with cAMP, Sephadex chromatography does not alter the activation process suggests that a more likely explanation is that a cAMP dependent protein kinase is involved. In fact, recent evidence has strongly implicated the involvement of a cAMP dependent protein kinase in the activation of tyrosine

TABLE 1

Effects of Electrical Stimulation and cAMP on the Kinetics of Striatal Tyrosine Hydroxylase

Treatment	Tyrosine Hydroxylase Activity+ (pmoles DOPA/mg Protein/min)	K_m Tyrosine (μM)	K_m BH_4 (mM)	K_i DA (mM)
None	22.6 ± 2.8 (6)	54.7 ± 5.1	0.42 ± 0.08	0.05 ± 0.01
Chloral Hydrate (400 mg/kg; 35 min.)	32.1 ± 3.1 (6)	41.5 ± 3.6	0.36 ± 0.09	0.06 ± 0.01
Stimulation* (15 Hz, 20 min.)	47.2 ± 2.1 (6)	17.1 ± 1.6	0.08 ± 0.01	0.29 ± 0.04
None + cAMP (50 μM)‡	40.1 ± 3.2 (6)	24.9 ± 1.7	0.05 ± 0.01	0.38 ± 0.01
Chloral Hydrate + cAMP (50 μM)‡	36.7 ± 2.8 (6)	26.1 ± 1.3	0.07 ± 0.02	0.34 ± 0.08
Stimulation* + cAMP (50 μM)‡	48.1 ± 1.7 (6)	20.2 ± 1.1	0.06 ± 0.03	0.39 ± 0.05

+Tyrosine hydroxylase activity was determined in 100,000 x g supernatants of rat corpus striatum at a tyrosine concentration of 10 μM and BH_4 concentration of 0.01 mM. Results are expressed as the mean ± S.E.M. Values in parentheses equal the number of separate experiments.

*Rats were administered chloral hydrate (400 mg/kg) 15 minutes prior to treatment.

‡cAMP was added to the high speed supernatant 10 min prior to initiation of the tyrosine hydroxylase reaction by addition of labeled substrate.

The K_m for tyrosine was determined according to the method of Lineweaver-Burk at a DMPH$_4$ concentration of 1 mM and 7 tyrosine concentrations ranging from 0.5 µM to 100 µM. K_m values are mean ± S.E.M. of K_m's generated from six separate lines.

The K_m for BH$_4$ was determined according to the method of Lineweaver-Burk at a tyrosine concentration of 100 µM and 7 BH$_4$ concentrations between 0.01 mM and 0.5 mM. The K_m values are the mean ± S.E.M. of the K_m's generated from six separate lines.

After determining the competitive nature of dopamine inhibition of tyrosine hydroxylase vs BH$_4$, the K_i was determined by the method of Dixon at BH$_4$ concentrations of 100, 10 and 1 µM and at 6 dopamine concentrations (0.01-0.5 mM). The K_i's are the mean ± S.E.M. of six determinations.

Data taken in part from Murrin et al., 1974.

hydroxylase produced by addition of exogenous cAMP to hippocampal homogenates (Morgenroth et al., 1975a).

Figure 4 presents a hypothetical schematic model illustrating a possible sequence of events by which neuronal depolarization could cause an activation of tyrosine hydroxylase via a cAMP dependent series of reactions. In this model the key events are as follows: An increase in impulse flow which leads to an increased rate of depolarization of the terminals of the dopaminergic neurons in the neostriatum and increased influx of calcium ions in the terminals. These changes by means of some calcium dependent reaction activate a presynaptic adenylate cyclase resulting in a local increase in the steady state levels of cAMP. The next step in this theoretical model is the activation of a presynaptic protein kinase by the increased levels of endogenous cAMP. This activated protein kinase could then directly phosphorylate tyrosine hydroxylase, converting it to a kinetically activated form. Alternatively the protein kinase may act to phosphorylate an unidentified protein acceptor which then serves as an activator of tyrosine hydroxylase. The latter possibility seems most likely since preliminary experiments indicate that addition of homogenates from the neostriatum on the stimulated side to control unstimulated neostriata results in a more than additive increase in tyrosine hydroxylase activity. This would not be expected if tyrosine hydroxylase were activated primarily by a direct phosphorylation of the enzyme but could be explained by the formation of a phosphorylated activator.

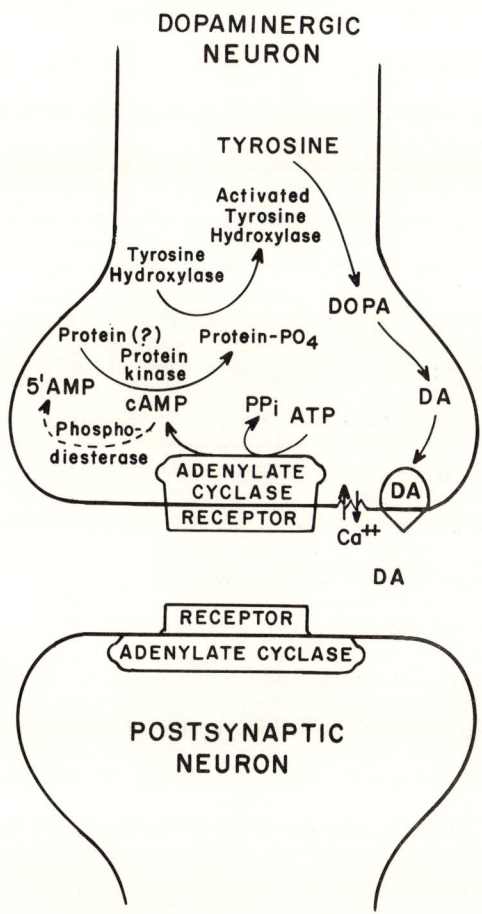

FIGURE 4. Schematic model of a dopaminergic neuron illustrating a proposed mechanism by which increased impulse flow may result in an activation of tyrosine hydroxylase. In this model the key events are the following: An increase in impulse flow results in an increase in the frequency of depolarization of the neuronal terminals with a consequent increase in the influx of calcium. The increase in calcium influx activates a presynaptic adenyl cyclase which results in an increase in the accumulation of cAMP. cAMP activates a protein kinase which then phosphorylates an as yet unidentified protein. This phosphorylated protein acts as an allosteric activator of tyrosine hydroxylase.

The observation that Sephadex chromatography of the tyrosine hydroxylase isolated from the striatum on the stimulated side does not remove the activator suggests that it may be a high molecular weight material such as a phosphorylated protein. If indeed electrical stimulation results in the phosphorylation of a protein distinct from tyrosine hydroxylase it would not be unrealistic to propose that it is this unidentified phosphorylated protein formed during periods of increased impulse flow which acts as an allosteric activator of neostriatal tyrosine hydroxylase. Experiments are currently in progress in our laboratory in an attempt to identify this activator.

Effects of inhibition of impulse flow on tyrosine hydroxylase

Numerous studies have now demonstrated that conditions which cause a cessation of impulse flow in the nigro-neostriatal pathway result in a rapid accumulation of dopamine in the neostriatum. This increase can be observed in the rat neostriatum after lesion of the substantia nigra or median forebrain bundle (Andén et al., 1971; Faull and Laverty, 1969; Nybäck, 1972; Walters et al., 1972), cerebral hemisection (Carlsson et al., 1972), intraventricular injection of 6-hydroxydopamine (Bell et al., 1970), and after administration of gamma-butyrolactone (GBL) (Aghajanian and Roth, 1970; Agid et al., 1974; Gessa et al., 1966; Roth and Surh, 1970; Stock et al., 1973; Walters and Roth, 1972) a precursor of gamma-hydroxybutyrate (GHB) which has been shown to inhibit impulse flow in the nigro-neostriatal neurons (Walters et al., 1972). Similar changes are also observed in the nucleus accumbens and olfactory tubercles after impulse flow is blocked in the dopamine neurons located in the ventral tegmental area (Aghajanian and Roth, 1970; Walters and Roth, unpublished observations). Thus the dopamine system when compared to other monoamine systems appears to respond in a rather unique fashion to an inhibition of impulse flow by rapidly increasing the transmitter content of its terminals. A similar increase in the steady state levels of norepinephrine or serotonin or an activation of the initial biosynthetic enzyme is not observed when impulse flow in these respective neuronal systems is interrupted either pharmacologically or by placement of a lesion in the locus coeruleus or median raphe (Carlsson et al., 1972; Herr and Roth, 1972; Korf et al., 1973). However, a rapid and marked increase in the steady state levels of acetylcholine in the hippocampus is observed when impulse flow is interrupted in the septohippocampal cholinergic pathway (Sethy et al., 1973).

The rapid increase in the accumulation of dopamine seen after pharmacological or mechanical interruption of impulse flow in the nigro-neostriatal pathway appears to be explainable in part by a marked increase in dopamine biosynthesis (Walters et al., 1973). The increased incorporation of labeled tyrosine into dopamine and the increased accumulation of dihydroxyphenylalanine (DOPA) after inhibition of DOPA decarboxylase are both suggestive that such treatments result in an increase in tyrosine hydroxylase activity. The observation that tyrosine hydroxylase activity is apparently increased during a time in which the endogenous levels of dopamine in the nerve terminals are rapidly increasing seems, however, quite paradoxical. Tyrosine hydroxylase is usually responsive to endproduct inhibition and thus small increases in endogenous dopamine or norepinephrine within the nerve terminal usually result in a reduction in tyrosine hydroxylase activity (Cooper et al., 1974). These unexpected results suggested to us that inhibition of impulse flow in dopaminergic neurons might somehow decrease the ability of endogenous dopamine to exert an inhibitory effect on the activity of tyrosine hydroxylase.

In an attempt to gain more insight into the mechanism involved we investigated the effects that pharmacological or mechanical blockade of impulse flow might have on the activity and kinetic properties of tyrosine hydroxylase isolated from the neostriatum of treated rats. When impulse flow was blocked by treatment with γ-butyrolactone (GBL, 750 mg/kg) or by placement of an electrothermic lesion in the nigro-neostriatal pathway the activity of the tyrosine hydroxylase measured in the presence of subsaturating concentrations of tyrosine and pterin cofactor was increased by about 300% (Table 2). In addition, the kinetic properties of the isolated enzyme were markedly altered. The tyrosine hydroxylase obtained from GBL treated rats or rats with unilateral electrothermic lesions in the nigro-neostriatal pathway had a marked increase in its affinity for tyrosine and pterin cofactor and a dramatic decrease in its affinity for

TABLE 2

Effect of Inhibition of Impulse Flow and Calcium Removal on Striatal Tyrosine Hydroxylase

Treatment	Tyrosine Hydroxylase Activity (pmoles/DOPA/mg protein/min.)	K_m Tyrosine (μM)	K_m DMPH$_4$ (mM)	K_i DA (mM)
Control	23.2 ± 2.6 (6)	53.9 ± 5.1	0.89 ± 0.03	0.11 ± 0.01
GBL Pretreatment (90 min, 750 mg/kg)	85.2 ± 4.6 (6)	8.9 ± .06	0.13 ± 0.01	73.9 ± 8.3
MFB Lesion (30 min)[+]	87.2 ± 6.1 (6)	7.8 ± 1.1	0.12 ± 0.01	75.6 ± 2.3
EGTA (50 μM)*	79.4 ± 8.1 (6)	9.1 ± 2.1	0.13 ± 0.03	73.9 ± 8.4
EGTA* + Calcium (100 μM)*	24.2 ± 3.1 (12)	52.7 ± 4.6	0.91 ± 0.06	0.15 ± 0.01
GBL Pretreatment + Calcium (100 μM)*	21.1 ± 3.6 (8)	57.2 ± 3.9	0.92 ± 0.05	0.14 ± 0.01
MFB Lesion[+] + Calcium (100 μM)*	21.5 ± 1.9 (6)	53.2 ± 5.1	0.86 ± 0.04	0.11 ± 0.02

Tyrosine hydroxylase activity and kinetic parameters were determined as described in Table 4. Data taken from Morgenroth, Walters and Roth, 1975.
*EGTA and calcium were added to the high speed supernatant 5 min prior to initiation of reaction by addition of labeled tyrosine.
[+]Unilateral electrothermic lesion of the median forebrain bundle.

the endproduct inhibitor, dopamine. No change was observed in the V_{max} for tyrosine or pterin cofactor.

Thus it appears as if a blockade of impulse flow in dopaminergic neurons leads to a change in the physical properties of preexisting enzyme molecules. The fact that the tyrosine hydroxylase obtained from the neostriatum of rats in which impulse flow is blocked has a marked decrease in its sensitivity to inhibition by dopamine may well explain why tyrosine hydroxylase activity appears to be enhanced even under conditions in which the endogenous levels of dopamine are rapidly increasing within the nerve terminals.

The question that then comes to the fore is: what is the molecular mechanism or event which triggers an alteration in the kinetic properties of tyrosine hydroxylase in response to a reduction or cessation of impulse flow? Previous studies conducted in brain slices suggested a possible answer to this question (Goldstein et al., 1970; Harris, 1971). These experiments in which dopamine synthesis was measured in slices of rat striatum also posed a paradoxical situation. In these experiments the formation of dopamine from tyrosine in slices of rat striatum incubated in Krebs-Ringer phosphate medium was enhanced when Ca^{++} ions were removed from the medium. However, synthesis of norepinephrine in slices of rat cerebral cortex or hippocampus remained unchanged under similar experimental conditions. Thus it appeared that Ca^{++} removal produced changes in striatal slices which led to an increase in dopamine formation.

These observations prompted us to investigate the effects of removal of Ca^{++} by means of Ca^{++} chelating agents on the activity of soluble preparations of tyrosine hydroxylase obtained from the rat striatum. In experiments in which we employed subsaturating concentrations of tyrosine and pterin cofactor we observed that addition of the calcium chelator, EGTA (50 µM) caused a marked increase in the activity of striatal tyrosine hydroxylase present in high speed supernatants (Morgenroth et al., 1974b) but was without effect on the tyrosine hydroxylase prepared from rat hippocampus (Roth et al., 1974a) or guinea pig vas deferens (Morgenroth et al., 1974a), tissues containing primarily noradrenergic neurons. The activation of tyrosine hydroxylase produced by addition of EGTA to the incubation medium is kinetically very similar to that produced by a cessation of impulse flow. Both treatments result in an enzyme which has an increased affinity for substrate and pterin cofactor and a dramatic decrease in affinity for dopamine (Table 2). In addition, these alterations in the kinetic properties of the enzyme are completely reversed in both instances by addition of Ca^{++} ions to the incubation medium.

These *in vitro* results suggest that changes in calcium fluxes in the dopaminergic nerve terminals might be responsible for altering tyrosine hydroxylase activity *in vivo*. A block of impulse flow in the nigro-neostriatal pathway would prevent depolarization of the dopamine containing nerve terminals in the neostriatum and the accompanying influx of calcium. This lack of calcium mobilization could result in an activation of tyrosine hydroxylase by causing a direct change in the physical properties of preformed enzyme molecules or by initiating the formation of an activator. The former possibility seems more likely since the effects are immediately reversible by addition of calcium to the medium. This change in the properties of tyrosine hydroxylase produces an enzyme that is less susceptible to endproduct inhibition by endogenous dopamine and which has a greater affinity for both substrate and pterin cofactor.

Figure 5 illustrates a schematic model of a dopaminergic nerve terminal depicting the possible mechanisms by which a cessation in impulse flow might regulate tyrosine hydroxylase activity. During periods of normal impulse flow (Figure 5A), tyrosine hydroxylase is susceptible to endproduct inhibition by dopamine, and a small change in a "strategic pool" of dopamine could conceivably influence tyrosine hydroxylase activity. This critical pool of dopamine is thought to be controlled by a balance between release, reuptake and synthesis. When increased demands are placed on the neuron and larger amounts of transmitter are utilized, the levels of this "strategic pool" of dopamine fall and tyrosine hydroxylase is activated. It is quite likely, as mentioned earlier, that changes in the concentration or fluxes of intracellular calcium which occur during depolarization may trigger an increase in the formation of cAMP which could then alter the physical properties of the enzyme (see previous section) resulting in a further activation of tyro-

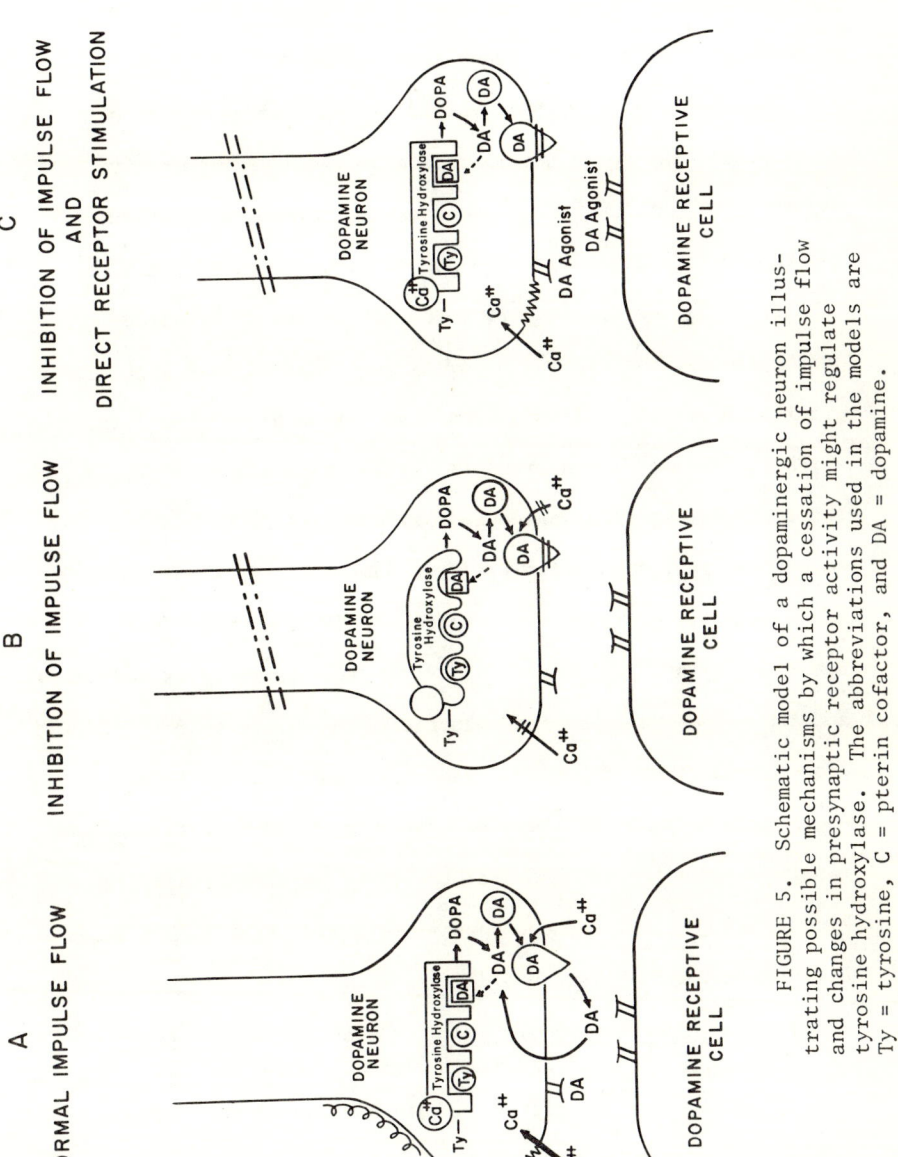

FIGURE 5. Schematic model of a dopaminergic neuron illustrating possible mechanisms by which a cessation of impulse flow and changes in presynaptic receptor activity might regulate tyrosine hydroxylase. The abbreviations used in the models are Ty = tyrosine, C = pterin cofactor, and DA = dopamine.

sine hydroxylase, in part, by making the enzyme less sensitive to feedback inhibition by endogenous dopamine.

When impulse flow is inhibited in dopaminergic neurons (Figure 5B), the nerve terminals are no longer periodically depolarized, calcium influx and dopamine release are retarded and the concentration of endogenous dopamine in the terminals rapidly increases due in part to an activation of tyrosine hydroxylase. This activation of tyrosine hydroxylase might occur as a result of this decrease in influx of calcium ions, which in dopaminergic neurons triggers a reversible change in the conformation of tyrosine hydroxylase causing the enzyme to have an increased affinity for tyrosine and synthetic cofactor and a dramatic decrease in the affinity for the endproduct inhibitor, dopamine. Thus tyrosine hydroxylase activity is increased and the enzyme has a marked reduction in sensitivity to inhibition by endogenous dopamine. Thus, although both an increase and a reduction in impulse flow in the nigro-neostriatal pathway result in an activation of striatal tyrosine hydroxylase, the kinetic alteration produced appears to differ from both a quantitative and mechanistic standpoint.

Presynaptic receptor modulation of the activation of tyrosine hydroxylase produced by increased impulse flow

Recent studies conducted on both peripheral and central noradrenergic systems have given rise to the concept that there may exist on the presynaptic side of the synapse a receptor sensitive to the amount of transmitter in the synaptic cleft and capable of somehow regulating the release of transmitter from the presynaptic terminals (Langer, 1974).

Experiments by Carlsson's group (Kehr et al., 1972) as well as our own (Roth et al., 1973, 1974; Walters and Roth, 1974, 1975; Walters et al., 1974) have suggested that such a presynaptic receptor might exist on central dopamine nerve terminals and in addition to regulating transmitter release might also be involved in the modulation of dopamine synthesis. If such presynaptic receptors exist and do indeed exert some modulatory influence on tyrosine hydroxylase it might be expected that administration of a dopamine receptor agonist would appreciably attenuate the post-stimulation increase in tyrosine hydroxylase activity observed following periods of increased impulse flow. Likewise, administration of dopamine receptor blockers would be expected to enhance the stimulus induced activation of tyrosine hydroxylase by removal of the braking effect exerted by the presence of endogenous synaptic dopamine interacting with the presynaptic receptor.

In an attempt to test the validity of the proposed modulatory role of presynaptic receptors on tyrosine hydroxylase we studied the influence of dopamine agonists and antagonists on the activation of neostriatal tyrosine hydroxylase induced by electrical stimulation of the nigro-neostriatal pathway.

In these experiments we observed that administration of dopamine receptor agonists such as trivastal (ET495) caused a significant reduction in the stimulus induced activation of tyrosine hydroxylase (Table 3). Administration of trivastal to chloral hydrate treated rats had no significant effect on tyrosine hydroxylase activity or on the kinetic properties of tyrosine hydroxylase isolated from the neostriatum in the absence of stimulation. However, trivastal significantly antagonized the increase in tyrosine hydroxylase activity and the kinetic alterations in tyrosine hydroxylase induced by stimulation of the nigro-neostriatal pathway (Table 3). When administered in a dosage of 10 mg/kg 15 minutes prior to stimulation, trivastal caused approximately a 50% block in the activation of tyrosine hydroxylase.

Administration of antipsychotic drugs such as haloperidol which appear to have potent presynaptic dopamine receptor blocking capabilities (Walters and Roth, 1975), causes an increase in the stimulation induced activation of tyrosine hydroxylase. This is reflected both by an increase in tyrosine hydroxylase activity and by an increased alteration in the kinetic properties of tyrosine hydroxylase when compared to stimulation alone (Table 3). Since stimulation of the nigro-neostriatal pathway was carried out for a time period and at a frequency which produced a maximal activation of tyrosine hydroxylase no further activation of tyrosine hydroxylase should be produced as a result of the feedback loop mediated postsynaptic blocking effects of haloperidol. Thus it seems possible that this enhanced activation might occur as a result of the removal of the normal braking effect

TABLE 3

Effects of Electrical Stimulation and Dopamine Receptor Stimulants and Blockers on the Kinetics of Striatal Tyrosine Hydroxylase

Treatment	Tyrosine Hydroxylase Activity[+] (nmoles DOPA/mg Protein/min)	K_m Tyrosine (μM)	K_m BH4 (mM)	K_i DA (mM)
None	22.6 $\pm$ 2.8 (6)	54.7 $\pm$ 5.1	0.42 $\pm$ 0.08	0.05 $\pm$ 0.01
Chloral Hydrate (400 mg/kg)	32.1 $\pm$ 3.1 (6)	41.5 $\pm$ 3.6	0.36 $\pm$ 0.09	0.06 $\pm$ 0.01
Trivastal* (10 mg/kg)	30.4 $\pm$ 2.7 (6)	44.6 $\pm$ 2.9	0.34 $\pm$ 0.07	0.05 $\pm$ 0.01
Haloperidol* (1 mg/kg)	48.9 $\pm$ 3.6 (6)	15.8 $\pm$ 0.8	0.16 $\pm$ 0.04	0.28 $\pm$ 0.01
Stimulation* (15 Hz, 20 min.)	47.2 $\pm$ 2.1 (6)	17.1 $\pm$ 1.6	0.08 $\pm$ 0.01	0.29 $\pm$ 0.04
Stimulation & Trivastal*	39.8 $\pm$ 2.9 (6)	27.2 $\pm$ 1.1	0.35 $\pm$ 0.05	0.11 $\pm$ 0.01
Stimulation & Haloperidol*	79.9 $\pm$ 3.2 (6)	6.5 $\pm$ 0.8	0.01 $\pm$ 0.004	0.38 $\pm$ 0.02

*Rats administered chloral hydrate (400 mg/kg) 15 minutes prior to treatment. Other drugs were administered 45 minutes prior to killing the animals.
[+]Tyrosine hydroxylase activity and kinetic parameters were determined as described in Table 1.

Data taken from Murrin, Morgenroth and Roth in preparation.

thought to be mediated by the presence of increased amounts
of synaptic dopamine interacting with the presynaptic receptor.
Haloperidol by blocking the interaction of dopamine with this
presynaptic receptor may effectively remove any modulatory
influence on tyrosine hydroxylase exerted by presynaptic receptor
activation, thus leading to the observed enhanced activation
of tyrosine hydroxylase. The actual mechanism through which
presynaptic receptor stimulation opposes the increase in tyrosine
hydroxylase activity which occurs with increased impulse flow
in the dopaminergic system is not known, but it appears to be
quite different from that mediating the effects of presynaptic
stimulation after blockade of impulse flow. Under conditions
of increased impulse flow, the effects of presynaptic receptor
stimulation are not mimicked by the in vitro addition of calcium
(Roth et al., 1975a).

Presynaptic receptor modulation of the activation of tyrosine hydroxylase produced by inhibition of impulse flow

Several studies have now shown that stimulation of dopamine
receptors also effectively counteracts the changes in dopamine
synthesis induced by a blockade of impulse flow in the nigro-
neostriatal pathway (Kehr et al., 1972; Roth et al., 1973, 1974;
Walters and Roth, 1974). Thus, administration of amphetamine,
apomorphine or trivastal prevents both the increase in endogenous
levels of neostriatal dopamine and the increase in DOPA accumulation following decarboxylase inhibition, which normally occurs
when impulse flow is blocked pharmacologically or by placement

of a lesion in the nigro-neostriatal pathway. Furthermore, the kinetic activation of tyrosine hydroxylase produced by a block of impulse flow can be completely reversed by administration of a dopamine agonist. For example, if rats are pretreated with GBL (750 mg/kg) and 50 minutes later administered a dopamine receptor stimulant such as apomorphine (2 mg/kg) or trivastal (10 mg/kg), the tyrosine hydroxylase isolated from the striatum of these rats has kinetic properties almost identical to the tyrosine hydroxylase isolated from the striatum of untreated rats (Table 4). Thus, in vivo administration of apomorphine or trivastal to GBL-treated rats causes a change in striatal hydroxylase from a form which has an increased affinity for substrate and cofactor and a decreased affinity for dopamine back to a form which has kinetic properties similar to those found in untreated animals. Administration of apomorphine (2 mg/kg) or addition of apomorphine (10^{-4}M) directly to the incubation medium is without significant effect on tyrosine hydroxylase activity measured in vitro. This ability of dopamine agonists to reverse the activation of tyrosine hydroxylase produced by a blockade of impulse flow can also be demonstrated in in vivo studies in which an estimation of tyrosine hydroxylase activity is obtained by following the short term accumulation of DOPA after administration of a decarboxylase inhibitor. For example, administration of apomorphine (2 mg/kg) or trivastal (10 mg/kg) alone normally causes about a 20 to 35% inhibition of in vivo tyrosine hydroxylase activity (Roth et al., 1974; Walters and

TABLE 4

Reversal by Dopamine Receptor Stimulants of the Activation of Tyrosine Hydroxylase Produced by a Cessation of Impulse Flow

Treatment[+]	Tyrosine Hydroxylase Activity (pmoles DOPA/mg/min)	K_m Tyrosine (μM)	K_m DMPH$_4$ (mM)	K_i Dopamine (mM)
Saline	23.1 ± 2.5 (18)	53.9 ± 5.1	0.89 ± 0.03	0.11 ± 0.01
Apomorphine (2 mg/kg; 40 min.)	21.5 ± 6.6 (6)	49.8 ± 4.5	0.90 ± 0.03	0.11 ± 0.01
Trivastal (10 mg/kg; 40 min.)	24.4 ± 3.1 (6)	55.5 ± 3.7	0.85 ± 0.02	0.13 ± 0.01
γ-Hydroxybutyrate (750 mg/kg; 90 min.)	85.2 ± 4.6* (6)	8.9 ± 0.6*	0.13 ± 0.01	73.9 ± 8.3*
γ-Hydroxybutyrate + Apomorphine	20.1 ± 3.0 (6)	50.4 ± 3.8	0.90 ± 0.05	0.12 ± 0.01
γ-Hydroxybutyrate + Trivastal	26.7 ± 4.1 (6)	52.6 ± 3.8	0.86 ± 0.06	0.10 ± 0.01

[+] γ-Hydroxybutyrate was administered in the lactone form (750 mg/kg, i.p.) 90 min prior to sacrifice. Apomorphine (2 mg/kg) and Trivastal (10 mg/kg) were administered 50 min after γ-hydroxybutyrate and 40 min prior to sacrifice. Results are expressed as the mean ± S.E.M.

Tyrosine hydroxylase activity was determined in the 100,000 x g supernatant of rat corpus striatum at a tyrosine concentration of 10 μM and a $DMPH_4$ concentration of 100 μM. Results are expressed as pmoles DOPA/mg protein/min ± S.E.M. Values in parentheses equal the number of separate experiments.

The K_m for tyrosine was determined by the method of Lineweaver and Burk (1934) according to the method described by Wilkinson (1961) at a $DMPH_4$ concentration of 1 mM and seven tyrosine concentrations ranging from 100 to 0.1 μM. Each value is the mean ± S.E.M. of the intercepts generated from six separate lines.

The K_m for $DMPH_4$ was determined by the method of Lineweaver and Burk (1934) at a tyrosine concentration of 0.1 mM and six $DMPH_4$ concentrations ranging from 1 to 0.01 mM. Each values is the mean ± S.E.M. of the intercepts generated from six separate lines.

The K_i was determined by the method of Dixon (1951) at $DMPH_4$ concentrations of 100, 10 and 1 μM and at 6 dopamine concentrations (0.01 to 0.5 mM). The K_i values are expressed as the mean ± S.E.M. of six determinations.

*Significantly different from saline control $P < 0.01$.

Data taken from Morgenroth, Walters and Roth, 1975.

Roth, 1975). However, if endogenous levels of dopamine are increased to a new steady state by causing a blockade of impulse flow by administration of GBL (a condition which, as indicated in Table 4, changes tyrosine hydroxylase to a form which is insensitive to inhibition by endogenous dopamine) then subsequent administration of either apomorphine or trivastal to these rats now causes a much more potent inhibition of DOPA formation. This enhanced inhibitory effect is presumably due to a conversion of the striatal tyrosine hydroxylase back to a form which is now sensitive to the elevated levels of dopamine. It is generally believed that these effects are mediated by the interaction of the dopamine receptor agonist with receptors on the presynaptic side of the synapse. However, it is premature to rule out the possibility that a trans-synaptic event mediated by an interaction of these dopamine receptor stimulants with postsynaptic dopamine receptors might also be involved.

If an interaction with dopamine receptors is indeed responsible for the ability of drugs like amphetamine, apomorphine and trivastal to block or reverse the increase in tyrosine hydroxylase activity observed during a cessation of impulse flow in dopamine neurons, then dopamine receptor blocking agents should be able to nullify the inhibitory effects of dopamine receptor stimulants. Administration of antipsychotic drugs such as haloperidol effectively reverse the inhibitory effects exerted by dopamine agonists on the increase in tyrosine hydroxylase activity observed after inhibition of impulse flow by

GHB administration or electrothermic lesions. Phenothiazines such as promethazine, devoid of antipsychotic effects and lacking dopamine receptor blocking capabilities, are ineffective in reversing the inhibitory effects of the dopamine receptor stimulants (Walters and Roth, 1974).

These experiments provided further evidence for the contention that activation of a dopamine receptor is responsible for the inhibitory effects exerted by the dopamine agonists on the increase in synthesis produced by a cessation of impulse flow. These observations also were suggestive that a presynaptic receptor mechanism may be involved since the effects of neuronal feedback and subsequent alterations in the firing rate of dopaminergic neurons normally produced by the antipsychotic drugs (Bunney et al., 1973) are prevented by the blockade in impulse flow produced by treatment of the rats with GHB (Walters and Roth, unpublished data). In fact this system has provided an excellent *in vivo* model in which it is possible to screen drugs for potential pre-synaptic receptor stimulating or blocking capabilities since inhibition of impulse flow in the dopamine neurons eliminates post-synaptically induced changes in tyrosine hydroxylase activity mediated by the neuronal feedback loop. In this system presynaptic receptor stimulants effectively block the activation of tyrosine hydroxylase produced by a cessation of impulse flow and agents with presynaptic blocking capabilities nullify the blocking effects of these dopamine receptor stimulants (Walters and Roth, 1975).

The idea that a presynaptic receptor may modulate dopamine synthesis raises questions about the possible mechanism(s) involved in this regulation and the relationship of this mechanism to the role presynaptic receptors play in the modulation of the activation of tyrosine hydroxylase produced by an increase in impulse flow. Iontophoretic application of dopamine onto the cell body of dopaminergic neurons in the zona compacta has recently been shown to inhibit the firing of these dopaminergic neurons (Aghajanian and Bunney, 1973a), and it was theorized that an interaction with the dopamine receptors on the cell body and the consequent alteration in membrane permeability may be responsible for the inhibitory effect of iontophoresed dopamine (Aghajanian and Bunney, 1973b). Furthermore, the suggestion was made that these receptors may be similar to the presynaptic receptors on the dopaminergic nerve terminals. If this is the case, it seems reasonable to suggest that stimulation of the presynaptic receptors in the synaptic cleft by dopamine or dopamine agonists might also affect ionic flow in the presynaptic terminals. Thus, one way in which the presynaptic receptor could control tyrosine hydroxylase activity would be by altering the permeability of the presynaptic membrane to ions or other substances that might influence tyrosine hydroxylase activity. Calcium may be a very important ion in this regard since as mentioned earlier removal of calcium activates striatal tyrosine hydroxylase producing an enzyme with the same kinetic parameters as those observed after inhibition of impulse

REGULATION OF TYROSINE HYDROXYLASE

flow. This activation as well as that caused by a cessation of impulse flow can be completely reversed by addition of calcium to the incubation medium (see Table 2). Thus, although the actual molecular mechanism by which presynaptic receptors modulate the activation of tyrosine hydroxylase produced by alterations in impulse flow remains unclear, dopamine receptors could regulate tyrosine hydroxylase activity by altering the permeability of the presynaptic membrane to calcium ions. Figure 5C illustrates a possible mechanism by which alterations in presynaptic receptor activity might modulate the activation of tyrosine hydroxylase produced by a blockade of impulse flow. In this model dopamine agonists activate the presynaptic dopamine receptor which in turn causes an increase in the permeability of the presynaptic membrane to calcium ions and effectively restores to normal the diminished influx of calcium due to impulse blockade. In the presence of normal intracellular calcium the physical properties of tyrosine hydroxylase revert back to normal in which the enzyme has kinetic properties similar to those found under untreated conditions.

SUMMARY

Electrical stimulation of central dopaminergic neurons in the nigro-neostriatal pathway results in a stimulus dependent increase in the formation of neostriatal dopamine from labeled tyrosine as well as an increase in the accumulation of endogenous DOPA following administration of a central decarboxylase inhibitor.

If tyrosine hydroxylase is isolated from the neostriatum on the stimulated side and its <u>in vitro</u> activity compared to the activity of tyrosine hydroxylase isolated from the unstimulated contralateral side, nearly a 50% increase in activity is observed. Ten minutes of continuous stimulation at 15 Hz is requred to obtain a maximal activation of tyrosine hydroxylase. This activation persists for about 15 minutes following termination of the stimulation period. The mechanism responsible for this activation of tyrosine hydroxylase appears to be related to alterations in the kinetic properties of the enzyme. The tyrosine hydroxylase isolated from the neostriatum on the stimulated side has an increased affinity for the substrate, tyrosine, an increased affinity for the pterin cofactor, and a decreased affinity for the natural end product inhibitor, dopamine.

The activation of striatal tyrosine hydroxylase produced by electrical stimulation is very similar to the activation produced by addition of cAMP to striatal homogenates suggesting that both treatments may be activating tyrosine hydroxylase by an identical mechanism. A possible mechanism by which increased impulse flow may activate striatal tyrosine hydroxylase is disccused.

A cessation of impulse flow in the nigro-neostriatal pathway also causes an activation of striatal tyrosine hydroxylase which appears to be mediated by changes in the affinity of the enzyme for substrate, pterin cofactor and dopamine. The most dramatic change is the greater than 700-fold increase in the K_i for dopamine. These kinetic alterations in contrast to those produced by an increase in impulse flow are completely reversed by addition of calcium to the incubation medium. It is postulated that the increase in tyrosine hydroxylase activity which occurs in the neostriatum during a cessation of impulse flow occurs as a result of a diminished influx of calcium ultimately resulting in an allosteric activation of tyrosine hydroxylase.

In this dopaminergic system as in others, presynaptic receptor stimulation appears to have a damping effect, opposing a marked increase in transmitter biosynthesis by attenuating the increase in tyrosine hydroxylase activity produced by an increase or a cessation of impulse flow in the nigro-neostriatal pathway.

ACKNOWLEDGMENTS

This work was supported in part by grants from N.I.H., MH-14092 and NS-10174 and the State of Connecticut. The authors wish to express their appreciation for the valuable technical assistance provided by Ms. Anne Morrison and Ms. Karen Brady and for the excellent typing assistance of Ms. Lynn Bon Tempo.

REFERENCES

G. K. Aghajanian and B. S. Bunney, "Central Dopaminergic Neurons: Neurophysiological Identification and Response to Drugs", In, Frontiers in Catecholamine Research, E. Usdin and S. H. Snyder (Eds.), Pergamon Press, New York, p. 643, 1973.

G. K. Aghajanian and B. S. Bunney, "Pre- and Postsynaptic Feedback Mechanisms in Central Dopaminergic Neurons, In <u>Neurotransmitters and Brain Function</u>, P. Seeman (Ed.), University of Toronto Press, p. 4, 1974.

G. K. Aghajanian, B. S. Bunney, and M. J. Kuhar, "Use of Single Unit Recording in Correlating Transmitter Turnover with Impulse Flow in Monoamine Neurons", In <u>New Concepts in Neurotransmitter Regulation</u>, A. J. Mandel (Ed.), Plenum Publishing Corp., New York, 1972.

G. K. Aghajanian and R. H. Roth, J. Pharmacol. Exp. Ther. <u>175</u>, 131, 1970.

Y. Agid, F. Javoy, and J. Glowinski, Brain Res. <u>74</u>, 41, 1974.

A. Alousi and N. Weiner, Proc. Natl. Acad. Sci. U.S.A. <u>56</u>, 1491, 1966.

N.-E. Andén, H. Corrodi, K. Fuxe, and U. Ungerstedt, Eur. J. Pharmacol. <u>15</u>, 193, 1971.

G. W. Arbuthnott, T. J. Crow, K. Fuxe, L. Olson, and U. Ungerstedt, Brain Res., <u>24</u>, 471, 1970.

L. J. Bell, L. L. Iverson, and N. J. Uretsky, Brit. J. Pharmacol., <u>40</u>, 790, 1970.

B. S. Bunney, J. R. Walters, R. H. Roth, and G. K. Aghajanian, J. Pharmacol. Exp. Ther. <u>185</u>, 560, 1973.

A. Carlsson, W. Kehr, M. Lindqvist, T. Magnusson, and C. V. Atack, Pharmacol. Rev. <u>24</u>, 371, 1972.

J. R. Cooper, F. E. Bloom and R. H. Roth, <u>The Biochemical Basis of Neuropharmacology</u>, Oxford University Press, New York, 1974.

J. T. Coyle, Biochem. Pharmacol. 21, 1935, 1972.

A. Dahlström and K. Fuxe, Acta Physiol. Scand. 64, Suppl. 247, 1, 1965.

M. Dixon, Biochem. J. 55, 170, 1953.

R. L. M. Faull and R. Laverty, Exp. Neurol. 23, 332, 1969.

G. L. Gessa, L. Vargiu, F. Crabai, C. C. Boero, R. Caboni, and R. Camba, Life Sci. 5, 1921, 1966.

M. Goldstein, T. Backstrom, Y. Ohi, and R. Frankel, Life Sci. 9, 919, 1970.

J. E. Harris, "Factors Controlling the Regulation of Catecholamine Biosynthesis in the Brain, Ph.D. Dissertation, Yale University Graduate School, 1971.

J. E. Harris, R. J. Baldessarini, V. H. Morgenroth, III, and R. H. Roth, Nature 252, 156, 1974.

B. E. Herr and R. H. Roth, Proc. Fifth International Congress on Pharmacology, p. 100, 1972.

S. Kakiuchi, T. W. Rall, and H. McIlwain, J. Neurochem. 16, 165, 1969.

W. Kehr, A. Carlsson and M. Lindqvist, Naunyn-Schmiedeberg's Arch. Pharmacol. 274, 273, 1972.

W. Kehr, A. Carlsson, M. Lindqvist, T. Magnusson, and C. V. Atack, J. Pharm. Pharmacol. 24, 744, 1972.

J. Korf, G. K. Aghajanian, and R. H. Roth, Eur. J. Pharmacol. 21, 305, 1973a.

J. Korf, R. H. Roth, and G. K. Aghajanian, Eur. J. Pharmacol. 23, 276, 1973b.

S. Z. Langer, Biochem. Pharmacol. 23, 1793, 1974.

H. Lineweaver and D. Burk, J. Amer. Chem. Soc. 56, 658, 1934.

V. H. Morgenroth, III, M. C. Boadle-Biber, and R. H. Roth, Proc. Natl. Acad. Sci. 71, 4283, 1974a.

V. H. Morgenroth, III, M. C. Boadle-Biber, and R. H. Roth, Trans. Amer. Soc. Neurochem. 5, 78, 1974b.

V. H. Morgenroth, III, L. R. Hegstrand, R. H. Roth, and P. Greengard, J. Biol. Chem., in press, 1975a.

V. H. Morgenroth, III, J. R. Walters, and R. H. Roth, Biochem. Pharmacol., submitted, 1975b.

L. C. Murrin and R. H. Roth, The Pharmacologist 15, 513, 1973.

L. C. Murrin, V. H. Morgenroth, III, and R. H. Roth, The Pharmacologist 16, 128, 1974.

H. Nybäck, Acta Physiol. Scand. 84, 54, 1972.

H. Nybäck and G. Sedvall, J. Pharmacol. Exp. Ther. 162, 294, 1968.

R. H. Roth, V. H. Morgenroth, III, and L. C. Murrin, "Effects of antipsychotic drugs and impulse flow on the kinetics of striatal tyrosine hydroxylase", Wenner-Gren Center International Symposium Series, Pergamon Press, Ltd., New York, 1975a.

R. H. Roth, V. H. Morgenroth, III and P. M. Salzman, Naunyn-Schmiedeberg's Arch. Pharmacol., submitted, 1975b.

R. H. Roth, P. M. Salzman, and V. H. Morgenroth, III, Biochem. Pharmacol. 24, 2779, 1974a.

R. H. Roth, L. Stjärne and U. S. von Euler, Life Sci. 5, 1071, 1966.

R. H. Roth, L. Stjärne and U. S. von Euler, J. Pharmacol. Exp. Ther. <u>158</u>, 373, 1967.

R. H. Roth and Y. Surh, Biochem. Pharmacol. <u>19</u>, 3001, 1970.

R. H. Roth, J. R. Walters, and G. K. Aghajanian, "Effect of Impulse Flow on the Release and Synthesis of Dopamine in the Rat Striatum", In <u>Catecholamine Research</u>, E. Usdin and S. H. Snyder (Eds.), Pergamon Press, New York, p. 567, 1973.

R. H. Roth, J. R. Walters, and V. H. Morgenroth, III, "Effects of Alterations in Impulse Flow on Transmitter Metabolism in Central Dopaminergic Neurons", In <u>Neuropsychopharmacology of Monoamines and Their Regulatory Enzymes</u>, E. Usdin (Ed.), Raven Press, New York, p. 369, 1974b.

G. C. Sedvall, "Effect of Nerve Stimulation of Accumulation and Disappearance of Catecholamines Formed From Radioactive Precursors In Vivo", In <u>Metabolism of Amines in the Brain</u>, G. Hooper (Ed.), Macmillan, p. 23, 1969.

V. H. Sethy, M. J. Kuhar, R. H. Roth, M. H. Van Woert, and G. K. Aghajanian, Brain Res. <u>55</u>, 481, 1973.

R. Shiman, M. Akino, and S. Kaufman, J. biol. Chem. <u>246</u>, 1330, 1971.

H. Shimizu, C. R. Creveling, and J. W. Daly, "Effect of Membrane Depolarization and Biogenic Amines on the Formation of Cyclic AMP in Incubated Brain Slices", In, <u>Role of Cyclic AMP in Cell Function</u>. Advances in Biochemical Psychopharmacology, Vol. 3, P. Greengard and E. Costa (Eds.), Raven Press, New York, p. 135, 1970.

G. Stock, T. Magnusson, and N.-E. Anden, Naunyn-Schmiedeberg's Arch. Pharmacol. 278, 347, 1973.

U. Ungerstedt, Acta Physiol. Scand., Suppl. 267, 1, 1971.

N. Weiner, Ann. Rev. Pharmacol. 10, 273, 1970.

J. R. Walters, G. K. Aghajanian and R. H. Roth, Proc. Fifth Cong. Pharmacol., p. 246, 1972.

J. R. Walters, B. S. Bunney, and R. H. Roth, "Peribidel and Apomorphine: Pre- and Post-synaptic Effects on Dopamine Synthesis and Neuronal Activity", in Advances in Neurology, D. Calne, T. N. Chase, and A. Barbeau (Eds.), Vol. 9, Raven Press, New York, in press, 1974.

J. R. Walters and R. H. Roth, Biochem. Pharmacol. 21, 2111, 1972.

J. R. Walters and R. H. Roth, J. Pharmacol. Exp. Ther. 191, 82, 1974.

J. R. Walters and R. H. Roth, "Pre- and Postsynaptic Actions of Antipsychotic Drugs", In Antipsychotic Drugs, Pharmacodynamics and Pharmacokinetics, Wenner-Gren Center International Symposium Series, Pergamon Press, Ltd., New York, 1975.

J. R. Walters, R. H. Roth, and G. K. Aghajanian, J. Pharmacol. Exp. Ther. 186, 630, 1973.

DISCUSSION

Dr. Everett wondered whether apomorphine had been tested in place of trivastal. Dr. Roth replied that this had been done, but at the dose used (2 mg/kg) apomorphine produced some kinetic alterations in the enzyme. This slight decrease in tyrosine hydroxylase activity is not observed with trivastal.

Dr. Meltzer was interested in the comparative effects of chronic electrical stimulation versus those of drugs but Dr. Roth replied that such chronic experiments had not been performed. In acute experiments, no changes in V_{max} were observed, for either tyrosine or tetrahydrobiopterin. Some preliminary experiments with long-term administration of antipsychotic drugs have shown very little change in V_{max}.

Dr. Costa wanted to know if the speaker was implying that dopamine receptor blockers did not work on presynaptic receptors. Dr. Roth said that some dopamine receptor blockers are very potent presynaptic receptor blockers, e. g., haloperidol and chlorpromazine. He then described a system used for screening the activity of pre- and postsynaptic blockers. In this model system, tyrosine hydroxylase activity is increased by blocking impulse flow in the dopamine system. Then the test drug is administered to see whether it will attenuate, or block the activation of tyrosine hydroxylase (as dopamine agonists do). If the drug nullifies the block, then it tends to have a presynaptic action. Whereas clozapine and pimozide have no presynaptic action (as shown in this system), the butyrophenones and many of the antipsychotic phenothiazines are very effective in nullifying the block produced by the dopamine agonist.

Dr. Gessa wondered whether Dr. Roth had studied the effect of gamma-hydroxybutyrate on tyrosine hydroxylase activity. The speaker replied that he had. GHB, by blocking impulse flow in the dopamine system, causes a marked activation of tyrosine hydroxylase and produces kinetic alterations in the enzyme. Most dramatically, it causes about a 750-fold change in the affinity of the enzyme for dopamine. The enzyme is no longer sensitive to inhibition by dopamine after blocking impulse flow either by placement of a lesion or by treatment with GHB. However, either of these effects (lesion or GHB) may be totally reversed by the addition of calcium to the medium. On the other hand, the effects discussed by Dr. Roth in terms of increased impulse flow are not affected by calcium ion.

RECEPTOR-MEDIATED CONTROL OF DOPAMINE METABOLISM

A. Carlsson

Department of Pharmacology
University of Göteborg
Göteborg, Sweden

I. INTRODUCTION

The concept that dopaminergic receptors may play a role in regulating the release, metabolism and synthesis of dopamine goes back to 1963, when we first reported on the ability of chlorpromazine and haloperidol to stimulate the metabolism and synthesis of brain catecholamines (1). We speculated that these antipsychotic agents by blocking dopamine receptors might influence a negative feedback mechanism leading to activation of dopaminergic neurons. A similar mechanism was postulated for noradrenergic neurons. These observations have been repeatedly confirmed and the concept of receptor-mediated regulation of catecholamine metabolism has been corroborated e.g. by the observation that dopaminergic and noradrenergic agonists cause inhibition of dopamine and noradrenaline turnover, respectively (see 2,3).

II. COMPLEXITY OF RECEPTOR-MEDIATED FEEDBACK CONTROL

Today we know that in the central nervous system the receptor-mediated feedback control of a transmitter such as dopamine is a complex phenomenon, involving at least 3 different, partly independent components:
1) Control of firing rate (see 4)
2) Control of transmitter release and metabolism; this phenomenon,

though dependent on nerve impulses, can still be demonstrated at constant firing rate and is thus not entirely secondary to component 1) (see 5,6).

3) Control of dopa synthesis; this mechanism can still be demonstrated after axotomy (see Fig. 1) and is thus not entirely secondary to component 1) or 2) (7,8).

While the feedback regulation is probably in part mediated via the classical postsynaptic receptors and neuronal loops feeding back the information to the cell bodies of the presynaptic neuron by impinging on its cell bodies or dendrites, it is evident that, in addition, a local feedback mechanism exists which can still operate after cutting the axons of the presynaptic neuron. While it cannot be excluded that also the local

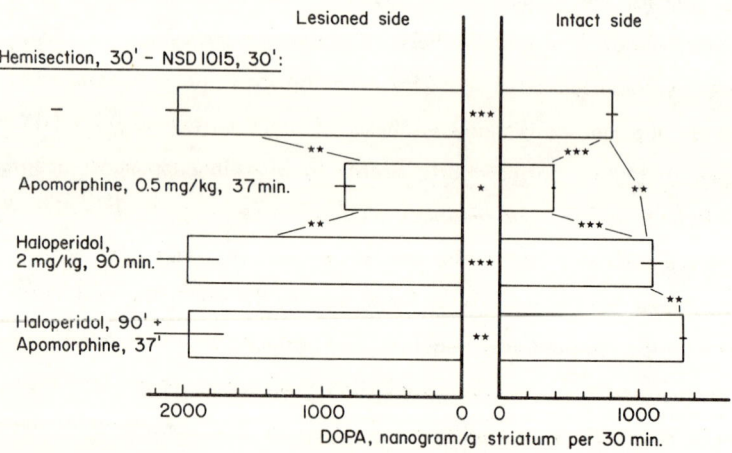

Fig. 1. Effect of a Dopamine Receptor Agonist (Apomorphine), of an Antagonist (Haloperidol), and of Both Drugs in Combination, on the Rate of Conversion of Tyrosine to Dopa in Rat Striatum: Evidence that Receptor-Mediated Feedback Control Persists after Axotomy.

Haloperidol, 2 mg/kg, and apomorphine, 0.5 mg/kg, were given i.p. 60 and 7 min, respectively, before a cerebral hemisection. NSD 1015, 100 mg/kg, was given at the time of hemisection. The animals were killed 30 min later, and striatal dopa levels were measured separately on the lesioned and on the intact side. - NSD 1015 (3-hydroxybenzyl-hydrazine HCl) is a potent inhibitor of the aromatic L-amino-acid decarboxylase and causes a rapid accumulation of dopa in brain from very low normal levels. (Unpublished data of this laboratory.)

feedback regulation is mediated via postsynaptic receptors, it seems at least as likely that presynaptic receptors are involved. In support of the latter alternative, it has been found in several instances, that the cell bodies of monoaminergic neurons show an inhibitory response to local application of the transmitter which they produce (see 4). It may thus be speculated that "presynaptic" receptors are widely distributed in all the different parts of the neuron. However, if this is so, the term "presynaptic receptor" is hardly adequate. It should perhaps be replaced by "autoreceptor", since the important feature is the neuron's sensitivity to its own transmitter substance, rather than the location relative to a synapse.

An important question which may possibly help to clarify the nature of "autoreceptors", is whether they, like postsynaptic receptor mechanisms, respond to surgical or pharmacological denervation by an increase in sensitivity. This question cannot be answered yet, but it has been found that the sensitivity to apomorphine-induced inhibition of dopamine synthesis is markedly increased during the first 24 h after a single dose of reserpine (Fig. 2). Further analysis of this phenomenon might prove fruitful, e.g. whether it also involves cell-body "autoreceptors".

III. POSSIBLE IMPLICATIONS OF PRESYNAPTIC RECEPTORS (OR "AUTORECEPTORS")

If autoreceptors occur and are widely distributed over the neuronal surface, the implications in physiology, pathophysiology and pharmacology may be great. Autoreceptors may help to explain some paradoxical phenomena, which are otherwise hard to explain, and they may open up new rationales in therapy. These aspects will be briefly discussed below.

A. Paradoxical Response to Axotomy

It has often been assumed that the synthesis of new transmitter is always positively correlated to the nerve impulse flow. This may be true in general, but we know of at least one striking exception to this rule.

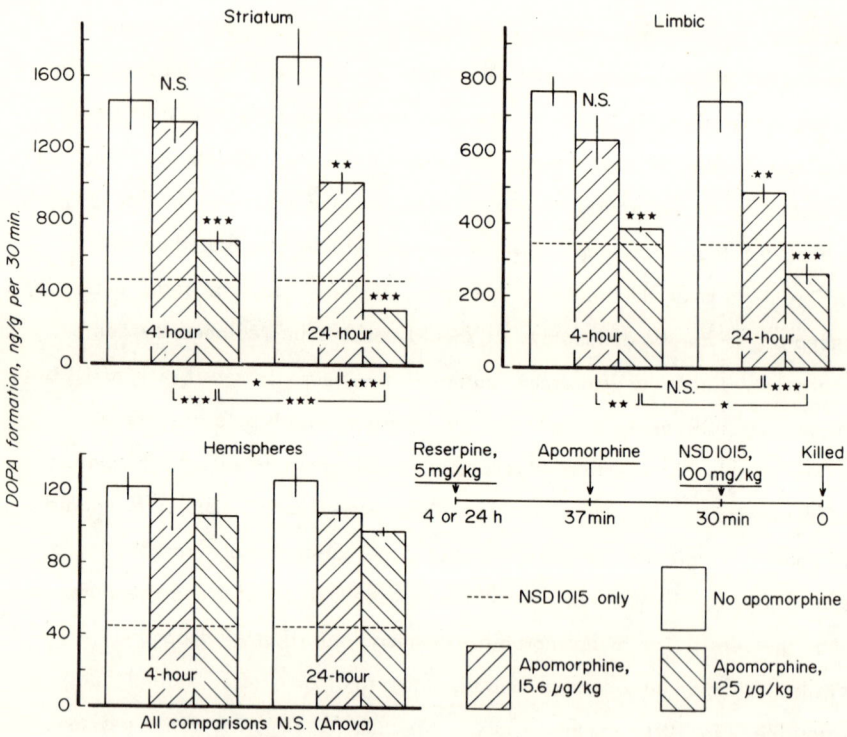

Fig. 2. Effect of Apomorphine on Dopa Formation in Rat Brain Parts after Pretreatment with Reserpine 4 or 24 Hours Previously. All animals were given an i.p. injection of NSD 1015 as indicated, 30 min before death. Injections of reserpine and apomorphine were given i.p. at the time intervals indicated, and the brain parts were analyzed for dopa.

Note. Treatment with reserpine (open columns) stimulated dopa formation as compared to animals treated with NSD 1015 only (broken horizontal lines) in all brain regions and about equally at both time intervals. The lower dose of apomorphine (15.6 μg/kg) was inactive when given 4 hours after reserpine but significantly reduced dopa formation in striatum and in dopamine-rich limbic regions 24 hours after reserpine. The larger dose of apomorphine was active at both time intervals but more active at the longer interval. Apomorphine caused no significant effects in the cerebral hemisphere portion, where noradrenaline predominates. (Unpublished data of this laboratory.)

When central dopaminergic axons are cut, the synthesis of dopamine in the terminal fibre system is not inhibited, but is instead markedly stimulated during an initial period lasting at least 30 min (9,10). Since, as mentioned, the receptor-mediated control of dopamine synthesis persists after axotomy, as indicated by agonist and antagonist induced responses, it is reasonable to assume that the marked stimulation of synthesis induced by axotomy is due to a virtually complete disappearance of the physiological agonist from dopaminergic synapses. This should have the same effect as depletion of dopamine by e.g. reserpine or blockade of dopamine receptors by e.g. chlorpromazine, i.e. a strong stimulation of dopamine synthesis.

It would thus appear that the nerve impulses have a dual influence on neurotransmitter synthesis: 1) a stimulating action via release of end-product inhibition or, probably more important, at least in some instances, through some more direct influence of nerve impulses on synthesis (cf. 7), 2) an inhibitory action via the receptor-mediated feedback mechanism. In central dopaminergic synapses, the second mechanism appears to be unusually well developed. It may, however, exist also in other synapses and may, for example, explain the remarkably slight effect of axotomy on transmitter synthesis in cerebral noradrenaline and 5-HT fibre systems (see 9,11).

B. Paradoxical Response to Dopaminergic Receptor Agonists

Perhaps the most fascinating possible implication of autoreceptors deals with paradoxical responses to low doses of agonists and antagonists.

As mentioned, dopamine receptor agonists have been shown to cause a marked inhibition of dopamine turnover. The inhibition of dopamine synthesis in rat or mouse brain occurs even in low doses (about 50 µg/kg i.p., see 12), i.e. an order of magnitude lower than the dose required for inducing excitation with typical stereotyped behavior. Interestingly, apomorphine in low doses or at early time intervals after larger doses, actually causes inhibition of locomotor activity, particularly striking during the initial phase of new environment exploration (13,24, Fig. 3). The dopamine agonist ET 495 (13) and dopa (14) behave similarly. It is tempting to suggest that dopamine agonists are capable of activating two

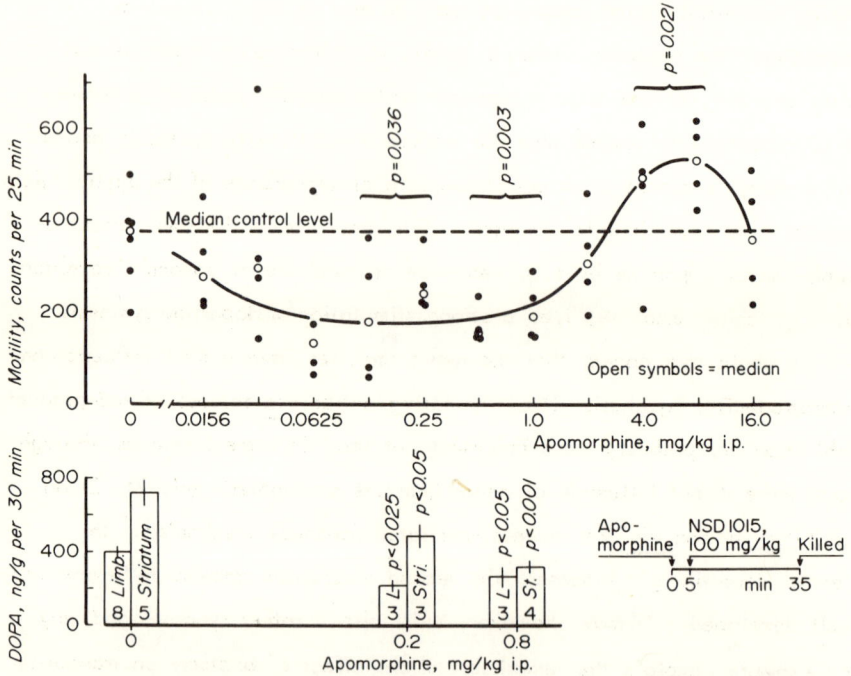

Fig. 3. Upper graph: Motility of Mice 20 to 45 min after Apomorphine. The animals were placed in the motility cage 5 min after the injection of apomorphine.

Lower graph: Dopa Formation in Dopamine-Rich Mouse Brain Parts 5 to 35 min after Apomorphine. NSD 1015 100 mg/kg was given i.p. 5 min after apomorphine, and the animals were killed 30 min later (24).

types of dopaminergic receptor, resulting in motor inhibition and stimulation, respectively, and that the former type of receptor is an autoreceptor. A possible reason why autoreceptors appear to be more sensitive than the ordinary postsynaptic receptors to exogenous agonists could be that the former have a more wide spread distribution than the latter. The reverse situation should prevail when dopamine is released by the nerve impulse into the synaptic cleft: here the postsynaptic receptors should predominate.

Preferential activation of autoreceptors by e.g. exogenous dopamine agonists may have clinical implications. Apomorphine has been used for many years in the treatment of alcoholism. Apomorphine is said to reduce the craving for alcohol, and the effect has been claimed to be not merely due to conditioning, induced by apomorphine's emetic action (see 15). Some experimental support for this view has been obtained by the demonstration that the stimulant action of ethanol is accompanied by a stimulation of catecholamine metabolism in the brain and that the stimulant and euphoriant action of apomorphine in animals and in man can be prevented by the tyrosine hydroxylase inhibitor α-methyltyrosine (see 16). Moreover, the stimulant action of ethanol in animals has been shown to be prevented by apomorphine or ET 495 (13). It is tempting to suggest that this action of dopamine agonists is due to inhibition of dopaminergic neurons, mediated via autoreceptor activation.

C. Response to Dopaminergic Receptor Antagonists

If the ordinary postsynaptic receptors predominate in the synaptic cleft, as suggested above, and if this is the chief site of transmitter release, one would hardly expect a diphasic dose-response curve of dopamine antagonists, as was found with the agonists. However, stimulant actions of low doses of certain dopamine receptor antagonists have been observed (see 17) and the possibility thus exists that blockade of dopaminergic autoreceptors may lead to some stimulation of dopaminergic neurons.

In general, the doses of a dopamine receptor antagonist required for stimulation of dopamine synthesis and for behavioral inhibition, respectively, are approximately the same, even though more precise and extensive measurements in the future may disclose differences (Table 1). Thus the receptors involved in behavioral inhibition and in stimulation of dopamine synthesis show no marked differences in sensitivity to the dopamine receptor antagonists investigated so far. Neuroleptic agents appear to have differential actions on different dopaminergic systems, and thus on different brain functions. For example, while pimozide, haloperidol and chlorpromazine stimulate dopamine synthesis more strongly in the striatal than

TABLE 1

Approximate Threshold Doses of Neuroleptic Agents Required for Stimulation of Dopa Synthesis in Dopamine-Rich Rat Brain Regions and for Suppression of Food-Reinforced Lever-Pressing Behavior.

Agent	Threshold Dose, mg/kg i.p.	
	Dopa Synthesis [a]	Inhibition of Behavior [b]
Haloperidol	0.05	0.05 (0.02)
Pimozide	0.1	0.08 (0.04)
Chlorpromazine	0.25 - 0.5	1 (0.5)
Thioridazine	2	3 (1.5)
Clozapine	6	2 (1)

a) Data taken from Fig. 4.
b) Figures in brackets refer to threshold doses of neuroleptic agents in rats pretreated with α-methyltyrosine (20, 21 and unpublished data).

in the limbic dopamine-rich areas, this difference is very slight after clozapine and thioridazine (Fig. 4, Table 2). Since the latter two agents appear to cause fewer extrapyramidal side effects than the former in doses which are equipotent with respect to antipsychotic activity, the data support Andén's suggestion (18,19) that antipsychotic and extrapyramidal actions reside in different brain regions, i.e. in limbic areas and in the striatum, respectively. Threshold doses for stimulation of dopamine synthesis are, however, about equal in the two regions even though, as mentioned, the amplitude of response may be different.

IV. FUNCTIONAL SIGNIFICANCE OF RECEPTOR-MEDIATED FEEDBACK CONTROL OF TRANSMITTER SYNTHESIS

As mentioned, control of transmitter synthesis is only one aspect of the complex receptor-mediated feedback control of dopaminergic neurons.

How much does this component contribute to the overall feedback response? This contribution is probably significant, because it has been found that a dopaminergic receptor antagonist, when given in a dose which is subthreshold with respect to behavior, will cause marked behavioral inhibition when given together with a subthreshold dose of the tyrosine hydroxylase inhibitor α-methyltyrosine (20,21). These observations in animals have been confirmed in schizophrenic patients. Thus it has been found that the antipsychotic action of phenothiazines is markedly potentiated by α-methyltyrosine, given in a dose which reduces the concentration of homovanillic acid in the cerebrospinal fluid by about 80 per cent but has no detectable antipsychotic activity per se (22,23). These observations have recently been confirmed in a study using a double-blind crossover design (Fig. 5). Thus, in the presence of a subthreshold concentration of a neuroleptic agent, schizophrenic symptomatology can be profoundly influenced by changes in tyrosine hydroxylase activity. It may be speculated that schizophrenia may result from dopaminergic predominance, perhaps in the limbic system, either due to an excessive activation of dopaminergic receptors or to insufficient activation of an antagonistic (GABA ?) pathway.

V. CONCLUDING REMARKS

The evidence in favor of dopaminergic presynaptic receptors, perhaps preferably called "autoreceptors", may be summarized as follows:

1) A local receptor-mediated feedback control mechanism exists in the dopaminergic terminal region.

2) Dopaminergic cell bodies and/or dendrites possess dopaminergic receptors (4).

3) The dopaminergic agonist apomorphine has a biphasic dose response curve with respect to behavior, inhibition occurring in the lower dose range. The threshold doses for inhibition of behavior and for inhibition of dopa formation are approximately the same, which would fit the hypothesis of

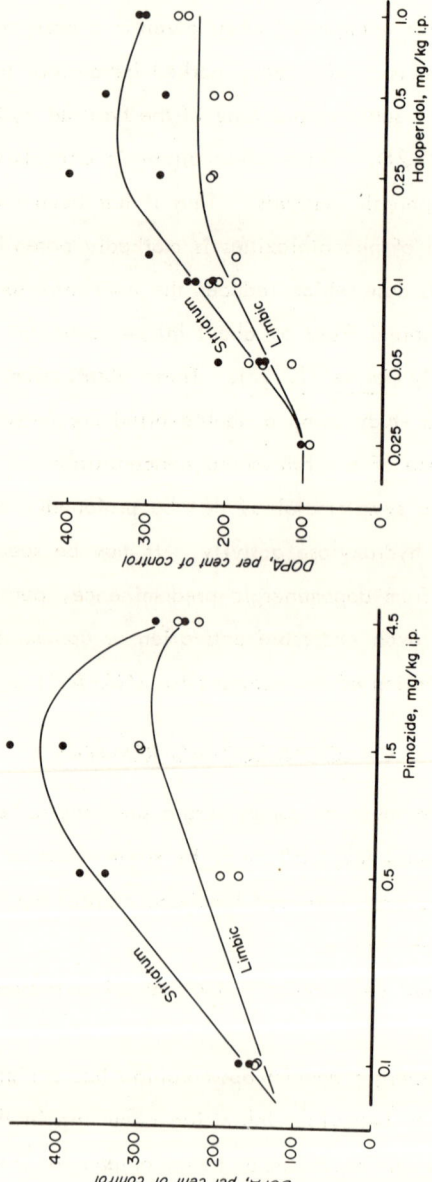

CONTROL OF DOPAMINE METABOLISM

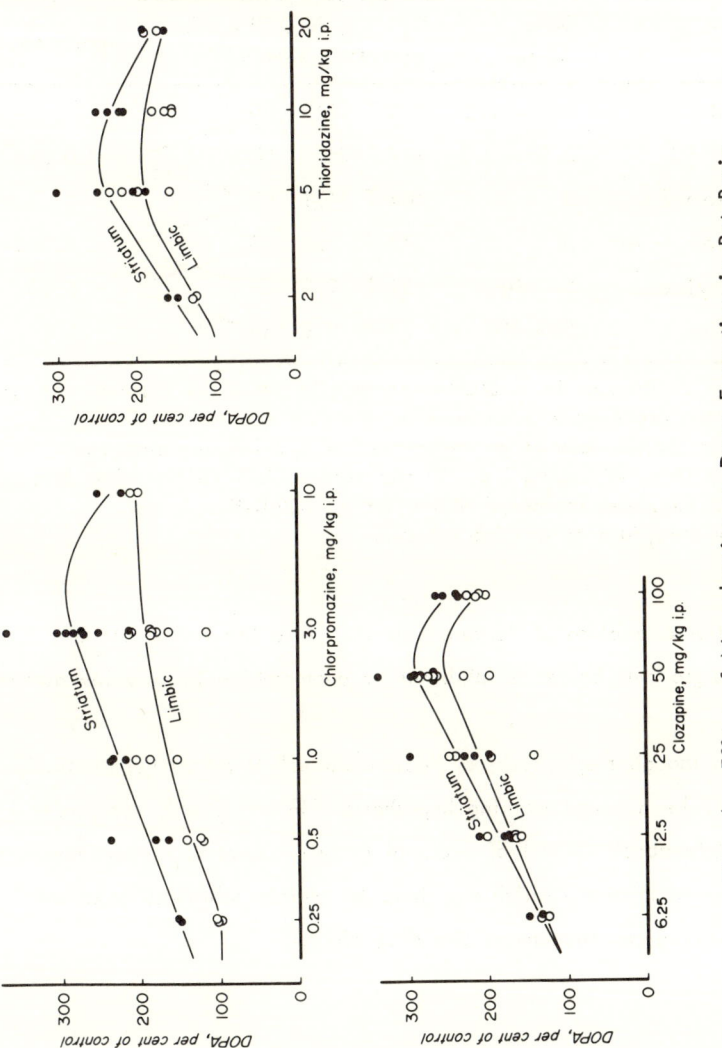

Fig. 4. Effect of Neuroleptics on Dopa Formation in Rat Brain Regions Rich in Dopamine. The neuroleptics were given 60 min before NSD 1015 (100 mg/kg i.p.) and the animals were killed after another 30 min. (Unpublished data of this laboratory.)

TABLE 2

Differential Action of Antipsychotic Drugs
on DOPA Formation in Striatum vs. Limbic Regions

Drug	Dose, mg/kg	Diff. in % DOPA incr., striatum − limbic	Significance
Pimozide	0.5 − 1.5	153 ± 18.3 (4)	
Haloperidol	0.25 − 0.5	117 ± 26.1 (4)	$p < 0.025$
Chlorpromazine	3	104 ± 11.1 (8)	
Chlorprom. + Atr.	3	73 ± 9.2 (5)	$p < 0.005$
Thioridazine	5 − 10	51 ± 9.3 (8)	$p < 0.05$
Clozapine	50 − 100	37 ± 8.8 (10)	

The differences in % DOPA increase between the striatum and the limbic areas were obtained from the data represented in Fig. 4 and from similar data of an experiment with chlorpromazine and atropine (Atr. 40 mg/kg i.p. 10 min before NSD 1015). The data refer to the doses indicated in the table. Statistics: t-test. (Unpublished data of this laboratory.)

preferential activation of "autoreceptors". Also the firing rate of dopaminergic cell bodies is inhibited by apomorphine in very low dosage (4).

Even though the concept of "autoreceptors" is partly hypothetical, it appears to be a useful working hypothesis. In any event, receptor-mediated feedback control of neuronal activity seems to be an important regulatory mechanism, which may help to explain otherwise puzzling pathophysiological phenomena and drug effects.

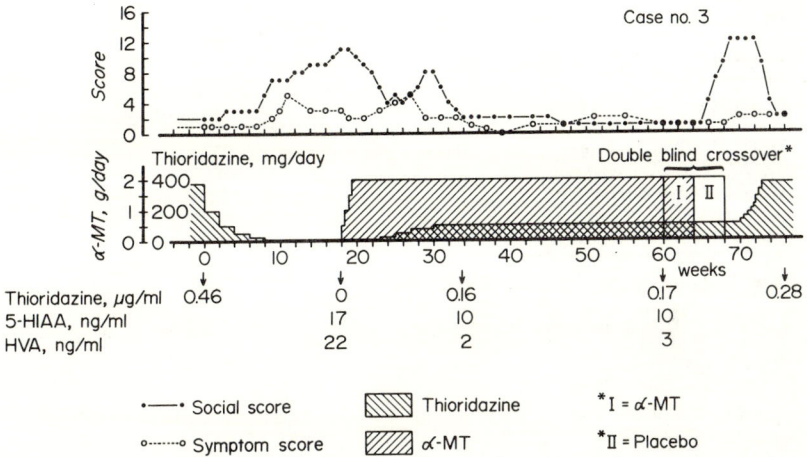

Fig. 5. Potentiation of the Antipsychotic Action of Thioridazine by α-Methyltyrosine (αMT) in a Schizophrenic Patient.

The patient, a 44-year-old male, had suffered from schizophrenia with stationary symptomatology for more than six months. He had been hospitalized and treated with thioridazine as the only antipsychotic drug in constant dosage for more than six months. The trial was started by rating the symptoms verbally by a psychiatrist and behaviorally by the head nurse. Then the dosage of thioridazine was reduced stepwise until the care of the patient became difficult. At this time the scores were markedly elevated. α-Methyltyrosine therapy was now started, the dosage being gradually increased to 2 g/day, while keeping the thioridazine dosage at a constant low level. This dose regimen was insufficient to control the condition, and thus the dose of thioridazine was gradually increased until the pretrial symptomatology level was attained. This occurred at a thioridazine dosage of 100 as compared to the pretrial dosage of 375 mg/day. The dose regimen was kept for 30 weeks. During this period the patient tended to be in an even better mental condition than before the trial.

At the termination of the trial α-methyltyrosine was replaced by placebo or α-methyltyrosine, using a double-blind crossover design. During the blind α-methyltyrosine period, which in this case came first, there was no change in the ratings, but during the placebo period a rapid deterioration occurred. The dosage of thioridazine was then gradually increased to the original level, and the pretrial symptomatology level was re-attained.

Similar results were obtained in 3 additional schizophrenic patients (25).

REFERENCES

1. A. Carlsson and M. Lindqvist, Acta pharmacol. et toxicol., 20, 140-144 (1963).

2. N.-E. Andén, A. Carlsson, and J. Häggendal, Annu. Rev. Pharmacol., 9, 119-134 (1969).
3. W. Kehr, A. Carlsson, and M. Lindqvist, Adv. in Neurology, Vol. 9, Raven Press, New York, 1975 (in press).
4. G.K. Aghajanian and B.S. Bunney, in Frontiers in Neurology and Neuroscience Research 1974 (P. Seeman and G.M. Brown, eds.), The University of Toronto Press, Toronto, 1974, Chap. 2.
5. L.-O. Farnebo and B. Hamberger, Acta physiol. scand., Suppl. 371, 35-44 (1971).
6. L.-O. Farnebo and B. Hamberger, in Frontiers in Catecholamine Research (S.H. Snyder and E. Usdin, eds.), Pergamon Press, New York, 1973, pp. 589-594.
7. W. Kehr, A. Carlsson, M. Lindqvist, T. Magnusson, and C. Atack, J. Pharm. Pharmacol., 24, 744-747 (1972).
8. A. Carlsson, W. Kehr, and M. Lindqvist, in Neuropsychopharmacology of Monoamines and Their Regulatory Enzymes (E. Usdin, ed.) Raven Press, New York, 1974, pp. 135-142.
9. A. Carlsson, W. Kehr, M. Lindqvist, T. Magnusson, and C.V. Atack, Pharmacol. Rev., 24, 371-384 (1972).
10. W. Kehr, J. Neural Transmission, 1974 (in press).
11. P. Bédard, A. Carlsson, and M. Lindqvist, Naunyn-Schmiedeberg's Arch. Pharmacol., 272, 1-15 (1972).
12. A. Carlsson, W. Kehr, and M. Lindqvist, "Receptor-Mediated Control of Dopamine Synthesis", presented at C.I.N.P. Meeting, Paris, 1974.
13. A. Carlsson, J. Engel, U. Strömbom, T.H. Svensson, and B. Waldeck, Naunyn-Schmiedeberg's Arch. Pharmacol., 283, 117-128 (1974).
14. U. Strömberg, Psychopharmacologia (Berl.), 18, 58-67 (1970).
15. E.K.E. Schlatter and S. Lal, Quart. J. Stud. Alcohol., 33, 430-436 (1972).

16. S. Ahlenius, A. Carlsson, J. Engel, T. Svensson, and P. Södersten, Clin. Pharmacol. Ther., 14, 586–591 (1973).
17. S. Ahlenius and J. Engel, J. Pharm. Pharmacol., 23, 301–302 (1971).
18. N.-E. Andén, J. Pharm. Pharmacol., 24, 905–906 (1972).
19. N.-E. Andén and G. Stock, J. Pharm. Pharmacol., 25, 346–348 (1973).
20. S. Ahlenius and J. Engel, European J. Pharmacol., 15, 187–192 (1971).
21. S. Ahlenius and J. Engel, J. Pharm. Pharmacol., 25, 172–174 (1973).
22. A. Carlsson, T. Persson, B.-E. Roos, and J. Wålinder, J. Neural Transmission, 33, 83–90 (1972).
23. A. Carlsson, B.-E. Roos, J. Wålinder, and A. Skott, J. Neural Transmission, 34, 125–132 (1973).
24. U. Strömbom, unpublished data, 1974.
25. J. Wålinder, A. Skott, A. Carlsson, and B.-E. Roos, unpublished data, 1974.

DISCUSSION

Dr. Moore asked for a clarification of the limbic areas in which Dr. Carlsson had reported on DOPA synthesis. Dr. Carlsson replied that included were the olfactory tubercle, the nucleus accumbens, part of the cingulate gyrus, the paleocortex and the amygdala - the anterior commisure was used as a landmark.

Dr. Gessa was concerned with the type of behavior measured by the speaker since it is known that 100 mg of haloperidol per kg will show an increase in dopamine turnover but will not produce any signs of catalepsy. Dr. Carlsson agreed with Dr. Gessa that the behavioral parameter had to be selected with care. In his lab, Dr. Carlsson has observed a paradoxical effect on behavior with low doses of haloperidol; within a very narrow dose range, stimulant or amphetamine-like behavior is observed.

Dr. Aghajanian reinforced the suggested usage of the term "autoreceptors" as being very useful. He felt this was particularly apt in the case of dopamine neurons since there is probably no catecholaminergic synaptic input to the dopamine neurons. It is very confusing to speak about presynaptic receptors to a transmitter substance when there is no synaptic input to the neuron in question utilizing that transmitter. He thought it might be very useful to adopt the term "autoreceptors".

Dr. Langlais wondered if the biphasic behavioral responses seen with apomorphine correlated with the presynaptic mechanism. He suggested that rather than Dr. Carlsson's explanation based on the more diffuse distribution of the presynaptic receptors, the results could be explained as the result of increased sensitivity of presynaptic receptors as compared to postsynaptic receptors. Dr. Carlsson agreed that it was possible that the affinity conditions for the two types of receptors might be different.

Dr. Iversen mentioned that Dr. Langer has evidence that noradrenaline neurons in the periphery have autoreceptors with dopaminergic activity. He wondered whether Dr. Carlsson had any evidence that apomorphine would affect noradrenaline in the CNS. Dr. Carlsson averred that it did, that one of his figures shows that if animals are pre-treated with reserpine, the effect of apomorphine on DOPA formation in noradrenergic areas completely disappears whereas in dopamine-rich areas it is actually enhanced.

Dr. Hornykiewicz remarked that since Dr. Carlsson had reported the inhibition of the locomotor-stimulation effect of ethanol by apomorphine, he must have tried the combination of dopamine receptor blockers and ethanol or reserpine and ethanol. Dr. Carlsson was not sure whether or not his laboratory had done this, but he had no doubt that these antagonists would block this phenomenon.

PHYSIOLOGICAL ASSESSMENT OF PRE- AND POSTSYNAPTIC RECEPTORS

F. E. Bloom

Laboratory of Neuropharmacology
Division of Special Mental Health Research, IRP
National Institute of Mental Health
Saint Elizabeths Hospital
Washington, D.C. 20032

I. INTRODUCTION

The psychopharmacologist who seeks to analyze the electrophysiological basis for drug receptor interactions finds himself in a "binding" predicament. His concepts of the cellular organization of the nervous system contrast with the "pure" electrophysiologist who may prefer to ignore the complexities of the central monoamine pathways. At the same time, electrophysiological methods of attack seem painfully detailed, because these methods demand excessively meticulous controls compared to biochemists who can simultaneously assess multiple drug actions on millions of neurons. As a result, electrophysiological methods applied to psychopharmacological problems are usually poorly regarded by electrophysiologists and far behind the latest emerging concepts of drug-neuron interactions advanced by the biochemists.

Having devoted several laborious years to the demonstration of norepinephrine as a central inhibitory transmitter in the cerebellum and hippocampus (1-5) and to the molecular mechanisms by which this inhibition is mediated intracellularly by cyclic adenosine monophosphate (cAMP; 6-9), my colleagues and I again find that we are behind the times in psychopharmacology where the existence of central monoamine synaptic pathways were assumed long before our demonstrations. No longer are drugs which affect human and animal behavior merely considered as potential agonists or antagonists of the monoamine synaptic transmitters, or as modifiers of the release or re-accumulation of the transmitter amine. These drugs are now viewed as acting through local or long distance "pre-synaptic feedback" circuits to regulate the synthesis and turnover of the transmitter and its synthetic and catabolic enzymes (see 10-12).

In the present discussion I intend to reflect upon the problems facing a detailed analysis of these "pre-synaptic" drug actions on the diffusely distributed, slowly conducting, long acting central monoamine pathways (13-15). I do so not as a critic, but as one who regards the pharmacological analysis of drug effects on central monoamines as a fundamental tool for the elucidation of the function of these pathways in the normal brain and as a clue to the dysfunctions which may occur in psychiatric illnesses. Implicit in such a quest is the assumption that a more clearcut understanding of the changes which drugs can produce in normal animals will illuminate the etiology of possible pathophysiological states which such drugs can treat. Perhaps these drug fortuitously act only on the small number of neurons whose neurotransmitter chemicals we now have methods to study. Perhaps these cells are affected only as epi-phenomena of the actions initiated at some other interconnected nucleus. Nevertheless, such electrophysiological studies on psychopharmacological agents can be heuristic by dissecting the chains of responsive neurons and their roles in the regulation of normal behavior.

II. PRESYNAPTIC RECEPTORS

Let us first consider the more "classical" concepts of receptors which could mediate pre-synaptic drug actions. In reviewing the pharmacological properties of pre-synaptic

PHYSIOLOGICAL ASSESSMENT

terminals (16), Eccles' earliest citation is that of Masland and Wigton who observed in 1940 (17) that intravenous injection of the anticholinesterase agent prostigmine initiated depolarizations of motor nerve fiber terminals which would propagate antidromically as well as cause the muscular twitches, which had been observed with eserine and prostigmine by Langley and Kato in 1915 (18). Further work by Eccles, Katz and Kuffler (19) led to the concept that acetylcholine liberated from motor nerve terminals in the presence of anticholinesterase inhibitors could generate impulses both in muscle endplate and in the nerve terminal. Volle and Koelle (20) later extended this concept of prepsynaptic action of synaptically released acetylcholine to the sympathetic pre- ganglionic cholinergic terminals. These studies suggested the pharmacological principle that a nerve terminal could also respond to the transmitter which it releases without specifying the nature or extent of the intra-synaptic responses.

The concept of pre-synaptic transmitter action in the central nervous system arose with the observations by Frank and Fuortes (21), who showed that spinal motorneurons exhibited reduced excitatory responses to primary afferents if the test stimulus was preceded by stimuli to the muscle afferent nerve. This effect occurs with no alteration in the resting membrane potential or in the resting membrane conductance of the motorneuron, and is now interpreted as the existence of an axo-axonic terminal which can depolarize the primary sensory afferent terminal and reduce the amount of transmitter which is released by the test stimulus onto the motorneuron. Furthermore, Nicoll and Barker (22) and Davidoff (23) have recently suggested that GABA, normally considered to be exclusively an inhibitory hyperpolarizing agent, could be also responsible for the pre-synaptic "inhibitory" depolarization.

Electron microscopic evidence of presumptive "pre-synaptic" synapse arrangements have been reported for a wide variety of CNS regions (see 24). However, in many of these regions, especially the subcortical sensory relay nuclei of the thalamus, it now appears that the "triadic" synaptic interneuronal dendrites interposed between the sensory afferent terminal and the principal post-synaptic relay neuron. This same arrangement may well apply to the "dendro-dendritic" synapses of the retina and the olfactory bulb as well (see 25).

A. Short-Loop Pre-Synaptic Receptors

The most recent work on "pre-synaptic" receptor mechanisms returns to the earlier intra-synaptic pre-terminal actions of acetycholine (see above). In sympathetically innervated organs such as the heart, nictitating membrane and spleen, alpha adrenergic receptor antagonists were observed to increase the amount of norepinephrine which could be released into a bath or superfusate by sympathetic nerve stimulation (26, 27). From such work, the concept arose that a pre-synaptic alpha receptor could control the amount of adrenergic transmitter released. Although the mechanisms of this pre-synaptic adrenergic negative receptor remain unknown, it is clearly separate from the site at which prostaglandins of the E series (28) or muscarinic cholinergic receptors (29) also operate to inhibit norepinephrine release. Because antagonism of the receptor leads to increased release, the un-antagonized receptor would be assumed to inhibit its own release by negative feedback. The electrophysiological mechanisms for this negative feedback of relase could simply involve some hyperpolarizing action of these substances, such as norepinephrine and acetylcholine can exert in other post-synaptic receptors, or a prevention--by the prostaglandins--of the Ca^{++} influx required for transmitter release. Thus, here the electrophysiological sign of the pre-synaptic receptor need not be the same as that of post-synaptic receptor. To test the assumption that their pharmacological responsiveness is similar requires: 1) that the pathway can be selectively activated and 2) that release and pre-synaptic activity can be monitored as well as post-synaptic responses during reversible drug actions.

PHYSIOLOGICAL ASSESSMENT

The pre-synaptic alpha receptor, the pre-synaptic cholinergic muscarinic receptor and the pre-synaptic prostaglandin receptor on catecholamine nerve terminals which decrease transmitter output may be termed short-loop negative feedback controls. These receptors may be called into play in the former two cases by the release of the transmitter or in the latter case by the actions of the transmitter on its post-synaptic receptor, the adenylate cyclase (28). Although not yet subjected to an extensive search, these three types of pre-synaptic receptors would appear to be "intra-synaptic," in that axo-axonic triadic structures have not been identified in any case. That minor omission leaves both the glia around such synapses as well as the nerve terminal as possible sites for the interaction. Presumably these sites are still separate from those regulating neurotransmitter re-uptake or vesicular storage. However, experiments are needed to clarify the functional importance of these intra-synaptic regulatory effects, and to determine whether release can ever be so suppressed by these receptors as to countermand the activity of the neuronal perikaryon, or whether these biochemical changes in transmitter dynamics represent any functional gradations in transmission efficiency.

B. Long-loop Pre-Synaptic Receptors

A separate conceptual "pre-synaptic" form of feedback control which now is repeatedly invoked in the explanation of metabolic changes following psychoactive drugs is better termed a long-loop feedback. This hypothesis was proposed by Carlsson and Lindqvist (12) to account for the increased amounts of CNS catecholamine catabolites observed in the presence of unchanged catecholamine levels after treatment with the neuroleptic drugs, chlorpromazine and haloperidol. The explanation offered for these drug effects came from experiments in animals pretreated with a monoamine oxidase inhibitor, the actions of which the neuroleptics blocked. The primary action as a receptor antagonist was envisioned to result in a "compensatory activation of the monoaminergic neurons" (12). In turn, the assumed feedback activation could increase release as well as synthesis, thereby accounting for increased catabolites and relatively unchanged catecholamine levels. If, then, the non-drug situation is considered, the explanation would seem to call for a tonic functional suppression of monoamine neurons by their post-synaptic target neurons. This loop could be a single or multicellular loop which is opened (or disinhibited) by the neuroleptics. Subsequently several groups have suggested that this loop can also be revealed by administration of monoamine agonists (or receptor activators) which then increase the tonic feedback inhibition (13, 30, 31). Alternatively, this "loop" could be wholly intraneuronal if recurrent axon collaterals or local metabolic factors could be influenced by receptors similar to those intra-synaptic receptors discussed above.

III. REFLECTIONS OF THE LONG-LOOP FEEDBACKS IN NEURONAL DISCHARGE RATES

While the hypothesis of Carlsson and Lindqvist (12) offers a simple explanation for a wide collection of neurochemical and fluorescence histochemical data, the hypothesis was considerably strengthened by the recent observations made by Aghajanian and his colleagues through the use of single unit recordings and parenteral and iontophoretic drug tests (13, 32, 33). When recording within either of the three major monoamine-containing nuclei (the raphe nuclei containing 5-HT; the substantia nigra pars compacta containing dopamine, or the locus coeruleus containing norepinephrine) neurons were observed to decrease their discharge rates when the respective monoamine's levels were elevated by parenteral injections of monoamine oxidase inhibitors or precursor amino acids (12). In contrast, the neuroleptic

PHYSIOLOGICAL ASSESSMENT

drugs, such as phenothiazines and butyrophenones (34), which antagonize catecholamine receptors, produce opposite actions, activating the catecholamine neuron firing rate.

A. Further Considerations

However, in achieving the complementary interpretation of these interactions, much depends upon the definition of the way in which the presumed agonist or antagonist interacts with each of the parts of the presumed "feedback system". For example, if the concept of the long loop feedback were generally applicable to central 5-HT neurons, the following alternative interpretations could arise. LSD injected parenterally slows raphe metabolism (35) and raphe neuron discharge rate (36); parenteral tryptophan or monoamine oxidase inhibition acts similarly, as do tricyclics which are thought to impair active transmitter re-uptake. First, consider LSD as a 5-HT receptor "stimulator": in that case, all drugs which-- when given parenterally--slow raphe neuron discharge, could be considered as activating a long-loop negative feedback through 5-HT receptors on 5-HT target neurons. Alternatively, if LSD, tryptophan and the other drugs were to act directly on the raphe neurons as tests with iontophoretic 5-HT and LSD have indicated (37), then the effects could reflect local negative feedback, through a receptor which accepts either 5-HT or LSD. However, consider that LSD can antagonize the inhibitory synaptic actions of the raphe projection to hippocampal pryamidal neurons (38, 39) but not those to the suprachiasmatic nucleus (10). If LSD were a 5-HT antagonist, the same data could support the view that LSD could dis-facilitate the raphe, either by the long-loop or short-loop concepts (36, 40). As Aghajanian himself has cautioned (40), the lack of any anatomical or physiological evidence for the feedback loop suggests that such an interpretation in this case may be premature.

B. Amphetamines

The cellular and behavioral actions of amphetamine provide further useful insights into the problems which arise upon a diligent search for their receptor sites. In the case of the dopamine cells of the substantia nigra, Bunney and Aghajanian have observed that upon iontophoretic testing, both dopamine and amphetamine only depress discharge rate weakly (10). More recently, Bunney (34) has reported that surgical transection of the connections between the substantia nigra and the caudate nucleus eliminates the ability of parenteral amphetamine to depress substantia nigra neuron discharge rates. They conclude that dopamine cells and caudate neurons are linked in a closed loop negative feedback which can be activated by amphetamine through the release of synaptic dopamine in the caudate. On the other hand, the dopamine neurons of the substantia nigra do possess receptors which enable them to respond reproducibly to apomorphine which is generally accepted as a dopamine agonist (see 32). If amphetamine could also act covertly at this or other catecholamine "receptors," how then would the effects of parenteral amphetamine be interpreted?

Several lines of evidence suggested that amphetamine can in fact act directly on some dopamine receptors in addition to its effects on the release of synaptic dopamine (41). In the caudate nucleus of the cat (42) and rat (43), dopamine, amphetamine and apomorphine all similarly inhibit neuronal discharge. These actions persist even after caudate dopamine terminals have been destroyed by 6-hydroxydopamine, or after inhibition of synthesis with alpha methyl tyrosine and blockade of vesicular storage with reserpine (42). Similarly, iontophoretically administered amphetamine inhibits cerebellar Purkinje cells, as does norepinephrine, whether or not the cerebellar noradrenergic pathway has been destroyed (44). Purkinje cells are also inhibited by iontophoretically administered amphetamine when tested in a cerebellum transplanted to the anterior chamber of the eye (45, 46). The cervical sympathetic ganglion supplies noradrenergic inhibitory innervation to the cerebellar transplant; ganglionectomy eliminates the noradrenergic synaptic inhibition, but not the actions of iontophoretic amphetamine (47). On the other hand, the response of a neuron to a substance applied iontophoretically does not necessarily imply that the response observed is per se meaningful to the actions of the drug when given systemically.

Among the many behavioral actions of amphetamine which have been reported, it is clear that effects on rodent behavior can be detected at parenteral doses of 0.1 to 0.5 mg/kg (48, 49). In the analysis of repetitive self-stimulation evoked from rats with stimulating electrodes implanted in the substantia nigra (48), or in the locus coeruleus (49), a small dose of amphetamine will markedly increase self-stimulation rates, but only if the electrodes are directly in these nuclei or in their axonal projections through the medial forebrain bundle (see 50). If the feedback actions of parenteral amphetamine on the catecholamine neurons through the long-loop or short-loop mechanisms were the crucial interaction, then it would be diffucult to explain how this behavioral facilitation occurs, since slowing of these source neurons would imply they have been hyperpolarized and thus harder to activate by the stimulating electrode. If the amphetamine acts only to release more dopamine or norepinephrine from synaptic terminals (41) and these terminals also can react to their own transmitter by decreasing release and by decreasing local synthesis, then these latter metabolic effects must be overshadowed functionally by the facilitation of impulse-induced release at least as it is observed in brain slices (41). What appears quite clear, however, is that the actions of parenteral amphetamine are probably not due to direct interaction with post-synaptic catecholamine receptors. This has been suggested, for example, by the findings of Hoffer et al., in the anterior chamber cerebellar transplants (47), that parenteral amphetamine does not inhibit Purkinje cell discharge at low doses after sympathetic denervation of the iris and transplant. Similarly, if the actions of dopamine and apomorphine on caudate neurons are mediated intracellularly by cyclic AMP as the activation of the cyclase (51-53) and the effectiveness of iontophoretic cyclic AMP (43) would suggest, then it is important to realize that amphetamine does not seem to be able to activate directly the adenylate cyclase (54) of caudate nucleus homogenates.

Even more perplexing to the formulation of testable electrophysiological hypotheses are the recent observations by Harris et al. (55), which bear upon the possible intracellular mechanisms underlying the intra-synaptic dopamine receptors responsible for negative "feedback" control of tyrosine hydroxylase. Harris and her associates (55) found that monobutyryl cyclic AMP and 3 other phosphodiesterase resistant derivatives of cyclic AMP would increase dopamine synthesis at the tyrosine hydroxylase step. Yet, if dopamine synthesis is regulated by dopamine feedback through a receptor which is also linked to a dopamine-activated adenylate cyclase, then cyclic AMP should--like dopamine--suppress intra-synaptic synthesis. Clearly, more date will be required in order to compare the physiological and pharmacological properties of pre- and post-synaptic receptors to the same molecular transmitter.

C. Phenothiazines

The adenylate cyclase receptor paradigm of central catecholamine actions is also useful in the consideration of the sites of action of the anti-psychotic phenothiazines. Several groups have confirmed the observations of Greengard and Kebabian that these drugs inhibit the ability of dopamine to activate adenylate cyclases in sympathetic ganglia (56), caudate nucleus (51-52) and limbic cortex (53) and that the drugs block the dopamine responses of caudate neurons (51-52) as well as retina (57). Phenothiazines also show similar ability to antagonize the

PHYSIOLOGICAL ASSESSMENT

actions of norephinephrine (58) and of norepinephrine activated adenylate cyclase (59). All of these actions require only post-synaptic sites of action. This interpretation stands in marked contrast to the recent proposals of Seeman and Lee (60) who studied the effects of phenothiazines in impairing the release of H^3-dopamine from field stimulated striatal slices in vitro, and interpreted the actions as exclusively pre-synaptic. Using what appear to be similar methods for the analysis of stimulus induced release, Farnebo (see 41) has, on the other hand, reported that phenothiazines facilitate release, perhaps through their ability to inhibit re-uptake.

IV. DESCRIPTIVE LEVELS OF ANALYSIS

Let us stipulate the goal of our psychopharmacological research to be a better understanding of the ways in which the nervous system executes behavior and how drugs can modify these systematic programs. When trying to apply electrophysiology to the analysis of drug actions on behavior, a primary consideration in the selection of the point of attack is the organization of the neuronal systems controlling such behaviors. Experimental analysis of rodent behavior has led to the concept that the limbic system together with its olfactory and mesencephalic inputs are the most relevant primary brain regions to study (see 25), but exactly how these regions regulate emotionality remains unknown. In considering the analysis of such a "system" there are at least four general levels which can be described with increasing density of information: 1) overall functional behavior; 2) elementary units or subfunctions of behaviors within this overall group; 3) the step-by-step identification of the interconnected nuclei and cortical regions within the elementary units; 4) the detailed analysis of the local circuitry and function of each of the involved areas.

A few examples may clarify how each of these levels has been applied in other physiological analyses. For example,

Szenthagothai and Arbib (25) proposed a functional analysis of binocular stereoptical vision. Here the level one function is to locate objects in space, but most current work is pitched at level three, namely, how visual information in each retina is reflected in the responses of units in the visual cortex. The missing links in the analysis here are at levels two and four: none of the known interconnections between the retina and the cortex explains how cortical neurons respond to the geniculate or other visual relays and work together to yield stereopsis or the transmitter chemicals involved. Tebecis (61) has, however, made recent important studies on this latter aspect. Alternatively, we can consider the cerebellum and its role in movement. Here the solid understanding of the cellular and chemical interconnections in the cortex, and between the cortex and the nuclei with which it is connected (levels 3 and 4), contrast markedly with the vague but emerging concepts of the overall function of the cerebellum in movement control (level 1) and the sub-routines in spinal cord and motor cortex (level 2) which the cerebellum can coordinate (see 25).

If we consider these tactical levels in the roles of monoamines in any type of behavioral control modified by drugs, most of our present knowledge may be seen to lie at level 4: through histochemistry (see 62, 63) and cellular electrophysiology (1, 12), we know mainly where the monoamine-containing cells are located, the target cells to which they send their synapses, and what kinds of effects those synapses can mediate. What we lack is some hypothesis to dissect any behavior into terms which anatomical and physiological probes can test. Even at level 4, there is little knowledge of the neuronal systems which project to the monoamine neurons, a level of local circuit knowledge which would be extremely helpful in assessing the topic of pre-synaptic versus post-synaptic actions of drugs. For example, the substantia nigra possesses high GABA content (64) and GABA can be accumulated by a high proportion of

PHYSIOLOGICAL ASSESSMENT

nerve terminals in this region (65); furthermore, GABA will inhibit substantia nigra neurons (32). If GABA is the transmitter for the striato-nigral pathway (66, 67), and if this pathway functioned as the long-loop of the dopamine negative feedback system, it would be of value to test the effects of GABA antagonists, such as picrotoxin and bicuculline, on the ability of parenteral amphetamine and gamma hydroxy butyrolactone (33) to reduce substantia nigra discharge rates.

V. CONCLUSIONS

My take-home messages, which may be difficult to distill simply from the foregoing reflections are two: one simple and the other complex. First the simple: in order to define the relative importance of the various pre-synaptic and post-synaptic receptor sites at which transmitters and drugs can affect cellular behavior, we simply must learn a great deal more about the circuits which tie the monoamine neurons into the brain. This trite axiom becomes even more crucial when parenterally injected drugs are relied upon for the initation of drug-induced changes because such forms of drug administration offer the widest possible range of receptive targets. The method of iontophoresis was devised especially to restrict the number of potential sites from which drugs can affect neurons (see 12), but this method cannot be relied upon unthinkingly to provide the final answer. Neurons may well respond to substances they never encounter or fail to respond to an appropriate substance when tested in the wrong point or with the wrong dose. Possible changes in blood pressure, respiration, and extracellular ion concentrations cannot be simply dismissed without verifacation. An alternate way to express this same point is that is far easier to document changes in neuronal firing after parenteral or iontophoretic drug administration than it is to explain the changes. To make tentative conclusions about the causes of drug-induced changes in neuronal firing requires knowledge of brain circuits and drug interactions beyond our present knowledge. Furthermore, distinctions need to be drawn between studying changes produced after a drug (i.e., in rate or metabolic pattern) and studying the points at which drugs begin to act in complex systems of interconnected neurons.

An appropriate analogy can be derived from consideration of the hypothalamic neurons of the supraoptic nucleus known to be target cells for noradrenergic synapses (see 62, 63, 68). These neurons respond to injections of hypertonic salt solutions, as would befit their presumed roles as "osmo-receptors." Do the norepinephrine cells ignore this change, participate in its generation or adapt to it through feedback from their hypothalamic synapses? How do neurons whose axons terminate in the pituitary "feedback" to the rest of the brain? Similar points could be raised about limbic cortical neurons whose rates repeatedly change in advance of small spontaneous fluctuations in blood pressure (69). Is this feedback or anticipation?

Now for the complex: in order to determine the relative importance of the concept of "feedback", we need more than just the anatomy of the underlying structures within the loops; we need some way to grasp the meaning of the presumed connections. If neurons only compensate neurochemically for drugs which mimic or antagonize their transmitter at post-synaptic receptors, we gain an impression of neuronal efficiency, but little understanding of how or when the brain uses these neurons. The problem here is closely reminiscent of the discussions of feedback in the regulation of movement.

In motor control physiology, the cybernetic concepts of feedback, and even feed forward, have been debated for many years (see 70). Clearly, controlling circuits between sensory and motor neuronal systems must exist in order to guide and control movements. When such systems are termed central efferent monitors, they are relatively easy to conceive. Teuber (71) has summarized an alternative interpretation of this control phenomenon (see also 25 and 70) under the term of corollary discharge which offers a relevant concept for extrapolation to monoamine neurons. In this conceptualization, the command to move a given set of muscles is also accompanied by a corollary command to sensing systems to prepare for the changes the motor effect will produce. The classical example used here is the voluntary movement of the eye which nevertheless does not disturb our spatial perception of the immobile world because the visual system has anticipated it; however, if the eye is passively displaced, the world seems to jump unexpectedly, because there was no forewarning corollary command.

The concept of the corollary discharge can be helpful in attempts to apply knowledge of the biochemical actions of psychotherapeutic compounds on the monoamine neurons to the nature of the disease in which such affected systems may be crucial. For example, if the monoamine neurons were to play an interneuronal role in a hierarchical sequence of neurons initiating behavioral interactions, the activation of turnover (and presumably synaptically-evoked transmitter release) after a receptor antagonist such as the phenothiazines could suggest that there has been a deficiency of catecholamine as perceived by one or more crucial catecholamine target neurons. Alternatively, if the post-synaptic antagonism is the crucial therapeutic action, then the untreated case might represent excessive catecholamine synapse activity. However, when considered under the general umbrella of the corollary discharge, and in the light of substantial behavioral work on animals which have recovered from virtually complete eradication of all telencephalic catecholamine pathways, upward or downward adjustment of the catecholamine nerve nest with drugs, could, for example, facilitate synchronization (or more abstractly "preparedness") between sensory perceivers, integrators and motor efferent units.

To come to grips more fully then with the concepts of feedback control in the regulation of central monoamines, we may now wish to inquire "what systems, sensory, motor or internuncial, call the monoamine neurons into play?". Are they internal assessors of some command operation as simple as "reward" or "attention"? Or are they part of a corollary discharge operation which may be a sub-routine such as "anticipate" or "remember"? Perhaps such lines of inquiry may help to clarify how the brain uses such diffusely distributed, slowly conducting, long acting inhibitory systems as the monoamines and of what significance to the normal brain their receptors are, be they pre-or post-synaptic. In any event, such clarifications are probably necessary in order to interpret the therapeutic effects of drugs given for long periods of time to mentally ill patients.

VI. REFERENCES

1. F. E. Bloom and B. J. Hoffer, in Frontiers in Catecholamine Research (E. Usdin and S. Snyder, eds.), Pergamon Press, New York, 1974, pp. 637-642.

2. B. J. Hoffer, G. R. Siggins, A. P. Oliver, and F. E. Bloom, J. Pharmacol. Exp. Therap., 184, 553 (1973).

3. G. R. Siggins, E. F. Battenberg, B. J. Hoffer, F. E. Bloom, and A. L. Steiner, Science, 179, 585 (1973).

4. M. Segal and F. E. Bloom, Brain Res., 72, 79 (1974).

5. M. Segal and F. E. Bloom, Brain Res., 72, 99 (1974).

6. B. J. Hoffer, G. R. Siggins, and F. E. Bloom, Brain Res., 25, 523 (1971).

7. G. R. Siggins, A. P. Oliver, B. J. Hoffer, and F. E. Bloom, Science, 171, 192 (1971).

8. G. R. Siggins, B. J. Hoffer, A. P. Oliver, and F. E. Bloom, Nature, 233, 481 (1971).

9. G. R. Siggins, B. J. Hoffer, and F. E. Bloom, Brain Res., 25, 535 (1971).

10. G. K. Aghajanian, B. S. Bunney, and M. J. Kuhar, in New Concepts in Neurotransmitter Regulation (A. J. Mandel, ed.), Plenum Press, New York, 1973, pp. 115-134.

11. N. E. Anden, K. Fuxe, and T. Hokfelt, Eur. J. Pharmacol., 1, 226 (1967).

12. A. Carlsson and M. Lindqvist, Acta Pharmacol. Toxicol., 20, 140 (1963).

13. F. E. Bloom, B. J. Hoffer, G. R. Siggins, J. L. Barker, and R. A. Nicoll, Fed. Proc., 31, 97 (1972).

14. F. E. Bloom, Life Sci., 14, 1819 (1974).

15. K. Fuxe, T. Hokfelt, and U. Ungerstedt, Intern. Rev. Neurobiol., 13, 93 (1970).

16. J. C. Eccles, The Physiology of Synapses, Academic, New York, 1964, p. 122.

17. R. L. Masland and R. S. Wigton, J. Neurophysiol., 3, 269 (1940).

18. J. W. Langley and T. Kato, J. Physiol. (London), 49, 410 (1915).

19. J. C. Eccles, B. Katz, and S. W. Kuffler, J. Neurophysiol., 5, 211, (1942).

20. R. L. Volle and G. B. Koelle, J. Pharmacol. Exp. Therap., 133, 223, (1961).

21. K. Frank and M. G. F. Fuortes, Fed. Proc., 16, 39 (1957).

22. J. L. Barker and R. A. Nicoll, Science, 176, 1043 (1972).

23. R. A. Davidoff, Science, 175, 331 (1972).

24. G. D. Pappas and S. G. Waxman, in Structure and Function of Synapses (G. D. Pappas and D. P. Purpura, eds.), Raven Press, New York, 1972, pp. 1-43.

25. J. Szentagothai and M. A. Arbib, Neurosciences Research Program Bulletin, 12, 307 (1974).

26. K. Starke, in Frontiers in Catecholamine Research (E. Usdin and S. S. Snyder, eds.), Pergamon Press, New York, 1973, pp. 561-565.

27. S. Z. Langer, in Frontiers in Catecholamine Research (E. Usdin and S. S. Snyder, eds.), Pergamon Press, New York, 1973, pp. 543-549.

28. P. Hedqvist, in Frontiers in Catecholamine Research (E. Usdin and S. S. Snyder, eds.), Pergamon Press, New York, 1973, pp. 583-587.

29. E. Muscholl, in *Frontiers in Catecholamine Research* (E. Usdin and S. S. Snyder, eds.), Pergamon Press, New York, 1973, pp. 537-542.

30. N. E. Anden, H. Corrodi, K. Fuxe, and T. Hokfelt, *Eur. J. Pharmacol.*, 2, 59 (1967).

31. H. Corrodi, K. Fuxe, and T. Hokfelt, Eur. J. Pharmacol., 1, 363 (1967).

32. R. H. Roth, J. R. Walters, and G. K. Aghajanian, in *Frontiers in Catecholamine Research* (E. Usdin and S. S. Snyder, eds.), Pergamon Press, New York, 1973, pp. 567-574.

33. J. Walters, R. H. Roth, and G. K. Aghajanian, *J. Pharmacol. Exp. Therap.*, 186, 630 (1973).

34. B. S. Bunney, J. R. Walters, R. H. Roth and G. K. Aghajanian, *J. Pharmacol. Exp. Therap.*, 185, 560 (1973)

35. G. K. Aghajanian, W. E. Foote, and M. H. Sheard, *Science*, 161 706 (1968).

36. G. K. Aghajanian, *Ann. Rev. Pharmacol.*, 12, 157 (1972).

37. G. K. Aghajanian, H. J. Haigler, and F. E. Bloom, *Life Sci.*, 11, 615 (1972).

38. M. Segal, *Brain Res*, in press.

39. M. Segal and F. Bloom, *Fed. Proc.*, 33, 299 (1974).

40. G. K. Aghajanian and H. J. Haigler, *Proc. 5th Intl. Congr. Pharmacol.*, San Francisco, 1973, Vol. 4, p. 269.

41. L-O. Farnebo, *Acta Physiol. Scand.*, Suppl. 371, 45 (1971).

42. P. Feltz and J. deChamplain, *Brain Res.*, 43, 601 (1972).

43. G. R. Siggins, B. J. Hoffer, and U. Ungerstedt, *Life Sci.* 15, 779 (1974).

44. B. J. Hoffer, G. R. Siggins, D. J. Woodward, and F. E. Bloom, *Brain Res.*, 30, 425 (1971).

45. L. Olson and A. Seiger, *Z. Zellforsch.*, 135, 175 (1972).

46. B. J. Hoffer, A. Seiger, T. Ljungberg, and L. Olson, *Brain Res.*, 79, 165 (1974).

47. B. J. Hoffer, A. Seiger, L. Olson, and F. E. Bloom, *J. Neurobiol.*, in press.

48. A. G. Phillips and H. C. Fibiger, Science, 179, 575 (1973).

49. S. Ritter and L. Stein, J. Comp. Physiol. Psychol., 85, 443 (1973).

50. D. C. German and D. M. Bowden, Brain Res., 73, 381 (1974).

51. J. W. Kebabian, G. C. Petzold, and P. Greengard, Proc. Nat. Acad. Sci. (U.S.A.), 69, 2145 (1972).

52. Y. C. Clement-Cormier, J. W. Kebabian, G. L. Petzold and P. Greengard, Proc. Nat. Acad. Sci. (U.S.A.), 71, 1113 (1974).

53. R. J. Miller, A. S. Horn, and L. L. Iversen, Molec. Pharmacol. 10, 759 (1974).

54. H. Sheppard and C. R. Burghardt, Molec. Pharmacol., 10, 721 (1974).

55. J. C. Harris, V. H. Morgenroth, R. H. Roth, and R. J. Baldessarini, Nature, 252, 156 (1974).

56. J. W. Kebabian and P. Greengard, Science, 174, 1346 (1971).

57. J. H. Brown and M. H. Makman, Proc. Nat. Acad. Sci. (U.S.A.), 69, 539 (1973).

58. R. Freedman and B. J. Hoffer, J. Neurobiol., in press.

59. P. Skolnick and J. Daly, personal communication.

60. P. Seeman and T. Lee, Proc. 4th Ann Meeting Soc. Neuroscience, St. Louis, 1974, p. 418.

61. A. Tebecis, Brain Res., 63, 31 (1973).

62. O. Lindvall and A. Bjorklund, Acta Physiol. Scand., Suppl. 412, 1974.

63. U. Ungerstedt, Acta Physiol. Scand., Suppl. 367, 1971

64. J. S. Kim, I. J. Bak, R. Hassler, and Y. Okada, Exp. Brain Res., 14, 95 (1971).

65. L. L. Iversen and F. E. Bloom, Brain Res., 41, 131 (1972).

66. H. J. W. Nauta, M. B. Pritz, and R. J. Lasek, Brain Res., 67, 219 (1974).

67. W. Precht and M. Yoshida, Brain Res., 32, 229 (1971).

68. B. A. Cross and J. D. Green, J. Physiol., 148, 554 (1959).

69. Y. Ben-Ari, G. LeGal LaSalle, and Champagnat, <u>Brain Res.</u>, <u>52</u>, 394 (1973).

70. E. Evarts, <u>Neurosciences Research Program Bulletin</u>, <u>9</u>, 86 (1971).

71. H. L. Teuber, <u>Handbook Neurophysiol.</u>, <u>III</u>, 1595 (1960).

DISCUSSION

Dr. Snyder wondered if you can record with micropipettes placed inside monoamine pathway target cells wouldn't the miniature inhibitory potentials reflect the status of presynaptic receptors and spontaneous release of monoamine transmitters? Dr. Bloom replied that most of the natural synaptic boutons containing monoamines are out on the dendrites so that recording with intracellular microelectrodes from perikarion could not provide any reasonable indication of spontaneous monoamine release.

Dr. Snyder then wanted to know if Dr. Bloom inferred that the monoamines do not have a prominent role in generating spontaneous firing rate. Dr. Bloom said that he did not wish to imply this; in fact, the only manipulation which has been found to alter the spontaneous firing of cerebellar Purkinje cells is the chronic elimination of catecholamine fibers through the use of 6-hydrxydopamine. It can do this through the cyclic AMP mediated system; only 1 impulse every 5 seconds is required to keep the cyclic AMP level up. This, then, places all the excitatory inputs over that particular 5 seconds at a different bias point on the threshold for activating any particular spontaneous discharge. Recording clearly spontaneous inhibitory miniature synaptic potentials from any central nerve cell other than the spinal motor neuron (and one or two others) and correlating it with spontaneous discharge of catecholamine-containing cells is not yet possible. The closest one can come to that is doing auto-correlations and cross-correlations between the discharge pattern of a locus coeruleus neuron and the discharge pattern of any of the target cells to which it projects.

Therefore, one can have independent monitors on the activity of the presynaptic and the postsynaptic cell and if there is tonic release of importance, then one should find that periods of spontaneous behavior which activate the locus coeruleus should have a corresponding opposite action on the target cells.

EVIDENCE FOR DRUG ACTIONS ON BOTH PRE- AND POSTSYNAPTIC CATECHOLAMINE RECEPTORS IN THE CNS

B. S. Bunney and G. K. Aghajanian

Depts. of Psychiatry and Pharmacology

Yale University School of Medicine and

Connecticut Mental Health Center

34 Park Street

New Haven, Connecticut 06508

I. INTRODUCTION

Concepts derived from studies in the periphery have often proved applicable to the central nervous system. A prime example of this is recent evidence which suggests that presynaptic catecholamine receptors may exist on catecholaminergic neurons in the brain as well as in the periphery. In the peripheral nervous system the evidence for adrenergic presynaptic receptors is derived from many sources. α-Adrenergic blocking agents (e.g., phenoxybenzamine) have been shown to increase outflow of norepinephrine (NE) from stimulated peripheral adrenergic nerves [16,85]. To explain this finding it was suggested that a local feedback mechanism acting within the synaptic gap leads to an increase in the amount of neurotransmitter released per nerve impulse [37,44].

This effect of α-adrenergic receptor blockers occurred at doses too low to be accounted for by NE neuronal uptake inhibition [32, 35,36] or an effect on postsynaptic receptors [55,76]. Conversely, α-adrenergic receptor stimulators have been shown to decrease the release of NE per nerve impulse [37,55,74,76]. The combined evidence would suggest a mode of regulation of neurotransmitter release in addition to that accounted for by changes in impulse flow. Two mechanisms for this regulation have been suggested. First, the postsynaptic (effector) cell might send a messenger across the synapse to control release. There is evidence that prostaglandins may be secreted by the effector cell and after diffusing across the synaptic cleft have an inhibitory effect on adrenergic terminals [47]. However, this cannot be the only mechanism involved as α-adrenergic antagonists increase and α-adrenergic agonists decrease nerve stimulation induced release of NE after inhibition of prostaglandin synthesis [82]. Second, peripheral adrenergic nerve endings might possess α-receptors which interact with NE and α-adrenergic stimulating and blocking agents to decrease or increase impulse coupled NE release respectively [32,52,54,74,78]. This latter possibility appears all the more likely as both α-receptor blocking and stimulating agents can have a marked influence on the release of NE at doses shown to have no effect on postsynaptic receptors [77].

II. BIOCHEMICAL STUDIES IN CNS

A. Biochemical Evidence For Catecholaminergic Presynaptic Receptors In The Central Nervous System

Recently biochemical evidence has suggested the presence of a presynaptic feedback mechanism in the central nervous system. Under certain conditions dopamine (DA) receptor blocking agents (e.g., antipsychotic drugs) have been shown to enhance the release of DA from terminals in neostriatal slices [25,36] whereas a DA agonist apomorphine, blocks DA release [36]. Clonidine and oxymetazoline, α-adrenergic agonists in the CNS, [6,79] as well as the periphery, [36,62,93] have been shown to decrease stimulation induced release of NE from cerebral slices [36]. Conversely, α-receptor blockers (e.g., phenoxybenzamine, phentolamine) and antipsychotic drugs increase NE release under the same conditions [78,79,80]. Thus, there is evidence in the CNS analogous to that in the periphery suggesting either a local transynaptic feedback mechanism involving the postsynaptic cell or a direct action of catecholamine agonists and antagonists on presynaptic receptors. All of these CNS studies, however, were done in vitro. The question as to whether these mechanisms obtain in vivo is more difficult to answer. Both catecholamine agonists and antagonists are thought to react with postsynaptic receptors and thereby exert an effect upon the neuronal activity of catecholaminergic neurons in the brain via a neuronal feedback pathway - a pathway which would be inactivated in in vitro preparations such as brain slices.

B. Biochemical Evidence For A Central Postsynaptic Neuronal Feedback Regulation of Catecholamine Metabolism and Release

1. Dopamine and Norepinephrine Receptor Blockers

A large body of evidence has accumulated suggesting that the antipsychotic drugs increase DA turnover and to a lesser extent the turnover of NE. Included in this evidence are the findings that antipsychotic drugs: 1) increase levels of catecholamine metabolites in the brain [5,11,24,31,56]; 2) increase the rate of disappearance of DA after inhibition of catecholamine synthesis with α-methyl-para-tyrosine [27,63]; and 3) increase the synthesis of DA from radioactive tyrosine and increase the disappearance of labelled DA [22,41,64,67,68].

The first suggestion that antipsychotic drug induced changes in catecholamine turnover might be due to alterations in neuronal activity was made by Carlsson and Lindqvist [24] in an attempt to explain an observed increase in O-methylated catecholamine metabolites induced by chlorpromazine and haloperidol following monoamine oxidase inhibition. They hypothesized that these antipsychotic drugs might block central postsynaptic catecholamine receptors which could in turn cause a compensatory increase in the activity of catecholaminergic neurons mediated through a neuronal feedback circuit. Indirect support for this hypothesis was obtained when it was shown that severing the DA pathway between the substantia nigra (zona compacta) and neostriatum prevented the usual increase in DA synthesis induced by antipsychotic drugs [7,25,65] thus suggesting that impulse flow was necessary for the antipsychotic drug induced increase in DA turnover. Another indirect piece of evidence was provided when Horn and Snyder [49] showed, using x-ray crystalography techniques, that the DA molecule could be superimposed upon part of the chlorpromazine molecule thus lending some credence to the hypothesis that chlorpromazine might be a competitive DA receptor blocker.

However, all of these effects are also compatable with the idea that antipsychotic drugs block presynaptic catecholamine receptors thereby increasing neurotransmitter release in a manner similar to that demonstrated in vitro.

2. Dopamine Receptor Stimulator

Apomorphine is thought to directly stimulate dopamine receptors [9,33,69]. Both the loss of DA after synthesis inhibition and the conversion of labelled tyrosine to DA are decreased after apomorphine administration [9,66]. It has therefore been suggested that apomorphine decreases the activity of DA neurons through stimulation of postsynaptic DA receptors possessed by cells which feedback onto DA neurons. However, again, stimulation of a presynaptic receptor which thereby decreases DA release could also explain these biochemical findings.

C. Two Biochemical Methods For Distinguishing Between Pre- And Postsynaptic Dopaminergic Receptors

1. Inhibition of Impulse Flow

In order to distinguish in vivo between pre- and postsynaptic effects a method is needed which eliminates the effect of any possible neuronal feedback loop but which still provides a means for measuring the effects of any presynaptic receptor that might be present. The discovery of an unexpected biochemical change seen within 30 minutes following blockade of impulse flow in the nigrostriatal dopaminergic pathway has provided the in vivo model needed to study the hypothesized presynaptic receptor. It has been found that interruption of impulse flow by any means (e.g. electrothermic lesions, mechanical transection, injection of local anesthetics, or the administration of gamma butyrolactone, a compound which has been shown to stop dopamine cell firing [89]) produces a marked increase in neostriatal dopamine levels [7,23, 71,72,89,92]. With impulse flow nonexistent in this preparation the effects of a neuronal feedback loop are eliminated and any drug induced alterations in the above effects must be mediated through a local synaptic effect. Thus it has been shown that the administration of DA agonists (e.g., apomorphine and ET495 - trivastal) or pretreatment with d-amphetamine, a DA releaser, prevent the increase in DA levels induced by cessation of impulse flow [51,71,72,90]. Many antipsychotic drugs (hypothesized postsynaptic DA receptor blockers) have been found to block the ability of DA agonists to inhibit the gamma butyrolactone induced increase in DA levels. However, one antipsychotic drug, clozapine, was found to be ineffective in this regard [91]. A biochemical feedback mechanism involving end product inhibition, seen under some circumstances, [28,50] could not explain this phenomenon as DA levels actually increase not decrease when DA neuronal impulse flow ceases. Consequently, it has been hypothesized that interruption of impulse flow leads to a decreased release of DA into the synaptic cleft resulting in a depletion of DA at receptor sites located on the presynaptic membrane. The resultant decrease in presynaptic DA receptor activation is then thought to cause an activation of tyrosine hydroxylase leading to an increase in intraneuronal DA levels [23,51,89,90,91]. The fact that known postsynaptic DA receptor agonists and antagonists interact in an identical manner in a system lacking the influence of a neuronal feedback loop greatly supports the concept of a presynaptic DA receptor.

2. Stimulation-induced Acceleration of Impulse Flow.

Further in vivo biochemical evidence for the existence of a presynaptic receptor has recently been provided in experiments analogous to the in vitro field stimulated brain slice experiments described earlier. It has been found that electrical stimulation of the nigrostriatal pathway results in a frequency dependent increase in tyrosine hydroxylase activity which reaches a maximum

(15 Hz for 10 min) that persists for 15 minutes following cessation of stimulation [70]. Pretreatment with a dopamine agonist (trivastal) attenuated the post stimulus increase of tyrosine hydroxylase activity whereas the administration of a potent DA receptor blocker, haloperidol, produced a marked augmentation of the stimulus induced activation of this enzyme [70]. It is hypothesized that this may be due to the removal of an inhibitory effect on tyrosine hydroxylase activity mediated by increased quantities of DA in the synaptic cleft. The increase in DA concentration in the synaptic cleft, by stimulating presynaptic DA receptors, would exert a modulating effect on the stimulus-induced activity of tyrosine hydroxylase. Dopamine receptor blockers are hypothesized to remove this breaking effect and therefore potentiate the stimulation induced activation of tyrosine hydroxylase. Since stimulation was performed at a frequency and time period which produced a maximal increase in tyrosine hydroxylase activity any drug effect mediated by a postsynaptic feedback loop should be cancelled out.

Thus a large body of biochemical evidence derived from both the periphery and central nervous system suggests the presence of presynaptic catecholaminergic receptors in addition to the long known postsynaptic receptors. Does electrophysiological evidence exist to support these biochemical findings in the central nervous system?

III. PHYSIOLOGICAL STUDIES IN CNS

A. Central Dopaminergic Neurons: Electrophysiological Evidence For Drug Actions On Pre- And Postsynaptic Receptors

Based on the biochemical findings mentioned above there appear to be at least two types of feedback mechanisms which potentially can modulate the physiological state of dopamine neurons: 1) a postsynaptic neuronal feedback circuit modulating the activity of the dopaminergic pathways; and 2) a local feedback mechanism at the dopaminergic synapse involving presynaptic dopamine receptors which can modulate transmitter synthesis and release independent of changes in impulse flow. Electrophysiological investigations of these two hypothesized feedback mechanisms have been made possible by the fluorescence histochemical mapping of the monoamine systems of the brain [5,30,40]. This permits biochemical and electrophysiological changes to be correlated with anatomically defined structures whose neurotransmitters are known. In a recently developed experimental approach a neurophysiological identification of DA neurons in the rat midbrain was made by means of combined histochemical and single unit recording techniques[21]. By recording the electrical activity of single dopaminergic neurons, it is possible to determine the effect on the activity of the nigrostriatal dopaminergic system of drugs and other substances given either systemically or applied locally by microiontophoresis to the soma and dendrites of DA neurons.

1. Electrophysiologically Determined Changes in Impulse Flow: Evidence for a Postsynaptic Receptor Mediated Neuronal Feedback Mechanism.

Direct support for the original neuronal feedback hypothesis [24] was obtained by the finding that the systemic administration of certain antipsychotic compounds including chlorpromazine and haloperidol cause an increase in the activity of dopaminergic neurons [21]. Thus, small intravenous doses (0.5 - 1.0 mg/kg) of chlorpromazine produce up to a doubling in the rate of firing of dopamine-containing cells [21]. Haloperidol accelerates the firing of dopaminergic cells to the same extent as does chlorpromazine [21]. When haloperidol is given after chlorpromazine it produces no further effect [1], suggesting that these drugs act upon a common set of receptors within the dopaminergic system. In contrast, when chlorpromazine is applied directly to dopaminergic neurons by microiontophoresis it has little or no effect [1].

Drugs that are believed to directly or indirectly stimulate DA receptors have been found to cause a decrease in the activity of dopaminergic neurons [20,21]. d-Amphetamine indirectly stimulates DA receptors by increasing the release and blocking the reuptake of DA [10,12,13,14,29,34,43,58,59,61,81,86,87]. By thus increasing the concentration of DA at the postsynaptic receptor it has been hypothesized that d-amphetamine may cause a neuronal feedback inhibition of catecholamine containing neurons [27]. As predicted, systemically administered d-amphetamine has been found to inhibit the firing of dopaminergic neurons [20,21] (Fig.

1, top trace). This effect is readily reversed by clinically proven antipsychotic drugs. α-Methyl tyrosine, an inhibitor of catecholamine synthesis, blocks and reverses the effects of intravenously administered amphetamine on DA neurons, suggesting an indirect mechanism of action [20]. Presumably amphetamine acts indirectly on postsynaptic cells by releasing DA from nigrostriatal terminals. However, in large concentrations amphetamine may also directly affect postsynaptic neurons [17,38]. A close correlation between the biochemical and electrophysiological effects of d-amphetamine is shown by the fact that the threshold doses of d-amphetamine (~0.25 mg/kg) for producing a significant depression of dopaminergic cell firing is approximately the same as that required to cause a detectable increase in striatal DA turnover.

Two pieces of evidence suggest that the ability of intravenous d-amphetamine to depress DA cells is mediated through an effect on postsynaptic DA receptors. 1) Microiontophoretically applied d-amphetamine was found to produce only a minimal slowing of DA neurons or to have no effect at all [17]. Increasing ejection currents do not significantly increase this effect and multiple application rapidly leads to an attenuation of the minimal depressant response. In many cases d-amphetamine at high ejection currents produces a local anesthetic effect as indicated by a decreasing spike amplitude in association with DA cell slowing. However, in low doses d-amphetamine administered intravenously has a marked inhibitory effect without any local anesthetic effect. 2) In contrast to the minimal response of DA cells to iontophoretic d-amphetamine,

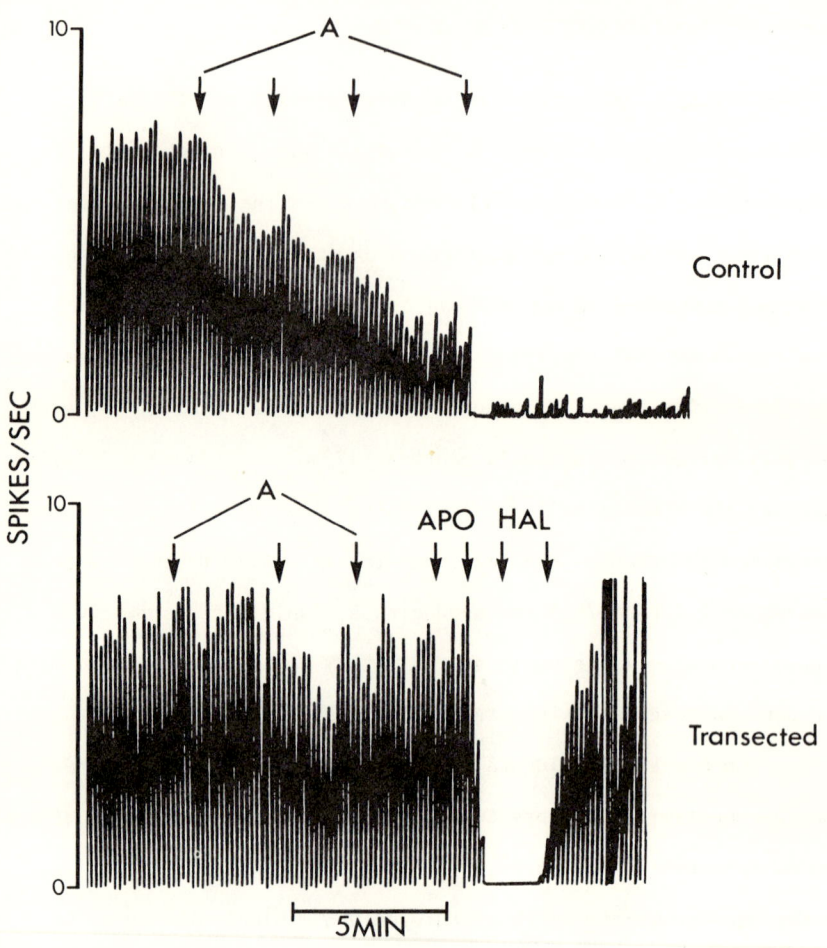

Fig. 1. Effects of intravenous d-amphetamine (A) on the rate of firing of dopaminergic neurons in the zona compacta (substantia nigra) in a control rat (upper trace) and in a rat with a diencephalic transection (lower trace) wich separates the substantia nigra from the neostriatum. In the upper trace, the typical depressant effect of A on dopaminergic cell firing can be seen. An initial dose of 0.25 mg/kg (i.v.) produces a partial slowing; a total inhibition occurs after a cumulative dose of 2.0 mg/kg has been given. In the transected preparation (lower trace) amphetamine in a cumulative dose of 3.2 mg/kg (i.v.) fails to produce significant slowing. However, intravenous apomorphine (APO) in a cumulative dose of 0.4 mg/kg totally inhibits firing of the cell. Haloperidol (HAL) (0.2 mg/kg, i.v.) rapidly reverses the apomorphine induced depression.

Methods as described in Ref. [17,20,21]. The figures are taken from direct, on-line, integrated-rate recordings. Reprinted from Ref. [2], P. 6, by courtesy of University Toronto Press.

postsynaptic cells in the caudate nucleus, accumbens nucleus, olfactory tubercles and certain cortical areas are markedly depressed by low ejection currents of d-amphetamine and/or DA [17,38, Bunney & Aghajanian, unpublished data]. No attenuation of response is observed with repeated applications. In neurons responsive to both DA and d-amphetamine local anesthetic effects of d-amphetamine were seen only at high ejection currents (> 20 nA).

Thus it would appear from the relative lack of response of DA cells to microiontophoretically ejected d-amphetamine that the inhibitory response of DA cells to systemically administered d-amphetamine is not through a direct effect on presynaptic receptors. However, these results do not provide positive proof for a postsynaptic non-dopaminergic feedback pathway. If such a pathway exists one should be able to abolish the inhibitory effect of systemically administered d-amphetamine on DA cells by destroying the pathway with a lesion. Accordingly, under chloral hydrate anesthesia, using a stereotaxically controlled fine retractable wire-knife, the diencephalon was transected at a level just anterior to the substantia nigra (A2970-A3290) [53]. Following this lesion almost all DA cells were firing abnormally fast (~10/sec) [17], suggesting a release from a tonic inhibitory input. One possible candidate for such an inhibitory input is the recently described GABAergic pallido-(paleo-striatal)-nigral pathway [46, 57]. Conceivably, if a GABAergic pathway was cut by the transection this could cause an acceleration of the DA neurons by releasing them from a striatal inhibitory influence. In any event, systemic administration of d-amphetamine in doses which are sufficient to cause total inhibition of most DA cells in unlesioned animals produces only a minimal or temporary slowing of DA cells in the transected preparation (Fig. 1, lower trace) [17]. Taken together the above evidence suggests that d-amphetamine depresses DA cell firing rate through an indirect effect on the postsynaptic DA receptors of a neuronal feedback pathway.

B. Electrophysiologically Determined Changes in Impulse Flow: Evidence For a Presynaptic Receptor Mediated Local Feedback Mechanism

The firing of dopaminergic neurons is depressed by the direct microiontophoretic application of DA at low ejection currents [1]. After repeated or prolonged application there tends to be an attenuation of the response to microiontophoretic DA. DA iontophoresed onto DA cells has a much greater depressant effect than d-amphetamine. DA does not produce a local anesthetic effect. These iontophoretic results suggest that a DA receptor may be present on the dendrites and/or cell bodies of DA neurons. However, it is unlikely that the minimal depressant effect observed with iontophoretic d-amphetamine has any physiological significance as the response is small even at concentrations many times that which would reach these cells when small doses of d-amphetamine are administdred intravenously. Moreover, the attenuation of response seen after repeated iontophoretic administration of d-amphetamine is not seen during a similar time period when d-amphetamine is administered intravenously. Taken together these results indicate that the small direct effect of iontophoretically applied d-amphetamine on DA cell firing rate is unrelated to the systemic action of the drug.

Apomorphine, a drug thought to stimulate DA receptors directly [9,33,69] has also been found to decrease the activity of dopaminergic neurons when it is administered systemically [20]. Apomorphine also has a powerful inhbitory effect when applied by microiontophoresis directly onto DA neurons [1]. Thus, in addition to its hypothesized effects upon "postsynaptic" DA receptors, apomorphine appears to mimic the action of DA on "presynaptic" DA receptors (i.e., receptors upon the dopaminergic neuron itself). These results correlate well with the biochemical finding that apomorphine can inhibit the increased DA synthesis seen in the neostriatum following interruption of the nigrostriatal pathway despite the fact that impulse flow can no longer be modulated by the action of a neuronal feedback pathway [51,71,90].

As indicated above, although amphetamine has a minimal direct action upon dopaminergic neurons, apomorphine is inhibitory when applied by microiontophoresis. This suggests that the inhibition of dopaminergic neurons by systemically administered apomorphine may be direct and therefore would not be blocked in the nigro-neostriatal-transected preparation. Indeed, despite little inhibition by amphetamine, dopaminergic neurons in transected animals are still readily inhibited by low intravenous doses of apomorphine (Fig. 1, lower trace) [2]. Of particular significance is the fact that haloperidol reverses the apomorphine inhibition. Since there is no anatomical communication between the pre- and postsynaptic neurons in this animal preparation it would appear that systemically administered apomorphine can directly inhibit dopaminergic neurons by acting upon presynaptic DA receptors (i.e., DA receptors upon the dopaminergic neurons). Moreover, haloperidol appears capable of blocking such presynaptic DA receptors since it reverses the apomorphine-induced depression in firing (Fig. 1, lower trace). These physiological results in transected preparations directly parallel the biochemical results in similarly transected animals with the exception that the biochemical measures were made upon DA terminals in the neostriatum whereas the recordings were made from dopaminergic soma and dendrites in the substantia nigra zona compacta. Allowing for this difference, the close correspondence of the biochemical and neurophysiological studies suggests that presynaptic DA receptors are present upon both the soma and terminals of dopaminergic neurons.

To further investigate the characteristics of presynaptic DA receptors experiments were carried out in which interactions between microiontophoretically applied DA and systemically administered haloperidol, chlorpromazine and clozapine were studied. The advantages of using the systemic route for the antipsychotic drugs are that local anesthetic effects are avoided [94] and direct comparisons can be made to biochemical studies in which the systemic route is also used. Microiontophoresis of DA at a low ejection current initially produces total inhibition of firing of dopaminergic neurons (Fig. 2, upper trace). Haloperidol (0.25 mg/kg) injected intravenously, produces a typical increase in baseline firing rate; such increases are even more prominent in unanesthetized animals than in the chloral hydrate anesthetized preparations used in these experiments [21]. Following the haloperidol, the microiontophoresis of DA no longer produced an inhibitory effect (Fig. 2, upper trace). Similar results were obtained with chlorpromazine except that a total blockade of DA could not be achieved even at doses 20 times that of haloperidol (Fig. 2, middle trace) [2].

Clozapine at doses 2 times that of chlorpromazine was ineffective in blocking DA induced inhibition of these cells (Fig. 1, lower trace). Thus there is a direct parallel between the relative efficacy of these three drugs in blocking DA depression of DA neuron activity and their efficacy in blocking the ability of DA agonists to inhibit impulse flow cessation induced activation of tyrosine hydroxylase [91].

C. Central Noradrenergic Neurons: Electrophysiological Evidence for Drug Action on Presynaptic Receptors

Clonidine, an imidazoline derivative with central α-adrenergic receptor stimulating properties, rapidly inhibits the norepinephrine containing cells of the locus coeruleus when administered intravenously in low doses (4-8 μg/kg) (Fig. 3, upper trace) [83].

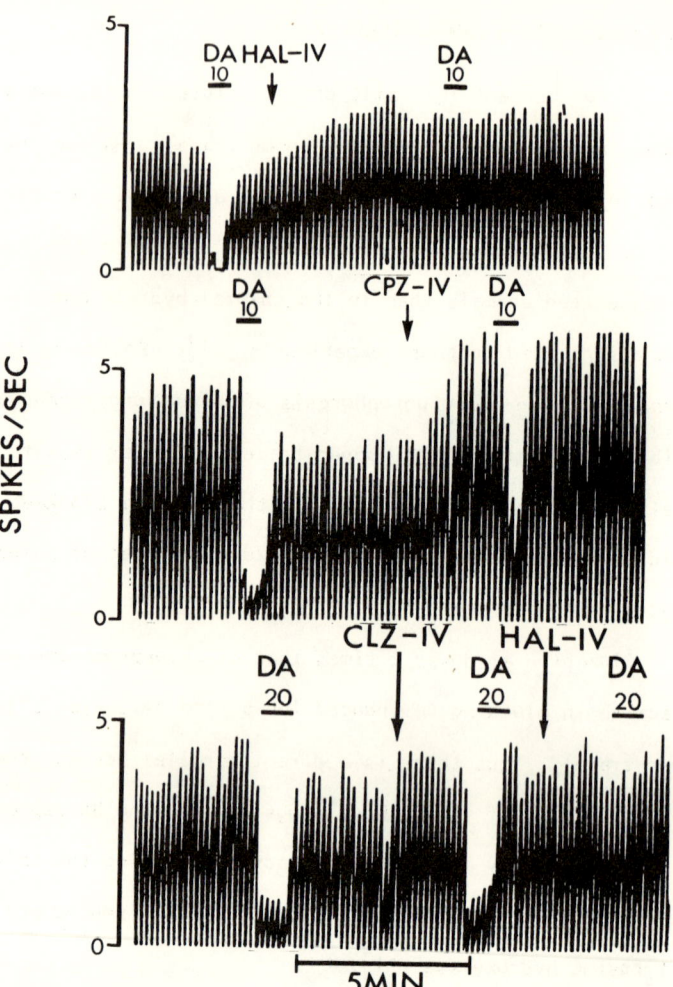

Fig. 2. The effect of intravenous haloperidol (HAL, upper trace), chlorpromazine (CPZ, middle trace), and clozapine (CLZ, lower trace) on the depression of dopaminergic neuron activity by microiontophoretically applied dopamine (DA). All these cells are inhibited by DA ejected at low iontophoretic currents (10-20 nA). HAL, in a dose of 0.25 mg/kg causes an increase in the baseline firing rate (upper trace). Following HAL, microiontophoretic DA is no longer effective in producing inhibition. CPZ, at a dose of 5.0 mg/kg attenuates but does not completely block the DA inhibition (middle trace). CLZ in a dose of 10.0 mg/kg has no effect on DA inhibition (lower trace). The subsequent administration of HAL, 0.25 mg/kg, completely blocks the DA induced depression of this cell.

Methods as in Ref. [1,4,45]. The bars above the tracings indicate duration of microiontophoresis and numbers above bars refer to ejecting currents in nA. The concentration of DA in the 5-barreled microiontophoretic electrodes was 0.2M (pH 4.0). Reprinted in part from Ref. [2], P. 7 by courtesy of University Toronto Press.

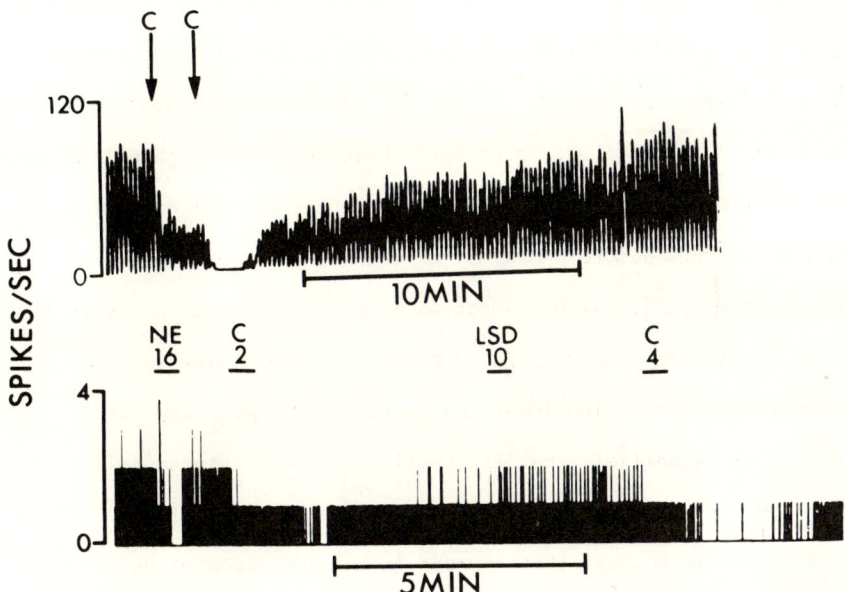

Fig. 3. Effect of intravenous (upper trace) and microiontophoretically applied (lower trace) clonidine (C) on noradrenergic neuron activity in the locus coeruleus. In the upper trace, the typical depressant effect of intravenous C can be seen. Total inhibition is achieved with a cumulative dose of 6 µg/kg (4 + 2 µg/kg). As shown in the lower trace both norepinephrine (NE) and C but not LSD inhibit these cells when applied directly by means of microiontophoresis. This cell was inhibited by NE (16 nA), C (2 and 4 nA) but not by LSD (10 nA).
Methods as described in [14,45]. The bars above the tracing indicate the duration of the ejection. The concentration of NE, C and LSD in the 5-barreled miroiontophoretic electrode was 0.1M, 0.01M, and 0.001M respectively. All were at pH 4.0.

The effect of clonidine on these cells was uniform and dose dependent - larger doses inhibiting locus coeruleus neurons for longer lengths of time. This was a specific effect in that the firing rate of non-catecholaminergic cells in the reticular formation and dopamine containing neurons in the substantia nigra zona compacta were unaffected.

Noradrenergic cells in the locus coeruleus are also inhibited by NE when applied microiontophoretically at low ejection currents (Fig. 3, lower trace) [83]. Similarly, clonidine when applied by means of microiontophoresis stopped these cells although unlike the immediate inhibition produced by NE there was often a delay of 30 - 90 seconds before a maximal effect was obtained, (Fig. 3, lower trace) [83]. As no reduction in spike amplitude was seen a local anesthetic effect is ruled out. Since clonidine was very effective in inhibiting locus coeruleus neurons when applied locally it is unlikely that its ability to inhibit these cells when administered intravenously is due to a systemic effect. These findings would suggest that neurons in the locus coeruleus possess presynaptic α-adrenergic receptors located on their soma and that an activation of these receptors sites by clonidine and NE may be responsible for their ability to inhibit the activity of these noradrenergic neurons.

These studies combined with the biochemical studies reviewed earlier would suggest that NE neurons, in the locus coeruleus, like DA containing cells in the substantia nigra zona compacta, possess catecholamine receptors on both their terminals and cell bodies.

IV. SUMMARY AND CONCLUSIONS

Clearly, there are many parallels between peripheral adrenergic neurons and central catecholamine neurons with regard to the possible functional role of presynaptic receptors activated by

DRUG ACTIONS ON RECEPTORS IN CNS   109

their respective neurotransmitters. Thus, catecholamine receptor blocking agents (e.g., the various antipsychotic drugs), under certain conditions, enhance the release of DA and NE from terminals in neostriatal and cerebral cortical slices respectively, [25,36] whereas apomorphine, a DA agonist and clonidine, a NE agonist, [77,80] block DA and NE release from their respective terminal areas.

We have presented electrophysiological evidence supporting the view that central catecholaminergic neurons possess presynaptic receptors for their respective neurotransmitters and that these receptors are responsive to specific agonists and antagonists. Stimulation of presynaptic catecholaminergic receptors through the microiontophoresis of DA or apomorphine onto the soma of DA neurons and NE or clonidine on to the soma of NE neurons inhibit the activity of these cells. If such presynaptic receptors exist on catecholaminergic terminals these inhibitory responses suggest that presynaptic receptors located there may be concerned with feedback inhibition of catecholamine synthesis and/or release. Certainly the results of our electrophysiological studies on DA and NE cell soma closely parallel biochemical studies involving the in vivo effects of DA agonists upon DA synthesis [51,71,90,91] and the in vitro release of DA and NE from their respective terminals in the neostriatum and cerebral cortex [25,36,77,79].

We have also presented electrophysiological evidence for the existence of postsynaptic receptors which, when stimulated, activate a neuronal feedback circuit responsible for modulating the rate of firing of cells in the dopaminergic nigrostriatal pathway. The increase in activity of dopamine neurons induced by some antipsychotic drugs is most likely mediated through this neuronal feedback circuit and is probably secondary to their ability to block postsynaptic dopamine receptors. Electrophysiological evidence in support of this hypothesis includes: 1) cells innervated by the dopamine system are inhibited by microiontophoretically applied dopamine [2,15,17,26,48,60]; 2) microiontophoretically applied chlorpromazine [94] and intravenous haloperidol [19] readily block the inhibitory effects of DA on cells in the caudate and accumbens nucleus respectively. The increase in DA turnover induced by all antipsychotic drugs has been attributed to their ability to block postsynaptic DA receptors thereby causing an increase in DA cell activity mediated via a neuronal feedback pathway [24]. However, such an action on postsynaptic DA receptors can not always explain the biochemical effects of antipsychotic drugs. Thus antipsychotic drugs increase DA turnover in a dose dependent fashion. Contrastingly, the increase in firing rate induced by many of these drugs rapidly reaches a maximum at low doses. In addition, some antipsychotic drugs (thioridazine and clozapine) that increase DA turnover do not increase DA cell activity, even at high doses [18]. The increase in turnover induced by antipsychotic drugs therefore, is not always accompanied by an increase in DA cell activity. A blocking effect on presynaptic receptors, however, would help explain these effects. Thus a blockade of these receptors, according to the biochemical evidence presented above, would cause an increase in dopamine release independent of changes in impulse flow. Unfortunately clozapine appears to lack such a presynaptic effect necessitating a further search for an explanation of its ability to increase DA turnover.

We have shown that d-amphetamine lacks a direct presynaptic effect on the activity of DA cells and instead depresses the firing of DA cells through a postsynaptic feedback loop. If depression of firing of DA neurons by d-amphetamine can thus be used as an index of postsynaptic DA receptor stimulation, then reversal or blockade of this depression by antipsychotic drugs presumably also reflects a postsynaptic phenomenon. Apomorphine, however, appears to act directly on both pre- and postsynaptic receptors. Since depression of DA neurons by iontophoretically applied DA and intravenous apomorphine can be blocked by systemically administered haloperidol or chlorpromazine, it would appear that these drugs are also effective antagonists at presynaptic DA receptors.

Interestingly, clozapine, an antipsychotic drug which appears to lack extrapyramidal side effects in man and does not increase the firing rate of DA neurons, is a very weak blocker of DA induced inhibition of both dopaminergic neurons in the substantia nigra zona compacta and postsynaptic cells in the striatum [Bunney and Aghajanian, unpublished data]. On the other hand drugs with a moderate to high incidence of extrapyramidal side effects (haloperidol and chlorpromazine) increase DA cell activity and are relatively good blockers of both pre- and postsynaptic DA receptors. The ability to weakly or strongly block postsynaptic DA receptors in the striatum may explain the difference in extrapyramidal side effects seen between various neuroleptics. The behavioral significance of the blockade of presynaptic receptors is much less clear as its effect would tend to oppose the postsynaptic receptor blocking actions of these drugs. It is conceivable that such a presynaptic blocking action might be important in the development of tardive dyskinesia. Thus, chronic treatment with antipsychotic drugs has been shown to produce postsynaptic dopamine receptor supersensitivity in animals [39,42,84] and is postulated to play a role in the development of tardive dyskinesia in man [73]. However, as drugs which are postsynaptic receptor blockers appear to also effectively block presynaptic receptors, it may be that the increased release of dopamine induced by this latter action is also important in the production of tardive dyskinesia.

In general it would now appear essential to assess the effect and relative potency of drugs on both pre- and postsynaptic receptors in order to fully understand the basis for their biochemical, physiological and behavioral actions.

ACKNOWLEDGMENTS

This research was supported by NIMH Grants (MH-17871; MH-14459), The Benevolent Foundation of Scottish Rite Freemasonry, Northern Jurisdiction, U.S.A., and The State of Connecticut.

REFERENCES

1. G.K. Aghajanian and B.S. Bunney, in Frontiers in Catecholamine Research (S.H. Snyder and E. Usdin, eds.), Pergamon Press, U.S.A., 1973, p. 643.

2. G.K. Aghajanian and B.S. Bunney, in Frontiers of Neurology and Neuroscience Research (P. Seeman and G.M. Brown, eds.), Univ. Toronto Press, Toronto, 1974.

3. G.K. Aghajanian and B.S. Bunney, Proc. 9th Int. Cong. Colleg. Int. Neuropsychopharmac., Excerp. Med. Found., 1974, in press.

4. G.K. Aghajanian, H.J. Haigler and F.E. Bloom, Life Sci., 11, 615 (1972).

5. N.E. Andén, A. Carlsson, A. Dahlstrom, K. Fuxe, N.A. Hillarp, and N. Larsson, Life Sci., 3, 523 (1964).

6. N.E. Andén, H. Corrodi, K. Fuxe, B. Hökfelt, T. Hökfelt, C. Rydin and T. Svensson, Life Sci., V. 9, P. 1, p. 513 (1970).

7. N.E. Andén, H. Corrodi, K. Fuxe, and U. Ungerstedt, Eur. J. Pharmacol., 15, 193 (1971).

8. N.E. Andén, B.E. Roos, and B. Werdinius, Life Sci., 3, 149 (1964).

9. N.E. Andén, A. Rubenson, K. Fuxe and T. Hökfelt, J. Pharm. Pharmacol., 19, 627 (1967).

10. A.J. Azzaro and C.O. Rutledge, Biochem. Pharmacol., 22, 2801 (1973).

11. H. Bernheimer and O. Hornykiewicz, Naunyn-Schmiedeberg's Arch. Exp. Path. Pharmak., 251, 135 (1965).

12. M.J. Besson, A. Cheramy, P. Feltz, J. Glowinski, Proc. Nat. Acad. Sci., 1969, 62, p. 741.

13. M. Besson, A. Cheramy, P. Feltz and J. Glowinski, Brain Res., 32, 407 (1971).

14. M. Besson, A. Cheramy, and J. Glowinski, J. Pharmacol. Exp. Ther., 177, 196 (1971).

15. F.E. Bloom, E. Costa and G. Salmoiraghi, J. Pharmacol. Exp. Ther., 150, 244 (1965).

16. G.L. Brown and J.S. Gillespie, J. Physiol. (Lond.), 138, 81 (1957).

17. B.S. Bunney and G.K. Aghajanian, in Frontiers in Catecholamine Research (S. Snyder and E. Usdin, eds.), Pergamon Press, New York, 1973, pp. 957-963.

18. B.S. Bunney and G.K. Aghajanian, in Predictiveness in Psychopharmacology (A. Sudilovsky, S. Gershon and B. Beer, eds.), Raven Press, New York, 1974, in press.

19. B.S. Bunney and G.K. Aghajanian, Wenner-Gren Center International Symposium Series, Pergamon Press, New York, 1974, in press.

20. B.S. Bunney, G.K. Aghajanian and R.H. Roth, Nature New Biol., 245, 123 (1973).

21. B.S. Bunney, J.R. Walters, R.H. Roth and G.K. Aghajanian, J. Pharmacol. Exp. Ther., 185, 560 (1973).

22. W.P. Burkard, K.F. Gey and A. Pletscher, Nature, 213, 732 (1967).

23. A. Carlsson, W. Kehr, M. Lindqvist, T. Magnusson, and C.V. Atack, Pharmacol. Rev., 24, 371 (1972).
24. A. Carlsson and M. Lindqvist, Acta Pharmacol. Toxicol., 20, 140 (1963).
25. A. Cheramy, M.J. Besson and J. Glowinski, Eur. J. Pharmacol., 10, 206 (1970).
26. J.D. Connor, J. Physiol. (Lond.), 208, 691 (1970).
27. H. Corrodi, K. Fuxe and T. Hökfelt, Eur. J. Pharmacol., 1, 363 (1967).
28. E. Costa and N.H. Neff, in Biochemistry and Pharmacology of the Basal Ganglia (E. Costa, L. Cote and M.D. Yahr, eds.), Raven Press, New York, 1966, p. 141.
29. J.T. Coyle and S.H. Snyder, J. Pharmacol. Exp. Ther., 170, 221 (1969).
30. A. Dahlström, and K. Fuxe, Acta Physiol. Scand., 64, suppl. 247, 1 (1965).
31. M. DaPrada and A. Pletscher, J. Pharm. Pharmacol., 18, 628 (1966).
32. M.A. Enero, S.Z. Langer, R.P. Rothlin and F.J.E. Stefano, Brit. J. Pharmacol., 44, 672 (1972).
33. A.M. Ernst, Psychopharmacologia, 10, 316 (1967).
34. L.O. Farnebo, Acta Physiol. Scand., 371, 45 (1971).
35. L.O. Farnebo and B. Hamberger, J. Pharm. Pharmacol., 22, 855 (1970).
36. L.O. Farnebo and B. Hamberger, Acta Physiol. Scand., 371, 35 (1971).

37. L.O. Farnebo and T. Malmfors, Acta Physiol. Scand., 371, 1 (1971).

38. P. Feltz and J. deChamplain, in Frontiers in Catecholamine Research (S.H. Snyder and E. Usdin, eds.), Pergamon Press, U.S.A., 1973.

39. B. Fjalland and I.M. Nielson, Psychopharmacologia (Berl.), 34, 105 (1974).

40. K. Fuxe, Acta Physiol. Scand., 64, 41 (1965).

41. K.F. Gey and A. Pletscher, Experientia (Basel), 24, 335 (1968)

42. G. Gianutsos, R.B. Drawbaugh, M.D. Hynes and H. Lal, Life Sci., 14, 887 (1974).

43. J. Glowinski and J. Axelrod, Pharmacol. Rev., 18, 775 (1966).

44. J. Häggendal, in Bayer-Symposium II, Springer-Verbag Heidelberg, 1970, p. 100.

45. H.J. Haigler and G.K. Aghajanian, J. Pharmacol. Exp. Ther., 188, 688 (1974).

46. T. Hattori, P.L. McGeer, H.C. Fibiger and E.G. McGeer, Brain Res., 54, 103 (1973).

47. P. Hedqvist, Acta Physiol. Scand., 345 (1970).

48. A. Herz and W. Zieglgänsberger, Int. J. Neuropharmacol., 17, 221 (1968).

49. A.S. Horn and S.H. Snyder, Proc. Nat. Acad. Sci. (U.S.A.), 68, 2325 (1971).

50. F. Javoy, Y. Agid, D. Bouvet and J. Glowinski, J. Pharmacol. Exp. Ther., 182, 454 (1972).

51. W. Kehr, A. Carlsson, M. Lindqvist, T. Magnusson and C.V. Atack, J. Pharm. Pharmacol., 24, 744 (1972).
52. S.M. Kirpekar and M. Puig, Brit. J. Pharmacol., 43, 359 (1971).
53. J.F.R. König and R.A. Klippel, The Rat Brain: A Stereotaxic Atlas, R.E. Krieger Publishing Company, Inc., 1970.
54. F.Z. Langer, E. Adler, M.A. Enero, J.F.E. Stefano, Proc. Int. Int. Union Physiol. Sci., 1971, 9, p. 335.
55. S. Langer, in Frontiers in Catecholamine Research (S.H. Snyder and E. Usdin, eds.), Pergamon Press, New York, 1973, p. 543.
56. R. Laverty and D.F. Sharman, Brit. J. Pharmacol., 24, 759 (1965).
57. P.L. McGeer, E.G. McGeer, J.A. Wada and E. Jung, Brain Res., 32, 425 (1971).
58. G.M. McKenzie and J.L. Szerb, J. Pharmacol. Exp. Ther., 162, 302 (1968).
59. J.R. McLean and M. McCartney, Proc. Soc. Exp. Biol. Med., 107, 77 (1961).
60. H. McLennan and D.H. York, J. Physiol. (Lond.), 189, 393 (1967).
61. K.E. Moore, J. Pharmacol. Exp. Ther., 142, 6 (1963).
62. M. Mujec and J.M. Van Rossum, Arch. Int. Pharmacodyn., 155, 432 (1965).

63. N.H. Neff and E. Costa, in Proc. First Int. Symp. Antidepressant Drugs (S. Garrattini and M.G. Dukes, eds.), Milan: Excerpta Medica Int. Cong., Series #122, 28 (1966).
64. H. Nybäck, G. Sedvall, J. Pharmacol. Exp. Ther., 162, 294 (1968).
65. H. Nybäck and G. Sedvall, J. Pharm. Pharmacol., 23, 322 (1971)
66. H. Nybäck, J. Schubert and G. Sedvall, J. Pharm. Pharmacol., 22, 622 (1970).
67. H. Nybäck, G. Sedvall and I.J. Kopin, Life Sci., 6, 2307 (1967).
68. T. Persson, Acta Pharmacol. (Kbh), 27, 397 (1969).
69. T. Persson, Acta. Pharmacol. Toxicol., 28, 387 (1970).
70. R.H. Roth, V.H. Morgenroth, III, and L.C. Murrin, Wenner-Gren Center Int. Symp. Series, Pergamon Press, New York, 1974, in press.
71. R.H. Roth, J.R. Walters and G.K. Aghajanian, in Frontiers in Catecholamine Research (S.H. Snyder and E. Costa, eds.), Pergamon Press, New York, 1973, p. 567.
72. R.H. Roth, J.R. Walters and V.H. Morgenroth, III, in Neuropsychopharmacology of Monoamines and Their Regulatory Enzymes (E. Usdin, ed.), Raven Press, New York, 1974, p. 369.
73. R. Rubovits and H.L. Klawans, Arch. Gen. Psychiat., 27, 502 (1972).
74. K. Starke, Naturwissenschaften, 58, 420 (1971).
75. K. Starke, Naunyn-Schmiedebergs Arch. Pharmac., 275, 11 (1972)
76. K. Starke, Naunyn-Schmiedebergs Arch. Pharmac. Exp. Path., 274, 18 (1972).

77. K. Starke, in Frontiers in Catecholamine Research (E. Usdin and S.H. Snyder, eds.), Pergamon Press, New York, 1973, p. 561
78. K. Starke and K.P. Altman, Neuropharmacology, 12, 339 (1973).
79. K. Starke and H. Montel, Naunyn-Schmiedebergs Arch. Pharmacol. 279, 53 (1973).
80. K. Starke and H. Montel, Neuropharmacology, 12, 1073 (1973).
81. L. Stein, Fed. Proc., 23, 836 (1964).
82. L. Stjärne, Nature New Biol., 243, 190 (1973).
83. T.H. Svensson, B.S. Bunney and G.K. Aghajanian, Submitted for publication, 1974.
84. D. Tarsy and R.J. Baldessarini, Nature New Biol., 245, 262 (1973).
85. H. Thoenen, A. Hürlimann, and W. Haefely, Helv. Physiol. Pharmacol. Acta, 22, 148 (1964).
86. H.A. Tilson and S.B. Sparber, J. Pharmacol. Exp. Ther., 181, 387 (1972).
87. P.F. VonVoigtlander and K.E. Moore, J. Pharmacol. Exp. Ther., 184, 542 (1973).
88. J.R. Walters, G.K. Aghajanian and R.H. Roth, Proc. Fifth Cong. Pharmacol., 1972, p. 246.
89. J.R. Walters and R.H. Roth, Biochem. Pharmacol., 21, 2111 (1972).
90. J.R. Walters and R.H. Roth, J. Pharmacol. Exp. Ther., 191, 82 (1974).
91. J.R. Walters and R.H. Roth, Wenner-Gren Center Int. Symp. Series, Pergamon Press, New York, 1974, in press.

92. J.R. Walters, R.H. Roth and G.K. Aghajanian, J. Pharmacol. Exp. Ther., 186, 630 (1973).

93. U. Werner, K. Starke and H.J. Schuman, Naunyn-Schmiedeberg's Arch. Exp. Path. Pharmacol., 266, 474 (1970).

94. D.H. York, Brain Res., 37, 91 (1972).

DISCUSSION

Dr. Everett wondered whether Dr. Bunney had done a dose-response study on amphetamine in the experiment where the formation of dopamine was inhibited and then added amphetamine was found to be ineffective in overcoming such a block. Dr. Bunney replied that the dose of amphetamine was pushed very high and still no effect could be observed.

Dr. Davis mentioned a clinical example which might implicate several different types of receptors. Normally pharmacologists assume that a pharmacological effect occurs when the concentration of a drug is at its maximum rather than 20 hours later when the concentration may have dropped to one-third of its maximum. For a pharmacokinetic study, Dr. Davis gave a single dose of the phenothiazine butaperazine to patients and then measured blood levels over time. Two of the patients had dystonias 19-26 hours after the administration of drug, when levels were down to 1/2 or 1/3 of the maximum. In searching for an explanation, Dr. Davis said that he realized that there is a catecholamine involvement in dystonias since a dystonia could be turned off by giving the patient Ritalin or an anticholinergic. One possible explanation would be that a

DRUG ACTIONS ON RECEPTORS IN CNS

phenothiazine not only blocks receptors but also increases synthesis; the resulting balance does not result in dystonia. However, later, when the phenothiazine leaves the receptors, it may leave the postsynaptic receptors slightly faster than the presynaptic receptors. A slight imbalance results in dystonia. In some cases, Dr. Davis has seen a dystonia which disappeared within 5 or 10 minutes; he assumes that a temporary imbalance was indicated. Dr. Bunney felt this would be a possible explanation if there was a difference between the pre- and postsynaptic receptor in terms of the concentrations for interaction.

Dr. Carlsson wondered if the speaker had tested the sensitivity of the cell body of the receptors at various intervals after reserpine. Dr. Bunney thought this an interesting suggestion but stated that he had not yet done this.

Dr. Bloom proposed that Dr. Bunney might have a system in which the question asked of him by Dr. Snyder might be tested. Thus, if haloperidol is given while recording from the dopamine target neuron, then if there is chronically-released dopamine inhibiting that cell, there would be an increase in the discharge rate of that target neuron. Dr. Bunney replied that one of the things that they had hoped to see in recording from the caudate nucleus was that treatment with a phenothiazine would show an increased firing rate; results so far seem inconclusive.

Dr. Fuxe was rather surprised at the rapid blockade observed after a low dose of alpha-methyltrosine. Dr. Bunney pointed out that although the dose was low (10 mg/kg), it was given i. v. He agreed that the response time (<2 min) was extremely rapid.

Dr. Hornykiewicz agreed that the autoreceptors on the dopamine cell bodies are clearly of major importance for drug effects, but he wondered about their physiological importance. Dr. Bunney thought there might be none since there is no known dopaminergic input in terms of the presynaptic receptor. This is reinforced by the fact that there are no fluorescent terminals in the area.

DOPAMINE-SENSITIVE ADENYLATE CYCLASE AND PROTEIN PHOSPHORYLATION

IN THE RAT CAUDATE NUCLEUS

Bruce K. Krueger, Javier Forn and Paul Greengard

Department of Pharmacology
Yale University School of Medicine
New Haven, Connecticut   06510

I.   INTRODUCTION

Work in several laboratories during the past ten years has implicated dopamine as a neurotransmitter in the mammalian brain, particularly in the basal ganglia [1-11]. In addition, a deficiency of dopaminergic transmission in the caudate nucleus, due to a degeneration of dopaminergic fibers from the substantia nigra to the caudate nucleus, appears to be involved in the etiology of naturally-occurring Parkinson's disease [2, 12]. Similarly, iatrogenic Parkinsonism, seen with high frequency in patients given antipsychotic drugs, would appear to be due to a blockade, by the antipsychotic drugs, of dopamine receptors in the caudate nucleus [1, 4, 10]. Other evidence suggests that some of the symptoms of schizophrenia may be the result of hyperactivity of dopaminergic pathways innervating certain regions of the limbic system of the brain [13-17]. In view of both the theoretical and practical importance of an increased understanding of the role of dopamine within the mammalian central nervous system, our laboratory has carried out investigations attempting to elucidate the mechanism by which dopamine exerts its biological effects in the mammalian brain.

Earlier studies in our laboratory [18-20] led to the hypothesis that cyclic AMP mediates dopaminergic transmission within the superior cervical ganglion. The data suggested the following sequence of events: dopamine, released from interneurons within the ganglion as a result of neural activity, diffuses across the synaptic cleft and activates a dopamine-sensitive adenylate cyclase in the membrane of the postganglionic neuron, leading to the formation of cyclic AMP in the postganglionic neuron; this newly formed cyclic AMP causes a hyperpolarization of the postganglionic neuron, and thereby modifies its excitability [20].

While it seems likely that many of the actions of the catecholamines, both in neuronal and in non-neuronal tissues, may be mediated by cyclic AMP, there is less evidence concerning the mechanism by which cyclic AMP exerts its biological effects. Evidence has accumulated in the past several years supporting the hypothesis [21] that cyclic AMP achieves its biological effects by regulating the activity of cyclic AMP-dependent protein kinases. Indeed, cyclic AMP-dependent protein kinases have been found in a wide variety of animal tissues, including mammalian brain [22]. The discovery that the specific activity of this enzyme is highest in synaptic membrane fractions [23] suggested that cyclic AMP-dependent protein kinase may play a role in synaptic transmission. Recently, specific endogenous protein substrates for cyclic AMP-dependent protein kinase have been found in synaptic membrane fractions from rat cerebrum [24, 25].

Within the framework of the hypotheses that dopaminergic transmission in the mammalian nervous system may be mediated by cyclic AMP, and that the actions of cyclic AMP may in turn be mediated by cyclic AMP-dependent protein kinases, we undertook a search for dopamine-sensitive cyclic AMP formation and cyclic AMP-dependent protein phosphorylation in homogenates and slices of rat caudate nucleus.

II. REGULATION OF ADENYLATE CYCLASE ACTIVITY IN CELL-FREE SYSTEMS

An adenylate cyclase activated by low concentrations of dopamine has been found in homogenates of rat caudate nucleus. The effect of various concentrations of dopamine, ℓ-norepinephrine and ℓ-isoproterenol on this adenylate cyclase is shown in Figure 1. A half-maximal increase in enzyme activity was achieved with about 4 μM dopamine and with about 28 μM ℓ-norepinephrine. The β-adrenergic agonist, ℓ-isoproterenol, had no significant effect on adenylate cyclase activity at concentrations as high as 300 μM. The effect of ℓ-norepinephrine on the adenylate cyclase activity of the caudate homogenate would appear to be due to activation by ℓ-norepinephrine of the dopamine-sensitive enzyme: the maximal stimulation of adenylate cyclase activity achieved with ℓ-norepinephrine was equal to that observed with dopamine;

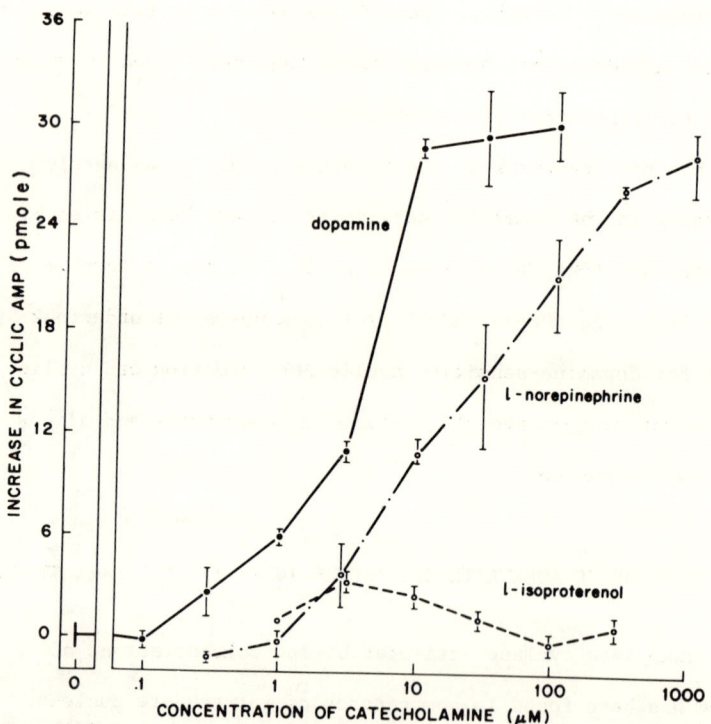

Fig. 1. Effect of catecholamines on adenylate cyclase activity in a homogenate of rat caudate nucleus. In the absence of added catecholamine, 27.1 ± 0.1 pmole (mean $\pm$ SEM, n = 6) of cyclic AMP were formed. The increase in cyclic AMP above this basal level is plotted as a function of catecholamine concentration. The data give mean values and ranges for duplicate determinations on each of two to five replicate samples. (Taken from [26].)

moreover, in the presence of optimal amounts of either dopamine or ℓ-norepinephrine, no further increase in adenylate cyclase activity was obtained by the addition of the other catecholamine.

Since the dopamine receptor of the mammalian caudate nucleus has been extensively characterized in many laboratories, through both clinical and animal studies, it was possible to compare the properties of the dopamine-sensitive adenylate cyclase found in homogenates of the rat caudate nucleus with the properties of the indirectly characterized dopamine receptor. The following properties of the dopamine receptor have been revealed by clinical, physiological and pharmacological studies: this receptor is stimulated by dopamine [5], as well as by the synthetic compound apomorphine [3]; ET-495 via a catechol metabolite also stimulates this receptor [7]; the effects of dopamine are blocked by a wide variety of antipsychotic drugs [1, 4, 11, 27], including representatives of the phenothiazine, butyrophenone, and dibenzodiazepine classes; compounds closely related structurally to these antipsychotic drugs, but which display neither antipsychotic efficacy nor the ability to produce a Parkinsonian syndrome, do not block the dopamine receptor. The properties of the dopamine-sensitive adenylate cyclase present in caudate homogenates are quite similar to the properties of the dopamine receptor observed in vivo, as the following results indicate.

Low concentrations of apomorphine stimulate adenylate cyclase activity in homogenates of rat caudate nucleus (Figure 2). Moreover, a metabolite of ET-495 has been demonstrated by Miller and Iversen [28] to stimulate the dopamine-sensitive adenylate cyclase of the caudate nucleus. Fluphenazine, a potent antipsychotic agent, competitively inhibited the stimulation of caudate adenylate cyclase by dopamine (Figure 3). The K_i value for fluphenazine was 8×10^{-9} M. The great potency of fluphenazine as an antagonist of the caudate enzyme suggests that this biochemical effect of fluphenazine may be responsible for the extrapyramidal side effects

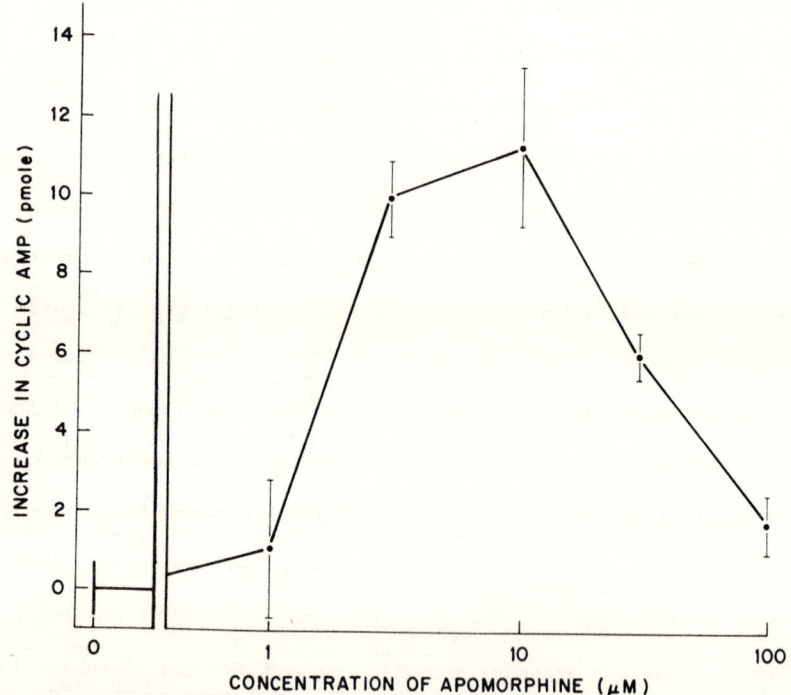

Fig. 2. Effect of apomorphine on adenylate cyclase activity in a homogenate of rat caudate nucleus. In the absence of added apomorphine, 26.5 ± 0.7 pmole (mean $\pm$ SEM, n = 4) of cyclic AMP were formed. The increase in cyclic AMP above this basal level is plotted as a function of apomorphine concentration. The data give mean values and ranges for duplicate determinations on each of two to four replicate samples. (Taken from [26].)

observed in patients given this drug. Several other antipsychotic drugs of various chemical classes were also found to inhibit the stimulation of adenylate cyclase activity by dopamine in caudate homogenates (Table I). The inhibition by these drugs was competitive with dopamine in all cases studied [29].

Interestingly, there was over a 1,000-fold difference in the potencies of various structurally-related phenothiazines as

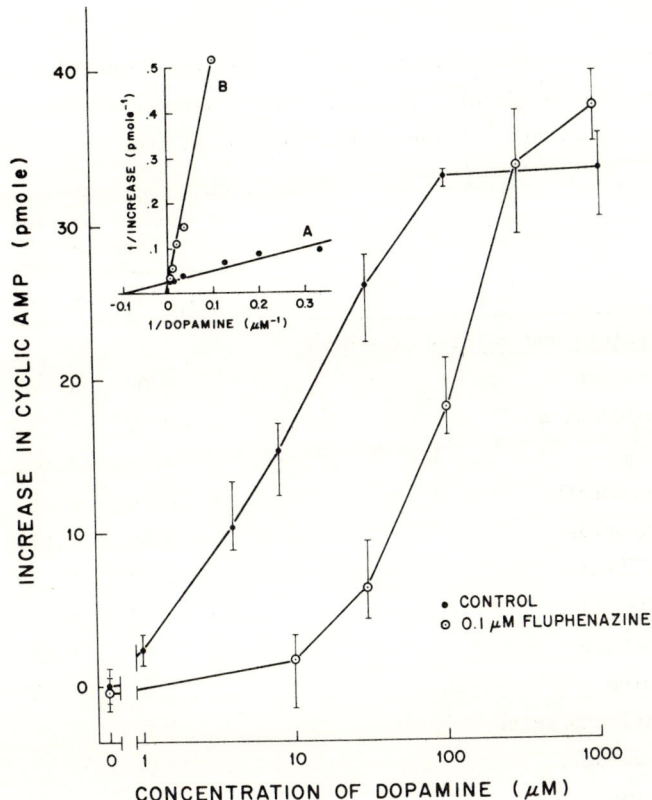

Fig. 3. Effect of various concentrations of dopamine, alone (●———●) or in combination with 0.1 μM fluphenazine (θ----θ), on adenylate cyclase activity in a homogenate of rat caudate nucleus. In the absence of added dopamine and fluphenazine, 46.0 ± 2.0 pmole (mean ± SEM, n = 6) of cyclic AMP were formed; in the presence of 0.1 μM fluphenazine (but without added dopamine), 45.9 ± 2.0 pmole (mean ± SEM, n = 6) of cyclic AMP were formed. The increase in cyclic AMP above the basal level (i.e. the level in the absence of both dopamine and fluphenazine) is plotted as a function of dopamine concentration. The data give mean values and ranges for duplicate determinations on each of three replicate samples. Inset: Double reciprocal plot of cyclic AMP increase as a function of dopamine concentration from 3 μM to 300 μM. A: control. B: 0.1 μM fluphenazine. (Taken from [29].)

antagonists of the stimulation by dopamine of caudate adenylate cyclase activity. Compounds closely related structurally to the

TABLE I

Calculated Inhibition Constant (K_i) of Several Phenothiazine Derivatives and Related Compounds for Dopamine-Sensitive Adenylate Cyclase of Rat Caudate Nucleus

Drug	Caudate nucleus enzyme	
	I_{50} (µM)	K_i (µM)
Phenothiazines and related compounds		
Fluphenazine	0.07	0.008
Trifluoperazine	0.10	0.011
Promazine	0.35	0.039
Triflupromazine	0.40	0.044
Prochlorperazine	0.50	0.055
Thioridazine	0.50	0.055
Chlorpromazine	0.60	0.066
Promethazine	15.0	1.67
Imipramine	27.0	3.00
Desmethylimipramine	28.0	3.11
Ethoproperazine	37.0	4.11
Diethazine	100.0	11.11
Butyrophenone and related compound		
Haloperidol	2.0	0.22
Pimozide	11.0	1.22
Dibenzodiazepine		
Clozapine	0.55	0.061

Data from experiments in which the concentration of dopamine was held constant, and the concentration of the test substance was varied. The K_i value was calculated from the relationship $I_{50} = K_i(1 + S/K_m)$, where I_{50} is the concentration of drug required to give 50% inhibition of the dopamine-stimulated increase in enzyme activity, and S is the concentration (40 µM) of dopamine. K_m is the concentration of dopamine required to give half-maximal activation of the enzyme. The mean value for K_m found in this series of experiments was 5 µM. (Taken from [29].)

psychoactive phenothiazines, but which have little or no antipsychotic or extrapyramidal actions clinically, had low relative potencies as inhibitors of dopamine-stimulated adenylate cyclase activity. Miller et al. [30] and Karobath and Leitich [31] have reported a similar order of efficacy for a number of antipsychotic compounds and inactive analogs with respect to their ability to inhibit dopamine-sensitive adenylate cyclase in homogenates of the rat caudate nucleus.

A dopamine-sensitive adenylate cyclase having properties similar to those of the enzyme in the rat caudate nucleus has been found in homogenates of rat olfactory tubercle and guinea pig nucleus accumbens, structures belonging to the limbic system [29, 32]. The finding that antipsychotic drugs prevent the stimulation by dopamine of adenylate cyclase activity in homogenates from both the caudate nucleus and the limbic system led to the suggestion that the extrapyramidal side effects of the antipsychotic drugs may be related to their ability to block the stimulation by dopamine of adenylate cyclase activity in the caudate nucleus, and that the therapeutic effects of the antipsychotic drugs may be related to a similar action on dopamine-sensitive adenylate cyclase in the limbic system [29].

The subcellular distribution of dopamine-sensitive adenylate cyclase activity was studied in the rat caudate nucleus (Table II). Subcellular fractions were prepared by differential centrifugation and discontinuous sucrose density gradient centrifugation as described by De Robertis et al. [33]. The highest specific

TABLE II

Distribution of Dopamine-Sensitive Adenylate Cyclase Activity in Subcellular Fractions of the Rat Caudate Nucleus

Fraction and ultrastructure	Protein	Adenylate cyclase activity			
		Total activity		Specific activity	
		−dopamine	+dopamine	−dopamine	+dopamine
	(mg)	pmol/2.5 min X 10^{-3}		pmol/mg protein/min	
A. Primary subfractions					
Nuclear	50.4	5.54	11.54	44.0	91.6
Mitochondrial	54.0	6.35	15.16	47.1	112.2
Microsomal	13.6	1.30	1.67	38.1	49.2
Cell Sap	3.2	N.D.*	N.D.*	N.D.*	N.D.*
Total	121.2	13.19	28.37		
Starting material (homogenate)	130.0	15.10	40.42	46.5	124.4
Recovery (%)	93.2	87.4	70.2		
B. Mitochondrial subfractions					
M-1 nerve ending membranes; myelin; mitochondria; membranes of various sizes	33.5	6.53	14.14	78.0	168.8
M-2 + M-3 synaptic vesicles; small smooth membranes	18.7	0.92	0.87	19.7	18.6

Total	52.2	7.45	15.01		
Starting material (mitochondrial)	54.0	6.35	15.16		
Recovery (%)	96.7	117.3	99.0		
C. Subfractions of M-1 separated by sucrose density gradient centrifugation					
M-1 (0.8) myelin	3.7	0.22	0.31	23.8	33.5
M-1 (0.9) nerve endings; myelin; membranes; mitochondria	2.5	0.55	1.09	88.0	174.4
M-1 (1.0) nerve endings and mitochondria	4.0	1.34	2.14	134.0	214.0
M-1 (1.2) nerve endings; mitochondria and small smooth membranes	11.9	3.43	5.05	115.3	169.7
M-1 (1.4) predominantly mitochondria; small smooth membranes; nerve endings	6.7	0.98	1.53	58.5	91.3
Pellet mitochondria	1.0	0.05	0.05	20.0	20.0
Total	29.8	6.57	10.17		
Starting material (M-1)	33.5	6.53	14.14		
Recovery (%)	89.0	100.6	71.9		

*Not detectable.

Subcellular fractions of rat caudate nucleus were prepared by the method of De Robertis et al. [33]. (Taken from [34].)

activity of dopamine-sensitive adenylate cyclase was found in subfractions M-1 (0.9), M-1 (1.0) and M-1 (1.2), all of which are enriched in synaptic membranes. Recent evidence indicates that the adenylate cyclase activity of the caudate nucleus has an increased sensitivity to dopamine after lesioning of the dopaminergic neurons in the substantia nigra [35]; the results are compatible with the hypothesis that at least part of the dopamine-sensitive adenylate cyclase is located postsynaptically.

III. REGULATION OF CYCLIC AMP LEVELS IN SLICES

Dopamine, as well as the dopamine agonist, apomorphine, was able to increase levels of cyclic AMP by 75-100% in slices of rat caudate nucleus (Figure 4A). The concentrations causing half-maximal stimulation were approximately 60 µM for dopamine and 150 µM for apomorphine. The effects of ℓ-isoproterenol and ℓ-norepinephrine on cyclic AMP levels are shown in Figure 4B. ℓ-Isoproterenol caused a 2- to 4-fold increase in cyclic AMP levels and the concentration of ℓ-isoproterenol causing a half-maximal stimulation was 0.03 µM. ℓ-Norepinephrine caused a 3- to 5-fold increase in cyclic AMP levels and the concentration of ℓ-norepinephrine causing a half-maximal stimulation was about 30 µM. The maximal stimulation by ℓ-norepinephrine was always greater than the maximal stimulation by ℓ-isoproterenol. Cocaine, a blocker of catecholamine uptake [37, 38], increased the sensitivity to ℓ-norepinephrine, so that the concentration of ℓ-norepinephrine

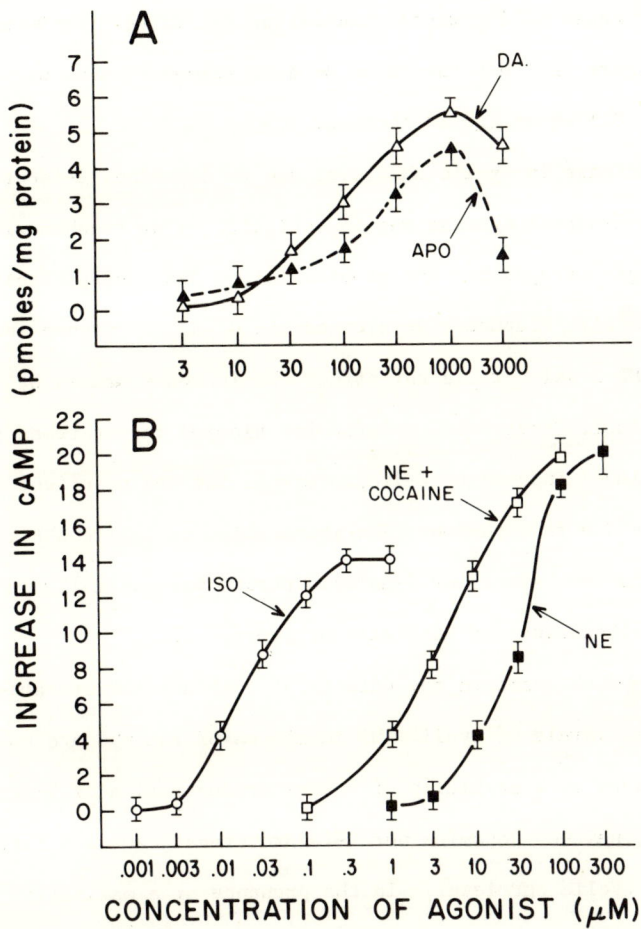

Fig. 4. Increase in cyclic AMP level in slices of rat caudate nucleus as a function of the concentration of (A) dopamine (DA) and apomorphine (APO) or (B) ℓ-isoproterenol (ISO) and ℓ-norepinephrine (NE). Concentration of cocaine, 0.1 mM. The data represent the mean ± SEM for 40 replicate samples (dopamine curve), 12 replicate samples (apomorphine curve), or 18 replicate samples (ℓ-isoproterenol and ℓ-norepinephrine curves). In the absence of added agonist, the level of cyclic AMP was 7.1 ± 0.3, 6.7 ± 0.5, and 6.0 ± 0.6 pmole/mg protein, respectively, for the dopamine, apomorphine, and isoproterenol-norepinephrine curves. (Taken from [36].)

required to cause half-maximal stimulation decreased from 30 µM to 4 µM (Figure 4B), but the dopamine dose-response curve was not affected by 0.1 mM or 1.0 mM cocaine.

The increase in cyclic AMP level due to dopamine, ℓ-isoproterenol and ℓ-norepinephrine was investigated using fluphenazine, a dopaminergic antagonist, and propranolol, a β-adrenergic antagonist (Figure 5). Fluphenazine blocked the dopamine-induced increase in cyclic AMP level but did not affect the increase caused by ℓ-isoproterenol. Conversely, propranolol blocked the increase in cyclic AMP level induced by ℓ-isoproterenol but had no effect on the increase due to dopamine. The stimulation of cyclic AMP levels in caudate nucleus slices by ℓ-norepinephrine was partially inhibited by fluphenazine and partially by propranolol.

We have also examined the effects of combinations of catecholamines on levels of cyclic AMP in slices of rat caudate nucleus. In the presence of a maximally effective concentration of ℓ-norepinephrine, neither dopamine nor ℓ-isoproterenol caused a further increase in cyclic AMP level. In the presence of a maximally effective concentration of ℓ-isoproterenol, dopamine caused a significant increase in cyclic AMP level, such that stimulation by the combination of ℓ-isoproterenol and dopamine was similar to that caused by ℓ-norepinephrine alone.

The results of these studies on the regulation of cyclic AMP levels in slices of the rat caudate nucleus suggest the existence, in the caudate nucleus, of two classes of catecholamine receptors, the stimulation of which results in an increased level

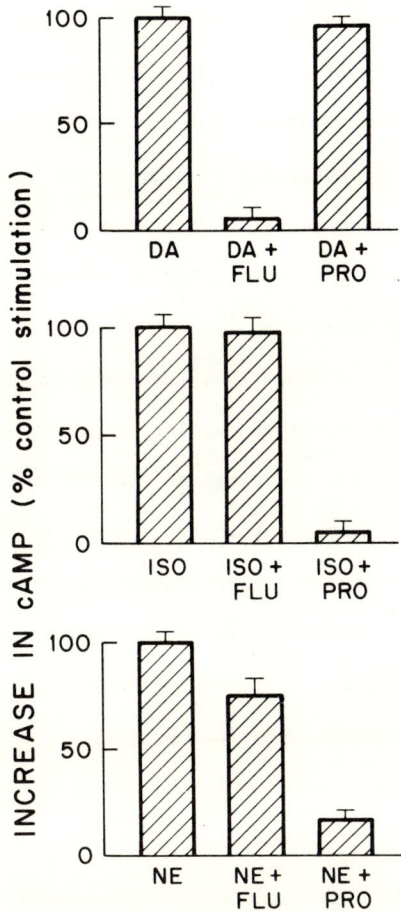

Fig. 5. Blockade by 100 μM fluphenazine (FLU) or 100 μM dℓ-propranolol (PRO) of catecholamine-induced increases in cyclic AMP levels in slices of rat caudate nucleus. In the absence of any blocking agent the increases in cyclic AMP induced by 100 μM dopamine (DA, top), 1 μM ℓ-isoproterenol (ISO, center), and 100 μM ℓ-norepinephrine (NE, bottom) were 4.2 ± 0.2, 15.4 ± 0.8, and 12.3 ± 0.6 pmole/mg protein, respectively. The basal level of cyclic AMP (absence of added agonist or blocking agent) was 6.8 ± 0.3 pmole/mg protein. At the concentrations studied, none of the blocking agents significantly altered this basal level of cyclic AMP. Each determination represents the mean $\pm$ SEM for 8 to 12 replicate samples. (Taken from [36].)

of cyclic AMP. One class of receptors is activated by either
dopamine, apomorphine or ℓ-norepinephrine, but not by ℓ-isoproterenol, and is blocked by fluphenazine but not by propranolol. These
properties of this receptor are similar to the properties of the
dopamine-sensitive adenylate cyclase found in homogenates of the
rat caudate nucleus. The other class of receptors in rat caudate
nucleus slices is activated by low concentrations of either ℓ-isoproterenol or ℓ-norepinephrine, but not by dopamine or apomorphine, and is blocked by propranolol but not by fluphenazine.
These data indicate that an adenylate cyclase sensitive to β-adrenergic agonists is present in the caudate nucleus *in vivo*.
Since it has not been possible to demonstrate ℓ-isoproterenol-sensitive adenylate cyclase activity in homogenates of the caudate
nucleus (*e.g.* see Figure 1), it would appear that the ℓ-isoproterenol-sensitive enzyme loses its hormonal sensitivity upon
homogenization of the tissue.

IV. REGULATION OF ENDOGENOUS PROTEIN PHOSPHORYLATION

The cyclic AMP-dependent phosphorylation of endogenous proteins in membrane fractions from the rat caudate nucleus was
studied by incubation of the membrane fractions with [γ-^{32}P]ATP,
in the absence or presence of cyclic AMP. Sodium dodecyl sulfate
was added to the incubation mixture to terminate the reaction
and to solubilize the membrane proteins, which were then subjected
to polyacrylamide gel electrophoresis [39]. Protein staining
and autoradiography were carried out in order to determine the

amount of radioactivity incorporated into individual protein bands [25]. As seen in Figure 6, cyclic AMP stimulated the endogenous phosphorylation of three protein bands in a fraction enriched in synaptic membranes. Two of these proteins (with apparent molecular weights of 85,000 and 80,000) were found only in those subcellular fractions containing synaptic membranes. (This pair of proteins corresponds to the broad band, designated "Protein I", which is observed when phosphorylated synaptic membrane preparations from rat cerebrum are subjected to polyacrylamide gel electrophoresis in the system of Fairbanks et al. [40].) The concentration of cyclic AMP causing half-maximal stimulation of the phosphorylation of these proteins by endogenous protein kinase(s) was about 1 μM. It was observed that this endogenous cyclic AMP-dependent protein phosphorylation was localized in the same subcellular fractions which contained the dopamine-sensitive adenylate cyclase. This observation is compatible with the idea that cyclic AMP-dependent membrane protein phosphorylation may mediate the effects of dopamine in the brain.

A third phosphoprotein was found in all subcellular fractions of the caudate nucleus studied, including the cytosol. This phosphoprotein had an apparent molecular weight of 59,000 in the electrophoresis system of Studier [39], and of 49,000 in the electrophoresis system of Fairbanks et al. [40]. In fact, cyclic AMP-dependent phosphorylation of a similar phosphoprotein has been demonstrated in soluble and particulate fractions of all vertebrate tissues studied [41].

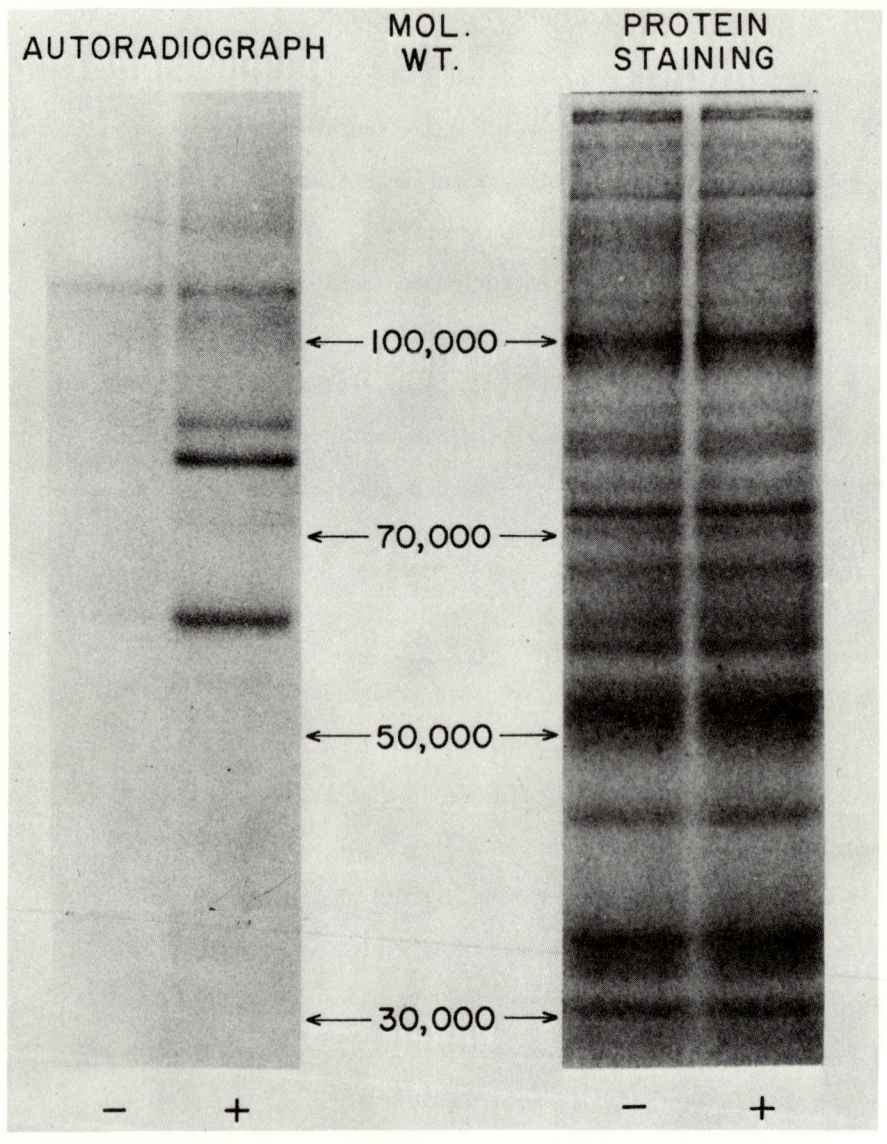

Fig. 6. Effect of cyclic AMP on endogenous protein phosphorylation in a synaptic membrane fraction from rat caudate nucleus. Subcellular fractions were prepared by the method of De Robertis et al. [33]. Fraction M-1 (0.9), which was enriched in synaptic membranes, was incubated for 15 sec at 30°, in a total volume of 0.1 ml containing 80 mM Tris-Cl, pH 7.4, 10 mM $MgCl_2$, 1 µM [γ-^{32}P]-ATP, in the absence (-) or presence (+) of 5 µM cyclic AMP. The reaction was terminated by the addition of sodium dodecyl sulfate, and an aliquot was subjected to sodium dodecyl sulfate-polyacrylamide gel electrophoresis as described by Studier [39]. The gels were stained, dried and subjected to autoradiography as described by Ueda et al. [25]. Left: phosphorylation of endogenous protein in the absence or presence of cyclic AMP. Right: protein staining.

The regulation of protein phosphorylation by cyclic AMP was also examined in slices of rat caudate nucleus. The slices were preincubated for 1 hour with [^{32}P]-orthophosphate, and then incubated for 15 min in the presence or absence of various test substances. Sodium dodecyl sulfate was then added to stop the reaction and to solubilize membrane proteins. Aliquots of the solubilized proteins were subjected to electrophoresis and autoradiography, as in the case of the membrane fractions described above. The phosphorylation of three proteins, of apparent molecular weights 85,000, 80,000 and 59,000, was selectively stimulated by incubation of the slices with a phosphodiesterase inhibitor, 3-isobutyl-1-methylxanthine (Figure 7), which also causes an increase in cyclic AMP levels in slices of caudate nucleus [36]. 8-Bromo cyclic AMP, a potent analog of cyclic AMP [42], was able to mimic the effect of 3-isobutyl-1-methylxanthine on endogenous protein phosphorylation, whereas N^6-monobutyryl cyclic AMP, $N^6,O^{2'}$-dibutyryl cyclic AMP, and cyclic AMP itself were without effect.

V. CONCLUDING REMARKS

The finding of dopamine-sensitive adenylate cyclase in homogenates of the caudate nucleus and of the limbic system, together with the effects of antipsychotic drugs on this enzyme, has provided a possible biochemical mechanism for the action of dopamine in the mammalian brain [26, 28-32, 35]. These studies have shown that the properties of dopamine-sensitive adenylate cyclase are similar to the properties of the dopamine receptor characterized

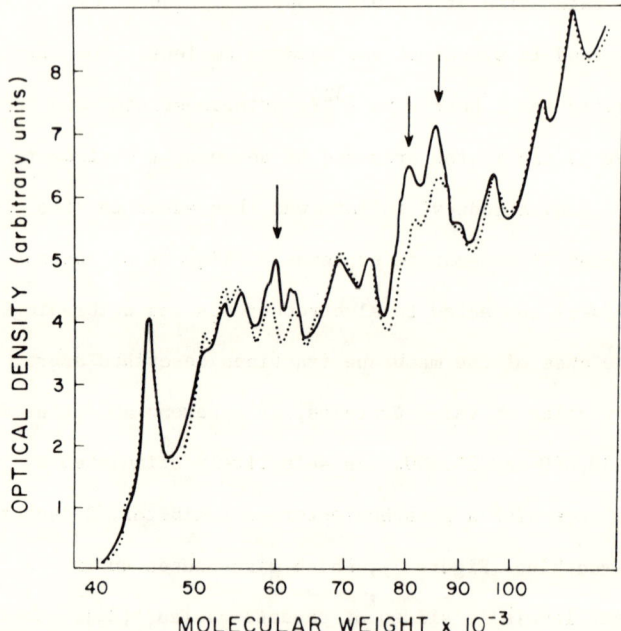

Fig. 7. Effect of 3-isobutyl-1-methylxanthine, a phosphodiesterase inhibitor, on protein phosphorylation in slices of rat caudate nucleus. Slices were preincubated for 15 min at 37° in Krebs Ringer bicarbonate buffer (pH 7.4) equilibrated with 95% O_2-5% CO_2. [^{32}P]orthophosphate was added (1 mCi/ml) and the preincubation was carried out for a further 60 min. Aliquots of the suspension of slices, containing 15 mg tissue, were then incubated in the absence (dotted line) or presence (solid line) of 1 mM 3-isobutyl-1-methylxanthine for 15 min. The incubation was terminated by addition of sodium dodecyl sulfate (final concentration, 3%), followed by incubation at 100° for 5 min to solubilize the tissue completely and to inactivate proteolytic enzymes. Aliquots (50 µl) were subjected to sodium dodecyl sulfate-polyacrylamide gel electrophoresis as described by Studier [39]. The gel was stained, dried and subjected to autoradiography as described by Ueda et al. [25]. The autoradiograph was scanned on a Canalco Model G II densitometer. The optical density of the various protein bands is proportional to the amount of radioactivity incorporated into these bands. The arrows indicate the proteins, with apparent molecular weights of 59,000, 80,000, 85,000, the phosphorylation of which was significantly increased by 3-isobutyl-1-methylxanthine.

by clinical, behavioral and pharmacological studies. Moreover, the properties of the dopamine receptor in the caudate nucleus, as characterized by studies on the regulation of cyclic AMP in tissue slices, are similar to those of the dopamine-sensitive adenylate cyclase previously characterized in homogenates of the caudate nucleus. The various results suggest that the therapeutic effects of the antipsychotic drugs may be due to their ability to block dopamine-sensitive adenylate cyclase in the limbic system, and that the Parkinsonian side effects of these drugs may be due to their ability to block dopamine-sensitive adenylate cyclase in the caudate nucleus.

Recent electrophysiological studies [43] are consistent with the conclusion that cyclic AMP mediates the actions of dopamine. Thus, the inhibition by dopamine of the spontaneous firing of neurons in the caudate nucleus [44, 45] is mimicked by cyclic AMP, potentiated by 3-isobutyl-1-methylxanthine, and blocked by chlorpromazine, a phenothiazine, but not by propranolol.

The studies with slices of rat caudate nucleus also indicate the presence of a β-adrenergic receptor in this tissue. This receptor was stimulated by ℓ-isoproterenol and ℓ-norepinephrine, but not by dopamine, and was blocked by propranolol, a β-adrenergic antagonist, but not by the antipsychotic drug fluphenazine. From the point of view of studying dopamine-sensitive adenylate cyclase in mammalian brain, the fact that the β-adrenergic adenylate cyclase is inactivated upon tissue homogenization is fortunate, since it has facilitated the study of the dopamine receptor in a cell-free system without interference from the adenylate cyclase sensitive to β-adrenergic agonists.

Our studies have provided some clues as to the mechanism by which cyclic AMP may mediate the effects of dopamine in the brain. One particularly interesting result was that the cyclic AMP-dependent phosphorylation of certain proteins was demonstrable only in those subcellular fractions enriched in synaptic membranes, i.e. the same fractions which contain the dopamine-sensitive adenylate cyclase. We have also found that the potent phosphodiesterase inhibitor 3-isobutyl-1-methylxanthine, as well as 8-bromo cyclic AMP, increases the phosphorylation of the same or similar proteins in tissue slices. These various lines of evidence suggest that cyclic AMP-dependent protein phosphorylation may mediate the effects of dopamine in the brain. We are currently investigating the effect of dopamine on protein phosphorylation in slices of rat caudate nucleus.

REFERENCES

[1]. A. Carlsson and M. Lindquist, Acta Pharmacol. Toxicol., 20, 1963, 140-144.
[2]. O. Hornykiewicz, Pharmacol. Rev., 18, 1966, 925-964.
[3]. N. E. Andén, A. Rubenson, K. Fuxe, and T. Hökfelt, J. Pharm. Pharmacol., 19, 1967, 627-629.
[4]. H. Nybäck and G. Sedvall, J. Pharmacol. Exp. Ther., 162, 1968, 294-301.
[5]. U. Ungerstedt, L. L. Butcher, S. G. Butcher, N. E. Andén, and K. Fuxe, Brain Res., 14, 1969, 461-471.
[6]. H. Nybäck, J. Schubert, and G. Sedvall, J. Pharm. Pharmacol., 22, 1970, 622-624.
[7]. H. Corrodi, K. Fuxe, and U. Ungerstedt, J. Pharm. Pharmacol., 23, 1971, 989-991.

[8]. O. Hornykiewicz, Contemp. Neurol., 8, 1971, 34-65.
[9]. N. E. Andén, J. Pharm. Pharmacol., 24, 1972, 905-906.
[10]. H. Nyback and G. Sedvall, Psychopharmac., 26, 1972, 155-160.
[11]. B. S. Bunney, J. R. Walters, R. H. Roth, and G. K. Aghajanian, J. Pharm. Exp. Ther., 185, 1973, 560-571.
[12]. H. Ehringer and O. Hornykiewicz, Klin. Wschr., 38, 1960, 1236-1239.
[13]. A. Randrup and I. Munkvad, Orthomolec. Psychiat., 1, 1972, 2-7.
[14]. S. Matthysse, Fed. Proc., 32, 1973, 200-205.
[15]. S. H. Snyder, Arch. Gen. Psychiat., 27, 1972, 169-179.
[16]. S. H. Snyder, S. P. Banerjee, H. I. Yamamura, and D. Greenberg, Science, 184, 1974, 1243-1253.
[17]. J. Stevens, Arch. Gen. Psychiat., 29, 1973, 177-189.
[18]. D. A. McAfee, M. Schorderet, and P. Greengard, Science, 171, 1970, 1156-1158.
[19]. J. W. Kebabian and P. Greengard, Science, 174, 1971, 2915-2918.
[20]. P. Greengard and J. W. Kebabian, Fed. Proc., 33, 1974, 1059-1067.
[21]. J. F. Kuo and P. Greengard, Proc. Nat. Acad. Sci. U.S.A., 64, 1969, 1349-1355.
[22]. E. Miyamoto, J. F. Kuo, and P. Greengard, Science, 165, 1969, 63-65.
[23]. H. Maeno, E. M. Johnson, and P. Greengard, J. Biol. Chem., 246, 1971, 134-142.
[24]. E. M. Johnson, T. Ueda, H. Maeno, and P. Greengard, J. Biol. Chem., 147, 1972, 5650-5652.
[25]. T. Ueda, H. Maeno, and P. Greengard, J. Biol. Chem., 248, 1973, 8295-8305.
[26]. J. W. Kebabian, G. L. Petzold, and P. Greengard, Proc. Nat. Acad. Sci. U.S.A., 69, 1972, 2145-2149.
[27]. H. Nyback, A. Brozecki, and G. Sedvall, Eur. J. Pharmacol., 4, 1968, 395-402.
[28]. R. J. Miller and L. L. Iversen, Naunyn-Schmiedeberg's Arch. Pharm., 282, 1974, 213-216.
[29]. Y. C. Clement-Cormier, J. W. Kebabian, G. L. Petzold, and P. Greengard, Proc. Nat. Acad. Sci. U.S.A., 71, 1974, 1113-1117.
[30]. R. J. Miller, A. S. Horn, and L. L. Iversen, Mol. Pharmacol., 10, 1974, 759-766.
[31]. M. Karobath and H. Leitich, Proc. Nat. Acad. Sci. U.S.A., 71, 1974, 2915-2918.
[32]. A. S. Horn, A. C. Cuello, and R. J. Miller, J. Neurochem., 22, 1974, 265-270.
[33]. E. De Robertis, R. De Lores Arnaiz, and M. Alberici, J. Biol. Chem., 242, 1967, 3487-3493.
[34]. Y. C. Clement-Cormier, R. G. Parrish, G. L. Petzold, J. W. Kebabian, and P. Greengard, J. Neurochem., 1975, in press.
[35]. R. K. Mishra, E. L. Gardner, R. Katzman, and M. H. Makman, Proc. Nat. Acad. Sci. U.S.A., 71, 1974, 3883-3887.
[36]. J. Forn, B. K. Krueger, and P. Greengard, Science, 1974, in press.

[37]. G. Herting, J. Axelrod, and L. G. Whitby, J. Pharmac. Exp. Ther., 134, 1961, 146-153.
[38]. E. Muscholl, Br. J. Pharmac. Chemother., 16, 1961, 352-359.
[39]. F. W. Studier, J. Mol. Biol., 79, 1973, 177-189.
[40]. G. Fairbanks, T. L. Steck, and D. F. H. Wallach, Biochem., 10, 1971, 2606-2616.
[41]. A. M. Malkinson, B. K. Krueger, S. A. Rudolph, J. E. Casnellie, B. Haley, and P. Greengard, Metabolism, 1975, in press.
[42]. J. P. Miller, K. H. Boswell, K. Muneyama, L. N. Simon, R. K. Robins, and D. A. Shuman, Biochemistry, 12, 1973, 5310-5318.
[43]. G. R. Siggins, B. J. Hoffer, and U. Ungerstedt, Life Sci., 15, 1974, 779-792.
[44]. F. E. Bloom, E. Costa, G. C. Salmoiraghi, J. Pharm. Exp. Ther., 150, 1965, 244-252.
[45]. J. D. Connor, J. Physiol., 208, 1970, 691-703.

DISCUSSION

Dr. Hess wondered if any inhibitors other than 3-isobutyl-1-methylxanthine had been tested. Dr. Greengard replied that none had been tried in the phosphorylation experiments.

Dr. Mandel asked about the phosphodiesterase inhibitors used in the adenyl cyclase experiments. Dr. Greengard suggested that this was not too critical, that theophylline or isomethylxanthine would be satisfactory. Dr. Mandel and Dr. Greengard then discussed experiments with minces and homogenates of brain tissue. Dr. Greengard pointed out that beta-adrenergic sensitivity is lost when tissue is homogenized, but Dr. Mandel felt that some recent results indicated this might not be so.

Dr. Langlais wondered if Dr. Greengard could correlate the response to dopamine (inhibition, excitation) of caudate cells to a particular type of cell. Dr. Greengard replied that the electrophysiological studies reported from Dr. Bloom's laboratory and the biochemical studies from his laboratory agreed with the concept proposed by Dr. Carlsson and others that dopamine inhibits the postsynaptic cell. Dr. Greengard was not certain which excitatory effects of dopamine Dr. Langlais was referring to. Dr. Langlais referred to some studies where dopamine was iontophoretically applied to different populations of cells; not all cells were inhibited, some were facilitated. Dr. Greengard pointed out that since the percentage of cells showing facilitation was very low, it would not be possible to show this in a study using homogenates. He then mentioned that there is a cyclic AMP system in adrenergic terminals. Work done by several investigators has shown that cyclic AMP activates tyrosine hydroxylase and this activation is mediated by bradykinin - indicating clearly that it is presynaptic.

Dr. Everett asked for information on the effects of amphetamine and methamphetamine in relation to cyclic AMP. Dr. Greengard replied that he, as well as Drs. Iversen and Shepherd, had found that amphetamine was absolutely ineffective in stimulating adenyl cyclase.

Dr. Weiner was interested in blocking in the caudate nucleus. Dr. Greengard said that he had not made a comparative study of alpha blockers on his two enzymes, but that the sensitivity of the caudate enzyme and the sensitivity of the ganglion enzyme are quite different with respect to antipsychotic drugs. He felt that it was quite advantageous to patients that the antipsychotic drugs have virtually no effect on the dopamine-sensitive adenyl cyclase of the ganglia.

MECHANISMS OF RECEPTOR MEDIATED REGULATION OF CATECHOLAMINE
SYNTHESIS IN BRAIN

Walter Lovenberg and Eleanor A. Bruckwick

Section on Biochemical Pharmacology
Hypertension-Endocrine Branch
National Heart and Lung Institute
National Institutes of Health
Bethesda, Maryland 20014

I. INTRODUCTION

Catecholamines serve as neurotransmitter substances in the brain, spinal cord, and peripheral sympathetic nervous system. In brain dopamine, norepinephrine and epinephrine are the specific transmitters for specific cell types. These cell types can be distinguished by their complement of aminergic biosynthetic enzymes. All of the aforementioned cell types contain tyrosine hydroxylase and aromatic L amino acid decarboxylase. Dopaminergic cells occur in many regions of the brain, although the corpus striatum contains an unusually high concentration of dopaminergic nerve endings. Noradrenergic cells are present in many brain regions and are distinguished by the presence of dopamine-β-hydroxylase but not phenylethanolamine N-methyltransferase. Localization of adrenergic cells which contain all four biosynthetic enzymes is less well defined. In each of the cell types the rate of synthesis of catecholamine is regulated by the initial biosynthetic enzyme, tyrosine hydroxylase. Transmitter synthesis is clearly coupled to neuronal activity, although it is not clear whether changes in synthesis lead to changes in neuronal activity. There currently appear to be 3 types of regulatory mechanisms that control the rate of tyrosine hydroxylation. As recently discussed by Costa et al. [1] tyrosine hydroxylase can be regulated on a long term basis by enzyme induction involving the synthesis of new enzyme molecules, and on a short term basis by either substrate and cofactor availability and end-product inhibition or enzyme modification. These latter two mechanisms appear to be related and will be the subject of the following brief review.

II. IN VIVO SYNTHETIC RATES AND SYNTHETIC CAPACITY

The rate of tyrosine hydroxylation in vivo has been estimated by several techniques, including synthesis inhibition [2], product formation following treatment with a decarboxylase inhibitor [3], and incorporation of radioactive precursors [4]. While these techniques do not yield identical quantitative results they yield somewhat similar values. Table 1 gives the regional activity of tyrosine hydroxylase measured in vitro under conditions that we assume to be nearly optimal for enzyme activity and gives a comparison with in vivo synthetic rates. Even allowing for errors in the various in vivo measuring techniques it is clear that at least in the rat striatum tyrosine hydroxylase is functioning at less than 5% its optimal rate. There are a number of factors which could account for the significant modulation of activity. These factors include:

1. substrate availability (tyrosine and oxygen)
2. cofactor availability

TABLE 1

Regional Distribution of Tyrosine Hydroxylase in Rat Brain (nmole/g/hr)*

Striatum	724	Mesencephalic Tectum	< 20
Septum	160	Mesencephalic Tegmentum	61
Hypothalamus	84	Pons Medulla	< 20
Forebrain	26	Spinal Cord	< 20

Estimated In Vivo Synthesis Rates of Catecholamines

Striatum	10-15 nmole/g/hr [16]
Brainstem	1-4 nmole/g/hr [4]

*These values were obtained from experiments done using a ^{3}H release assay [34]. Rat striata were homogenized in 0.2M sodium acetate, pH 6.0, containing 0.2% Triton X 100. The enzyme was assayed in the 40,000 x g supernatant fraction in reaction mixtures containing 0.1 mM tyrosine, 1 mM 6-methyltetrahydropterin, 0.1 mM ferrous ammonium sulfate, 10 mM 2-mercaptoethanol, and 0.2M sodium acetate. All reaction mixtures were adjusted to pH 6.0 before the start of the reaction. Total volume of the incubation was 0.1 ml.

3. end-product inhibition
4. natural occurring regulatory molecules
5. alternate molecular forms of the enzyme

It is clear that in order to fully understand this dramatic regulation of tyrosine hydroxylase in vivo an understanding of the molecular and regulatory properties of the isolated enzyme is needed.

III. MECHANISM AND KINETIC PROPERTIES OF BRAIN TYROSINE HYDROXYLASE

The majority of studies to date have been done using enzyme purified to varying extents from the striatal region because of the relatively high proportion of dopaminergic neurons in this region and consequently the high tyrosine hydroxylase activity. Although it has been shown that this enzyme is immunologically similar to the enzyme from adrenal glands [5], there appear to be distinct differences in its kinetic properties. The enzyme from brain like other aromatic amino acid hydroxylases [6] is a mixed function oxygenase requiring reduced pterin as an electron donor and molecular oxygen (Fig. 1). The affinity constants for the substrate have been determined and are compared in Table 2 with the constants measured for the bovine adrenal tyrosine hydroxylase. The affinity for tyrosine and oxygen are similar for the enzyme from these two sources; however, a significant difference in the K_m value for the reduced pterin cofactor exists. The reason for this difference is

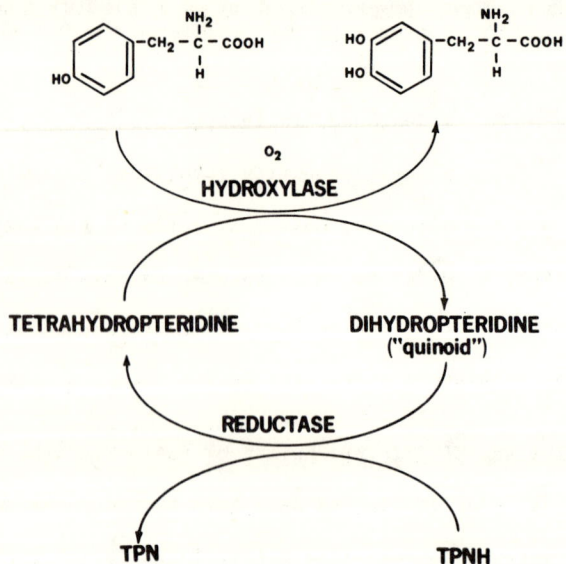

Fig. 1. Reaction mechanism of tyrosine hydroxylase.

TABLE 2

Comparison of Some Properties of Soluble Tyrosine Hydroxylase from Bovine Adrenal and Rat Brain*

	Central Nervous System	Adrenal Gland
Substrate K_m	0.07 mM	0.02 mM
Cofactor (6MPH$_4$) K_m	0.5 mM	0.06 mM
Oxygen K_m	2.5%	2.5%
Molecular Weight	150,000	150,000

*The substrate and cofactor values were taken from [10,22]. The molecular weight data is from [25,26].

not known, but since the enzymes are immunologically identical it would appear that a minor modification of one of the protein molecules has occurred and that this modification has altered the affinity of the enzyme for tetrahydrobiopterin. It should also be pointed out that the chemical identity of the cofactor in brain has not been resolved, although it is thought to be tetrahydrobiopterin. This compound has been positively identified as the natural cofactor for phenylalanine hydroxylase in liver [7].

IV. COFACTOR LEVELS

Several recent studies suggest the natural hydroxylase cofactor content in tissue may limit the rate of tyrosine hydroxylation. In adrenal tissue [8] the level of cofactor-like material is very low

(10 nmoles/g). Measurement of cofactor activity in brain tissue also indicates very low levels of cofactor in whole brain [9]. Kettler et al. [10] have recently estimated the rat striatum contains about 29 nmoles tetrahydrobiopterin equivalents per gram of tissue. Preliminary experiments in our laboratory using a hydrogen-platinum oxide reduction step to convert all the cofactor to the tetrahydro form have yielded similar results. If we arbitrarily assume that about 25% of the striatal tissue is aminergic and that the cofactor is limited to these cells then the cofactor concentration at the site of tyrosine hydroxylation could be as high as 10^{-4}M. This concentration is substantially below the apparent K_m of striatal tyrosine hydroxylase. The recent study of Kettler et al. [10] shows that following an intraventricular injection of tetrahydrobiopterin a four-fold increase occurs in the cofactor content of the striatum with a concomitant 2.5-fold increase in the rate of tyrosine hydroxylation. These results are entirely consistent with the above estimation of cofactor concentration in the dopaminergic neuron. If one then follows the same line of reasoning the dopamine concentration would be 0.2 mM and would cause 90 to 95% inhibition of tyrosine hydroxylase activity. As indicated in the discussion above the actual *in vivo* rate of hydroxylation appears to be less than 5% of the total potential of the tyrosine hydroxylase present in the cell. The relatively low activity in the striatum under control conditions can therefore be easily rationalized on the basis of classical kinetics, and cofactor and end-product concentration.

The in vivo rate of hydroxylation should therefore be very sensitive in an inverse manner to changes in the dopamine content of the tissue. Recently several experimental conditions have been reported in which both the dopamine content and rate of hydroxylation have increased simultaneously in the striatum suggesting that factors other than end-product inhibition are participating in the regulatory process.

V. EFFECT OF DOPAMINE AGONISTS AND ANTAGONISTS ON DOPAMINE TURNOVER

Following the original observations [11] that chloropromazine and haloperidol increase dopamine turnover in brain, many workers have observed that in general compounds which block dopamine receptors cause increases in dopamine turnover whereas receptor agonist such as apomorphine cause a significant decrease in dopamine turnover. Whether these effects were direct effects on nerve terminals or mediated through changes in impulse flow has yet to be resolved. It is clear that based on electrophysiologic studies [12,13,14] that peripheral administration of dopamine agonists decrease and dopamine antagonists increase dopaminergic cell activity in the substantia nigra. It is therefore possible that increased impulse frequency arriving at the terminal regions have a direct effect on the catecholamine biosynthetic machinery [14,15]. Recent evidence also suggests that presynaptic receptors are activated either by the released dopamine or a substance liberated from post-synaptic neuron after successful receptor activation by the neurotransmitter. Activation of the presynaptic receptor then results in an inhibition of the catecholamine synthetic machinery.

This mechanism is speculative but there are several lines of experimentation that support the presynaptic receptor mechanism. Walters and Roth [15] find that lesioning the nigro-striatal pathway or pharmacologically inhibiting impulse flow in this pathway results in an increase in dopamine synthesis which is blocked by prior administration of dopamine agonists.

VI. RECEPTOR MEDIATED FEEDBACK INHIBITION

Carlsson and his colleagues [14,16] have used the term receptor mediated feedback to describe the aforementioned phenomenon in the regulation of striatal tyrosine hydroxylase. The distinguishing feature of Carlsson's term is that it implies that either pre or postsynaptic dopamine receptor must be activated in order to get an inhibitory response. In these experiments it was shown that dopamine synthesis in the striatum is markedly enhanced after sectioning of the nigro-striatal pathway in spite of increased dopamine content of the nerve endings. It therefore seemed that tyrosine hydroxylase was released from its feedback inhibition when dopamine receptors were not activated just as it did when the receptors were blocked with neuroleptic compounds. In the same series of experiments it was shown that the apparent release from feedback inhibition could be largely prevented by treatment with apomorphine suggesting that it was lack of receptor stimulation that released the nerve terminals from feedback inhibition. Recently several advances in the understanding of biochemical events in synaptic transmission have permitted us to refine our concepts of how catecholamine synthesis is regulated in striatal nerve endings.

VII. NEUROTRANSMITTER SENSITIVE ADENYLATE CYCLASES

This subject is dealt with in depth elsewhere in this symposium and will only be summarized here. Basically tissues such as the striatum which contain a relatively large number of dopamine receptors have contained a dopamine sensitive adenylate cyclase. This enzyme has the properties of the dopamine receptor. Cyclic AMP production from ATP is dependent upon the presence of dopamine or other receptor agonist [17,18]. Conversely it has been observed that drugs thought to be dopamine receptor blockers are strong inhibitors of this dopamine sensitive adenylate cyclase [19-21]. The inhibitory efficacy of these compounds also appears to relate to their antipsychotic activity and as such represents one of the most interesting and important findings in molecular pharmacology. It also suggests that this adenylate cyclase may be the "dopamine receptor". This enzyme may therefore have a role in the molecular events that occur during receptor mediated feedback inhibition.

VIII. EFFECTS OF NEUROLEPTICS ON THE KINETIC PROPERTIES OF TYROSINE HYDROXYLASE

Several reports [1,22,23] have recently shown that when animals are treated with dopamine receptor blockers, there is a dramatic reduction in the affinity (K_m) of striatal tyrosine hydroxylase for the pterin cofactor. In these studies the <u>in vitro</u> enzyme activity had changed suggesting that the enzyme has been transformed by the drug from less active to a more active form. This type of transformation also appears to occur following administration of the anesthetic γ-hydroxybutyrate [24]. In both above experimental conditions and in the lesioning experiments of Carlsson et al. [16] the inability of dopamine to react with either the pre or post-synaptic dopamine receptor appears to cause a paradoxical increase in tyrosine hydroxylation which can in turn be blocked by a dopamine receptor agonist. The conversion of tyrosine hydroxylase from a form having high K_m for its cofactor to a form having a low K_m would in turn make the enzyme less sensitive to the competitive feedback inhibition by dopamine. If such a mechanism was operative in vivo then the paradoxical increase in catecholamine synthesis in the presence of elevated catecholamines could be explained.

If this line of reasoning is carried one step further it can be conjectured that since the dopamine receptor is an adenylate cyclase and is required for the interconversion of the forms of tyrosine hydroxylase then the formation of cyclic AMP participates in this conversion. Since all of the molecular mechanisms of the action of cAMP as a second messenger have been shown to be mediated by cyclic nucleotide dependent protein kinases, it is therefore necessary to determine whether a protein phosphorylation participates in the tyrosine hydroxylase interconversion.

IX. ATTEMPTS TO DEFINE MOLECULAR EVENTS THAT OCCUR DURING THE TRANSFORMATION OF TYROSINE HYDROXYLASE

The study of tyrosine hydroxylase from the central nervous system has been complicated by the variety of analytical and preparative procedures used by the various investigators. Tyrosine hydroxylase is thought to be a cytoplasmic enzyme although it has a tendency to aggregate or become associated with synaptosomes in nerve ending rich areas of the brain [25]. The enzyme also appears to exist in different molecular weight forms [26]. Kuczenski and Mandell [27] have shown that the kinetic properties of brain tyrosine hydroxylase change when the enzyme is aggregated or associated with membranes. This change appears to be analogous to the change observed when animals are treated with dopamine receptor blocking agents. Furthermore, it has recently been shown that heparin sulfate [27] and phosphatidyl serine [28] mimic these effects; i.e., a reduction in the K_m of the enzyme for its reduced cofactor and a concomitant decrease in the sensitivity to feedback inhibition by dopamine.

We have recently attempted to correlate the known regulatory and kinetic properties of brain tyrosine hydroxylase with the in vivo models of receptor mediated feedback inhibition. Figure 2 demonstrates the neuroleptic (haloperidol) effect on striatal tyrosine hydroxylase reported previously by Costa and coworkers [1,22,23]. In addition, we see that while rapid chromatography of each enzyme on Sephadex G-25 causes an activation, it is apparent that whatever neuroleptic treatment did to tyrosine hydroxylase was retained after this protein solution was separated from the small molecular species. A parallel line of experimentation was also done using rapid ammonium sulfate precipitation as a means to separate tyrosine hydroxylase from the ionic constituents of the cytoplasm. In this case, however, we found that the enzyme from both the control and haloperidol treated animals were activated or had similar reduction in tetrahydropterin K_m values (Fig. 3). In subsequent studies it was found that addition of 10% saturated ammonium sulfate

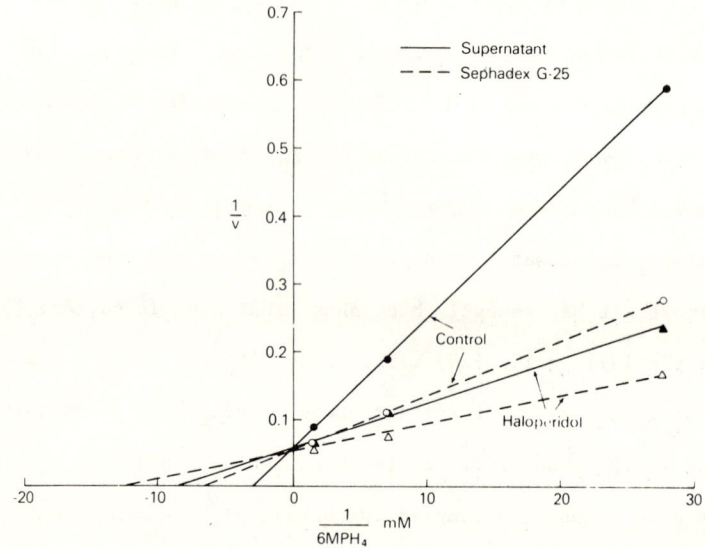

Fig. 2. Cofactor affinity following gel filtration of the tyrosine hydroxylase from control and haloperidol treated animals. Male Sprague-Dawley rats were treated with haloperidol (2 mg/kg) or saline 1 hour before sacrifice. The enzyme was assayed in duplicate by the procedure described in Table 1 and the data in this figure are representative of a number of similar experiments. The Sephadex chromatography was done on a 0.5 x 12 cm column of coarse G-25. The whole gel filtration procedure required about 5 minutes for each enzyme preparation.

to the tyrosine hydroxylase incubation mixture resulted in an effect very similar to that seen either with heparin sulfate [27] or phosphatidyl serine [28]; i.e., a marked activation of tyrosine hydroxylase at limiting cofactor concentration. Kuczenski and Mandell [29] have previously reported a stimulatory effect of ammonium sulfate, although their studies did not indicate an effect on the cofactor affinity.

Since the haloperidol effect appeared to be a molecular alteration of tyrosine hydroxylase, it was of interest to determine

CATECHOLAMINE SYNTHESIS REGULATION 161

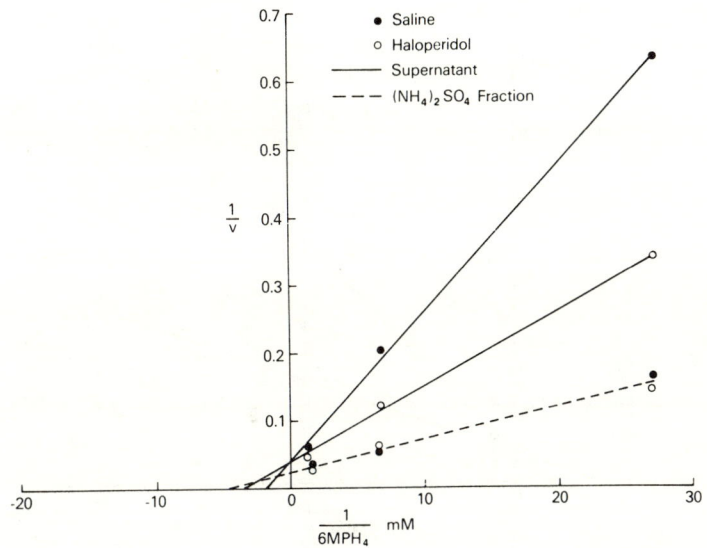

Fig. 3. The effect of ammonium sulfate precipitation on the cofactor affinity of striatal tyrosine hydroxylase from control and haloperidol treated rats. Aliquots of the respective supernatant fractions were mixed with an equal volume of saturated ammonium sulfate, centrifuged rapidly in a microfuge and resuspended in the original volume 0.2 M sodium acetate, pH 6.0.

whether tyrosine hydroxylase could be a substrate for a cAMP dependent protein kinase and whether phosphorylation or dephosphorylation could alter the kinetic properties of the enzyme. A 40,000 x g supernatant fraction was prepared from control rat striata and cAMP, ATP and other compounds necessary for optimal protein phosphorylation [30] were included in the standard tyrosine hydroxylase assay mixture. No exogenous cAMP dependent protein kinase was added since the brain is a rich source of this enzyme. The results of this experiment are shown in Figure 4. Clearly phosphorylating conditions cause the kinetic properties of the

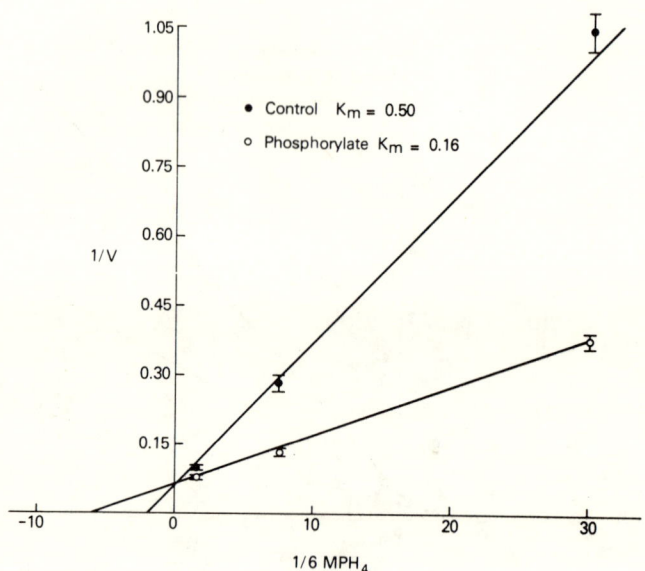

Fig. 4. The effect of phosphorylating conditions on the affinity of tyrosine hydroxylase for 6-methyltetrahydropterin. Experiments were done as described in Table 3.

enzyme to become similar to the enzyme isolated from haloperidol treated rats [22] or the control enzyme in the presence of either phosphatidyl serine [28] or heparin sulfate [27]. While ATP, cAMP, and Mg^{++} are with little effect on the <u>in vitro</u> assay in our system, there is a substantial dependency upon ATP, cAMP, and Mg^{++} for the effect on tyrosine hydroxylase (Table 3). This would suggest that the effect was being mediated by a protein phosphorylation, although actual phosphorylation of tyrosine hydroxylase cannot be inferred from the above experiments. We are currently pursuing other lines of experimentation to determine whether tyrosine hydroxylase is a substrate for cAMP dependent protein kinase and whether the putative

TABLE 3

Effect of Phosphorylating Conditions on Kinetic Properties of Tyrosine Hydroxylase

	Tyrosine Hydroxylase (nmole/hr/mg)	Apparent K_m for $6MPH_4$ (mM)
Control	0.93 ± 0.05	.50
Complete	2.60 ± 0.13	.16
" - ATP	0.89 ± 0.03	.57
" - cAMP	1.54 ± 0.02	.31
" - Mg^{++}	1.94 ± 0.01	.26

The enzyme was assayed in the supernanant fraction as described in Table 1 with an incubation volume of 0.15 ml. In addition to standard reaction ingredients in the complete system contained 0.5 mM ATP, 0.1 mM cAMP, 0.8 mM theophylline, 20 mM NaF, 0.12 mM EGTA, and 20 mM magnesium acetate.

phosphorylated form of the enzyme is the high cofactor affinity form seen after treatment with haloperidol.

It is interesting to note that Harris et al. [31] recently reported that dibutyryl cAMP stimulates tyrosine hydroxylation in synaptosomal preparations. These workers also reported that the addition of cAMP to soluble striatal tyrosine hydroxylase causes a shift in the kinetic properties to the more active form. We have not observed stimulation of soluble tyrosine hydroxylase by cAMP alone and in fact under our analytical conditions we find that cAMP is a weak competitive inhibitor with respect to the cofactor.

The reason for these differing results is not apparent although it probably resides in the somewhat different analytical techniques used in the two laboratories.

X. CONCLUDING REMARKS

From the studies recently reported in the literature and those presented here today there are emerging clues for the detailed mechanism of acute regulation of tyrosine hydroxylase. It has been about a decade since Nagatsu et al. [31] proposed a simple feedback inhibition of the enzyme by catecholamines in vivo. Recently the role of this end-product inhibition has been questioned by workers [11,24] who observed that in certain experimental situations one could observe both an increase in tissue catecholamine content and in the rate of tyrosine hydroxylation. This apparent paradox can now be explained by the observations that tyrosine hydroxylase can exist in at least two kinetic forms. The conversion of the form with high K_m for the cofactor to the low K_m form results in a marked decrease in the sensitivity of the enzyme to feedback inhibition.

The exact nature of these two forms of the enzyme remain to be determined. The fact that the interconversion of these two forms could be stimulated by dopamine receptor agonists and antagonists in vivo [22] and that these agents were also active as activators and inhibitors of dopamine sensitive adenylate cyclase suggested a role for cAMP in the interconversion. Furthermore, logic would suggest that if cAMP mediated its effect via protein kinase and subsequent phosphorylation of tyrosine hydroxylase then the phosphorylated form of the enzyme would be the less active.

The results of our experiments to date show the exact opposite; i.e., phosphorylation of tyrosine hydroxylase produces a more active species. This new finding of a molecular mechanism for the interconversion of the two forms of tyrosine hydroxylase may be very important to our understanding of neurotransmitter regulation in the central nervous system. However, one now has to invoke a more complex rationalization for the receptor mediated feedback inhibition.

It would thus appear that conditions of initial dopamine increase within the nerve ending (nigro striatal ligation [11] or γ-hydroxybutyrate treatment [24]) cause an initial increase in the rate of hydroxylation followed by a new level of feedback inhibition. Although more difficult to explain the receptor antagonist activation of tyrosine hydroxylase might be due to an increased amount of free dopamine activating a presynaptic receptor that was less sensitive than postsynaptic receptors to the antagonists. This line of reasoning however makes it difficult to explain the effects of the dopamine receptor agonist apomorphine.

Another approach that could be used is that levels of cAMP are regulated by the activity of phosphodiesterase. Weiss [32] has shown that multiple forms of phosphodiesterase exist in brain and that certain of these forms are activated by catecholamines. Thus, conditions which stimulate phosphodiesterase would tend to shift tyrosine hydroxylase into a less active form, whereas decreases in catabolism of cAMP would tend to activate tyrosine hydroxylase.

The above suggestions are highly speculative at this time. It is probable, however, that catecholamine synthesis is regulated by the interconversion of two forms of tyrosine hydroxylase, and that this interconversion probably involves a phosphorylation of a protein.

REFERENCES

[1]. E. Costa, A. Guidotti, and B. Zivkovic, Adv. Biochem. Psychopharm., 12, 1974, 161-175.

[2]. B. B. Brodie, E. Costa, A. Dlabac, N. H. Neff, and H. H. Smookler, J. Pharm. Exp. Ther., 154, 1966, 493-498.

[3]. A. Carlsson, J. N. Davis, W. Kehr, M. Lindqvist, and C. V. Atack, Naunyn-Schmiedeberg's Arch. Pharm., 275, 1972, 153-168.

[4]. H. Yamabe, W. de Jong, and W. Lovenberg, Eur. J. Pharm., 22, 1973, 91-98.

[5]. T. Lloyd and S. Kaufman, Mol. Pharm., 9, 1973, 438-444.

[6]. W. Lovenberg and S. J. Victor, Life Sci., 14, 1974, 2337-2353.

[7]. S. Kaufman, Oxygenase (O. Hayaishi, Ed.), New York, Academic Press, 1962, pp 129-180.

[8]. T. Lloyd and N. Weiner, Mol. Pharm., 7, 1971, 569-580.

[9]. G. Guroff, C. A. Rhoads, and A. Abramowitz, Anal. Biochem., 21, 1967, 273-278.

[10]. R. Kettler, G. Bartholini, and A. Pletscher, Nature, 249, 1974, 476-478.

[11]. A. Carlsson and M. Lindqvist, Acta Pharm. Toxicol., 20, 1963, 140-144.

[12]. B. S. Bunney, J. R. Walters, R. H. Roth, and G. K. Aghajanian, J. Pharm. Exp. Ther., 185, 1973, 560-571.

[13]. G. K. Aghajanian and B. S. Bunney (E. Usdin and S. H. Snyder, Eds.), Frontiers in Catecholamine Research, London, Pergamon Press, 1973, pp 643-648.

[14]. W. Kehr, A. Carlsson, M. Lindqvist, T. Magnusson, and C. Atack, J. Pharm. Pharmacol., 24, 1972, 744-747.

[15]. J. R. Walters and R. H. Roth, J. Pharm. Exp. Ther., 191, 1974, 82-91.

[16]. A. Carlsson, W. Kehr, and M. Lindqvist, Adv. Biochem. Psychopharm., 12, 1974, 135-142.

[17]. J. W. Kebabian, G. L. Petzold, and P. Greengard, Proc. Nat. Acad. Sci. USA, 69, 1972, 2145-2149.

[18]. J. W. Kebabian and P. Greengard, Science, 174, 1971, 1346-1349.

[19]. Y. C. Clement-Cormier, J. W. Kebabian, G. L. Petzold, and P. Greengard, Proc. Nat. Acad. Sci. USA, 71, 1974, 1113-1117.

[20]. M. Karobath and H. Leitich, Proc. Nat. Acad. Sci. USA, 71, 1974, 2915-2918.

[21]. R. J. Miller, A. S. Horn, and L. L. Iversen, Mol. Pharm., 10, 1974, 759-766.

[22]. B. Zivkovic, A. Guidotti, and E. Costa, Mol. Pharm., 10, 1974, 727-735.

[23]. B. Zivkovic and A. Guidotti, Brain Res., 79, 1974, 505-509.

[24]. R. H. Roth, J. R. Walters, and V. H. Morgenroth, Adv. Biochem. Psychopharm. 12, 1974, 369-384.

[25]. J. M. Musacchio, C. A. McQueen, G. L. Craviso (A. J. Mandell, Ed.), New Concepts of Neurotransmitter Regulation, New York, Plenum Press, 1973, pp 69-88.

[26]. T. H. Joh and D. J. Reis, Fed. Proc., 33, 1974, 535.

[27]. R. T. Kuczenski and A. J. Mandell, J. Biol. Chem., 247, 1972, 3114-3122.

[28]. T. Lloyd and S. Kaufman, Biochem. Biophys. Res. Commun., 59, 1974, 1262-1269.

[29]. R. T. Kuczenski and A. J. Mandell, J. Neurochem., 19, 1972, 131-137.

[30]. J. F. Kuo and P. Greengard, Proc. Nat. Acad. Sci. USA, 64, 1969, 1349-1355.

[31]. J. E. Harris, V. H. Morgenroth, R. H. Roth, and R. J. Baldessarini, Nature, 252, 1974, 156-158.

[32]. T. Nagatsu, M. Levitt, and S. Udenfriend, J. Biol. Chem., 239, 1964, 2910-2917.

[33]. B. Weiss (E. Usdin and S. Snyder, Eds.), Frontiers in Catecholamine Research, London, Pergamon Press, 1973, pp 327-333.

[34]. T. J. Cicero, L. G. Sharpe, E. Robins, and S. S. Grote, J. Neurochem., 19, 1972, 2241-2243.

DISCUSSION

Dr. Weiner asked about the purity of the tyrosine hydroxylase. Dr. Lovenberg replied that he was not using a pure enzyme but rather a crude high-speed super-natant fraction, although his laboratory is currently doing some studies with immunoprecipitation. He has observed that phosphorylation does not appreciably change the molecular weight of the enzyme.

Dr. Schanberg wondered if allopurinol had been added to the mixture in any studies but Dr. Lovenberg said this had not been done.

Dr. Iversen inquired whether Dr. Lovenberg had considered the possibility that dopamine inhibited the adenyl cyclase. Dr. Lovenberg replied that he had thought of the inverse - that dopamine stimulated phosphodiesterase; this was based on the fact that Weiss had shown a catecholamine-dependent phosphodiesterase. Dr. Lovenberg thought that Dr. Greengard's observations on the rapidity of dephosphorylation and on the role of cyclic AMP in the action of protein phosphatase were quite important.

Dr. Roth stated that he felt that the enzyme itself probably is not phosphorylated since he can take the preparations obtained from stimulated neostriatum and add them to non-stimulated neostriatum and get a very marked (much more than additive) potentiation of tyrosine hydroxylase activity. Dr. Lovenberg agreed that he had no evidence that the enzyme was phosphorylated.

Dr. Costa was interested in the relationship between protein kinase and Dr. Lovenberg's studies. Dr. Lovenberg mentioned that while in control animals there was a 50% to 70% dependency on cyclic AMP, in haloperidol-treated animals there was just about a 100% dependence for further activation, suggesting that perhaps cyclic AMP levels are lower or that protein kinase is less activated in the haloperidol-treated animals.

BEHAVIOURAL SEQUELAE OF DOPAMINERGIC DEGENERATION:
POSTSYNAPTIC SUPERSENSITIVITY ?

Ian Creese and Susan D. Iversen

Department of Pharmacology and Experimental Therapeutics
Johns Hopkins School of Medicine
Baltimore, Maryland
and
The Psychological Laboratory
University of Cambridge, England

The fluorescent histochemical delineation of the dopamine containing nigro-striatal pathway [1,2] has provided a model neuronal system for the study of the behavioural, pharmacological and electrophysiological properties of this central catecholamine neurotransmitter. Cell bodies in the pars compacta of the substantia nigra give rise to axons which run rostrally close to and within the classical medial forebrain bundle and innervate the caudate nucleus of the striatum (Figure 1). This uncrossed pathway contains the majority of the forebrain dopamine.

Selective lesions to this pathway can be made by the local, stereotaxic microinjection of 6-hydroxydopamine into either the substantia nigra or the caudate nucleus [2-4]. The success of the lesion can be assessed by the pharmacological assay of the remaining dopamine. 6-Hydroxydopamine is a chemical analogue of dopamine and is concentrated in catecholamine neurones by the selective catecholamine reuptake pump. The high concentration of this neurotoxic agent achieved inside dopamine and noradrenaline neurones leads to their degeneration, while non-aminergic neurones which do not concentrate 6-hydroxydopamine remain undamaged [4-7]. More widespread lesion to the central catecholamine neuronal systems can be made by the intraventricular injection of 6-hydroxydopamine which produces substantial depletions of both forebrain dopamine and noradrenaline [4,8].

The most noteworthy result of early experiments with intraventricular injections of 6-hydroxydopamine was the relatively minor changes in the behaviour of such lesioned rats, although they had a more than 50% depletion of their forebrain catecholamines [9-11]. This indicated that the catecholamine neurotransmitters

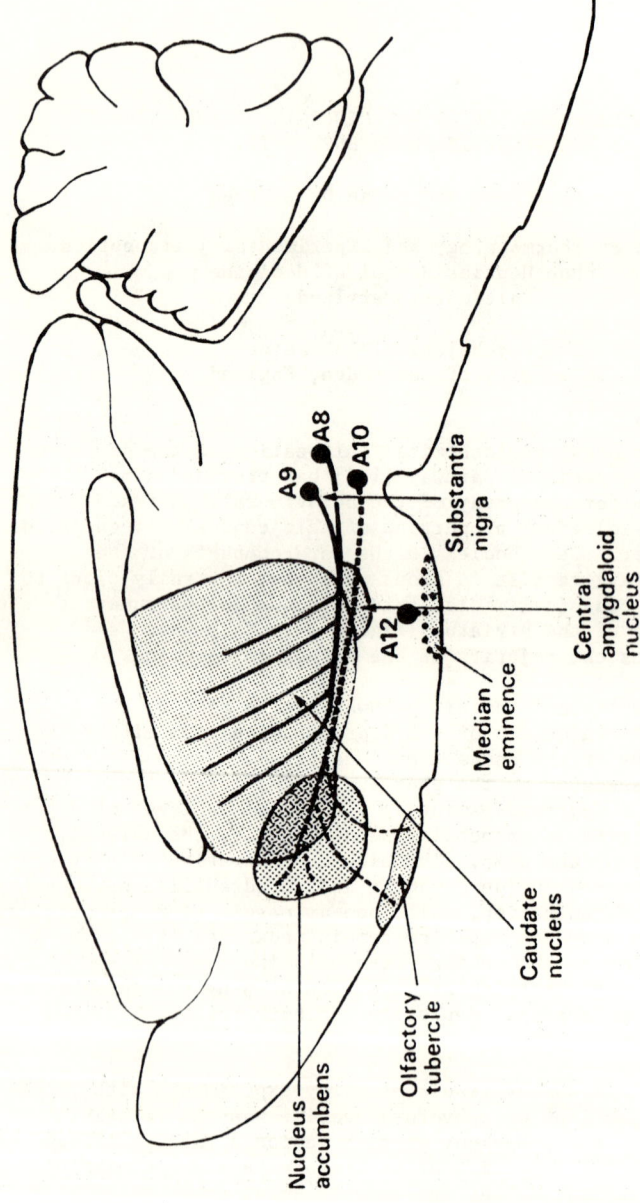

Fig. 1. Diagramatic representation of the major ascending dopamine pathways. The stippled areas indicate the projection regions. Modified from Ungerstedt [2].

were (i) little involved in the generation of overt behaviour, (ii) that the catecholamine neuronal systems contained massive redundancy in both quantity and function, or (iii) that a great deal of functional compensation could occur within the remaining catecholamine neurones or in other neuronal systems.

We investigated this problem by focusing our research on changes in the behavioural effects of drugs, which are known to influence catecholamine function, in rats following the bilateral lesion of the nigro-striatal dopamine system with 6-hydroxydopamine [12-16].

Amphetamine is a presynaptically acting sympathomimetic drug and when administered systemically in low doses (1.5mg/kg d-amphetamine sulphate) increases spontaneous locomotor activity in the rat. However, with increasing dose levels (5mg/kg) amphetamine induces stereotyped motor responses such as repetitive sniffing or gnawing. These behaviours are easily quantifiable: locomotor activity, automatically, by means of recording photocell beam interruptions, and stereotypy, observationally, by means of a rating scale. The stereotypy rating scale was developed from observations of the behaviour of normal rats exposed to increasing doses of amphetamine.

Stereotypy Rating Scale

Score	Behaviour
0	Asleep or stationary.
1	Active.
2	Predominantly active, but with bursts of stereotyped sniffing or rearing.
3	Stereotyped activity, such as sniffing along a fixed path in the cage.
4	Stereotyped sniffing or rearing, maintained in one location.
5	Stereotyped behaviour in one location with bursts of gnawing or licking.
6	Continual gnawing or licking.

6-Hydroxydopamine lesions to the nigro-striatal pathway either at the level of the substantia nigra [12] or the caudate nucleus [15], which result in the depletion of 85-90% striatal dopamine, completely abolished the stereotypy response to a high dose of amphetamine (Figure 2). Instead, the rats showed constant locomotor activity. The locomotor response to a low dose of amphetamine was enhanced over the first hour in the substantia nigra lesioned rats (Figure 3). However, a more complete lesion to the substantia nigra resulting in the almost total depletion (over 99%) of striatal dopamine abolished both the stereotypy and the locomotor responses to amphetamine [14]. A similar block of the amphetamine responses was obtained when such massive dopamine depletions were produced by

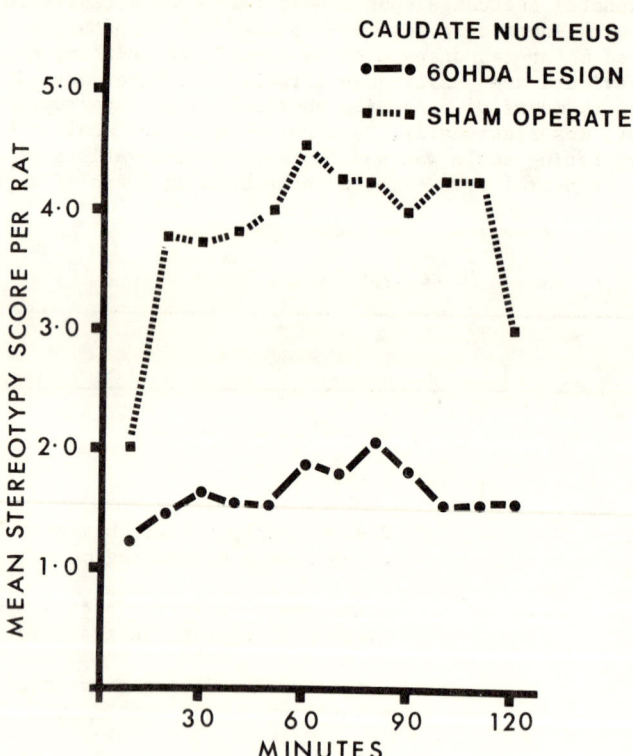

Fig. 2. Stereotypy response to 5 mg/kg d-amphetamine sulphate for bilateral caudate 6-hydroxydopamine (8 µg free base in 2 µl) lesioned rats and sham operates. The stereotypy response was rated every 10 min after drug injection. The sham operate group showed vigorous stereotypy throughout the session while the caudate lesioned rats (90% striatal dopamine depletion) maintained constant activity with no stereotypy.

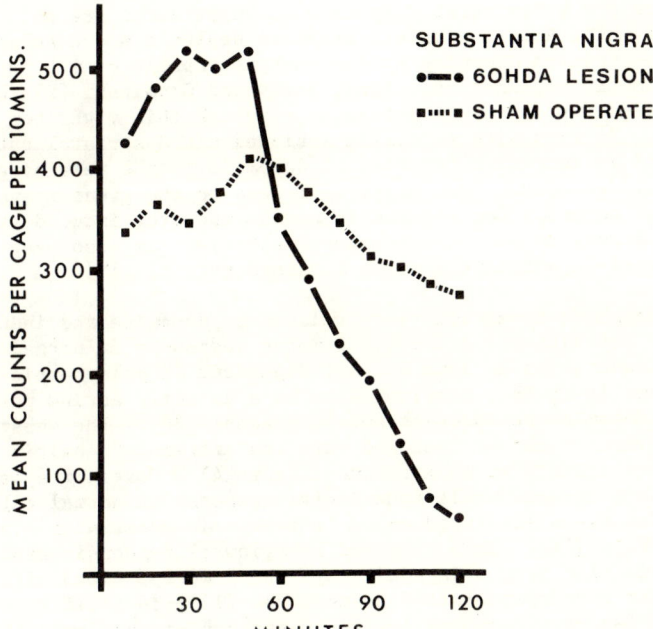

Fig. 3. Mean activity response to 1.5 mg/kg d-amphetamine sulphate for bilateral substantia nigra 6-hydroxydopamine (8 μ g free base in 2 μ l) lesioned rats and sham operates. The drug response was measured on days four, eleven and nineteen post-operation and did not change significantly over this period. Mean photocell beam interruptions/10 min were recorded after drug injection. The substantia nigra lesioned rats (85-90% striatal tyrosine hydroxylase depletion) showed enhanced locomotor activity over the first hour compared to the sham operate controls. Tyrosine hydroxylase is localized in catecholamine neurones and is used as an index of dopamine neurone destruction.

the treatment of neonate rats with intraventricular 6-hydroxydopamine. These rats were then tested, as adults, with amphetamine [13].

All these 6-hydroxydopamine lesions resulted in forebrain noradrenaline depletions as well as massive dopamine depletions. In view of this, control 6-hydroxydopamine lesions of the dorsal or ventral noradrenaline pathways were made in adult rats which achieved a similar spectrum of noradrenaline loss without affecting striatal dopamine levels. Such rats showed no change in their amphetamine responses [14]. These results indicated that the nigro-striatal dopamine pathway is, in fact, intimately involved in the production of the behavioural effects of amphetamine.

Since the behavioural responses to amphetamine are not abolished until almost complete dopamine depletions are achieved, the nigro-striatal dopamine system must be capable of a high degree of functional compensation. Agid, Javoy and Glowinski [17] have demonstrated a presynaptic mechanism by which this might be achieved. In rats with partially lesioned nigro-striatal pathways they found an increased turnover of dopamine in the remaining functional neurones. This might well lead to the greater availability of dopamine for release in normal and drug-induced states. However, a postsynaptic compensatory mechanism has also been demonstrated in substantia nigra lesioned rats [14,18].

Apomorphine is structurally related to dopamine and induces locomotor activity and stereotyped motor responses in normal rats [19]. However, its actions are not dependent on presynaptic dopamine release and it is thus considered to be a directly acting postsynaptic dopamine receptor stimulating agent [20]. The substantia nigra 6-hydroxydopamine lesioned rats are extremely sensitive to the stimulatory effects of apomorphine (Figure 4). Doses of apomorphine which elicit no observable behavioural response in normal rats give rise to intense stereotyped motor behaviour in substantia nigra lesioned rats [14]. This enhanced behavioural responsiveness to apomorphine also occurs in adult rats which were treated with intraventricular 6-hydroxydopamine as neonates [13], in adult rats following 6-hydroxydopamine lesion to the caudate nucleus [15], rats with unilateral substantia nigra lesions - which show vigorous contralateral rotation [18] and adult rats treated with intraventricular 6-hydroxydopamine [21].

Such enhanced behavioural supersensitivity is also seen to other dopamine agonists such as L-DOPA [18,22] and piribedil or its catechol metabolite S584 [16]. Rats with almost total striatal dopamine depletions respond to low doses of L-DOPA with increased locomotor activity and stereotypy (Figure 5). Their threshold for these behavioural effects is 10-25 mg/kg L-DOPA without a peripheral decarboxylase inhibitor. Control rats show very little stimulant effects of L-DOPA alone, even at massive 1 g/kg dose levels. With a peripheral decarboxylase inhibitor control rats do show an increase in locomotor activity and some stereotypy with L-DOPA 100-200 mg/kg. However, the 6-hydroxydopamine lesioned rats have a threshold of less than 1 mg/kg L-DOPA and show a vigorous, normal stereotypy response at 5-10 mg/kg L-DOPA (Figure 6). Higher doses of L-DOPA lead to a bizarre form of stereotyped gnawing, where the rat will actually gnaw off its own paws or bite into its abdomen.

L-DOPA does not appear to stimulate dopamine receptors directly as Ungerstedt [18] showed that high doses of peripheral decarboxylase inhibitor, which inhibit central decarboxylase activity as well, delay the onset of L-DOPA's behavioural effects. We have also confirmed this finding. Decarboxylase activity still exists in the striatum of these lesioned rats and L-DOPA is, in all probability, converted to dopamine in serotonin neurones or in the walls of cerebral blood vessels where DOPA-decarboxylase is present.

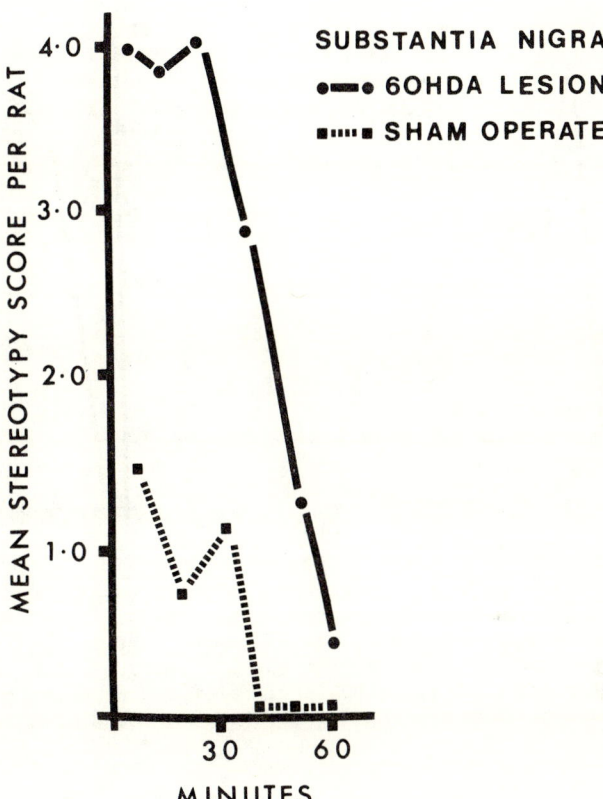

Fig. 4. Stereotypy response to 0.5 mg/kg apomorphine for bilateral substantia nigra 6-hydroxydopamine lesioned rats and sham operates twelve days post-operation. The substantia nigra lesioned rats (over 99% striatal tyrosine hydroxylase depletion) showed enhanced stereotyped behaviour compared to the sham operate controls.

Biochemical [23,24] and behavioural [25,26] evidence indicates that piribedil (ET495) may have a potential use in the treatment of Parkinson's disease through its interaction with the nigro-striatal dopamine pathway. However, the addition of piribedil to homogenates of rat striatum incubated with ATP did not evoke the increase in the rate of cyclic AMP production which followed the addition of dopamine [27,28]. This system may reflect drug interactions with dopamine receptors [29,30] - vide infra. However, the addition of S584, a catechol metabolite of piribedil, was effective in stimulating cyclic AMP production [27,28]. This suggested that the dopaminergic effects of piribedil may be mediated through its active metabolite S584. We have shown [16] that piribedil is capable of

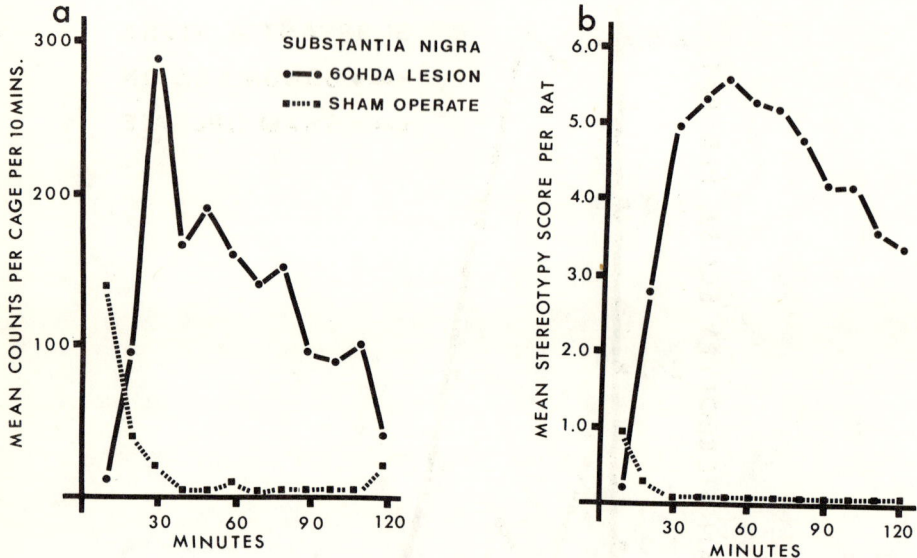

Fig. 5. a: Activity response, mean photocell beam interruptions/ 10 min and b: Stereotypy response, to 5 mg/kg L-DOPA (+ RO4-4602 50 mg/kg 30 min previously) for bilateral substantia nigra 6-hydroxydopamine lesioned rats and sham operate controls. The substantia nigra lesioned rats (over 99% striatal tyrosine hydroxylase depletion) showed a significantly enhanced response on both measures.

inducing enhanced stereotyped behaviour and locomotor activity in the rats which were treated with intraventricular 6-hydroxydopamine as neonates, when compared to their vehicle injected controls (Figure 7). As the presynaptic dopamine terminals have been destroyed, it would thus appear that the mode of action of piribedil is postsynaptic in origin. The fact that S584 also induced enhanced stereotypy and locomotor activity in these rats indicates that this catechol metabolite of piribedil is behaviourally as well as pharmacologically active and supports the hypothesis that the dopaminergic action of piribedil may be mediated via this active metabolite.

In the peripheral nervous system denervation of adrenergically innervated tissues gives rise to an increase in sensitivity of the tissues to the application of exogenous agonists [31]. Trendelenburg [32,33] has elegantly demonstrated that such degeneration supersensitivity is the result of two separate mechanisms, one pre- and the other post-synaptic. The pre-synaptic phase develops rapidly and is associated with the loss of amine uptake sites consequent on the degenerating adrenergic terminals. Thus the application of exogenous noradrenaline in the denervated tissue results in much higher functional levels of noradrenaline at the receptor sites, producing

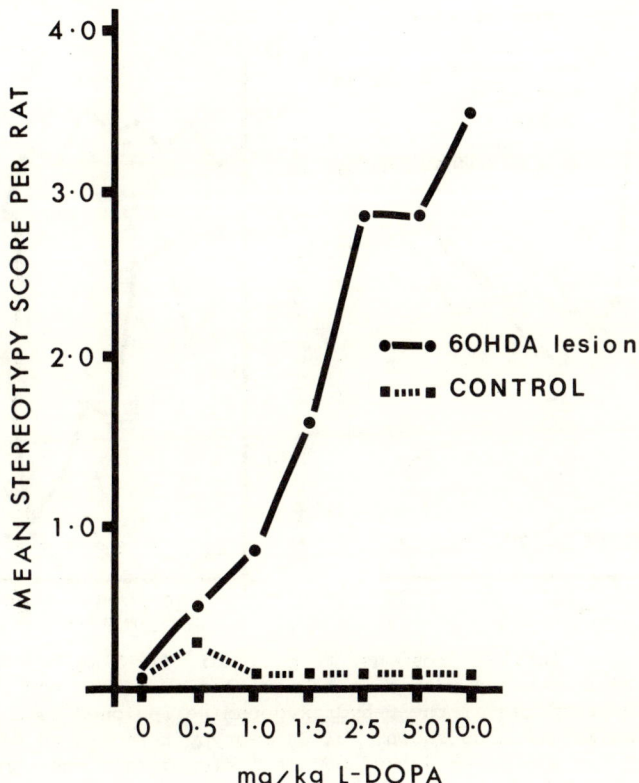

Fig. 6. Mean stereotypy response to increasing doses of L-DOPA (+ RO4-4602 50 mg/kg 30 min previously) for adult 6-hydroxydopamine neonate lesioned rats and sham operate controls. Stereotypy responses were measured over a 2 hr period following L-DOPA injection. The 6-hydroxydopamine lesioned rats (98% striatal tyrosine hydroxylase depletion) showed enhanced stereotyped behaviour, responding to doses of L-DOPA which were subthreshold for control rats.

the greater "supersensitive" response. The more slowly developing post-synaptic change occurs over a much longer time period and results in a much greater quantitative change in sensitivity. Both forms of supersensitivity move the agonist dose-response curve to the left as lower doses of the agonist are required to achieve the same biological response.

The increased behavioural response of the 6-hydroxydopamine lesioned rats to L-DOPA could thus be explained, in part, by a presynaptic mechanism. The degenerating dopamine terminals would decrease the number of dopamine uptake sites thereby increasing

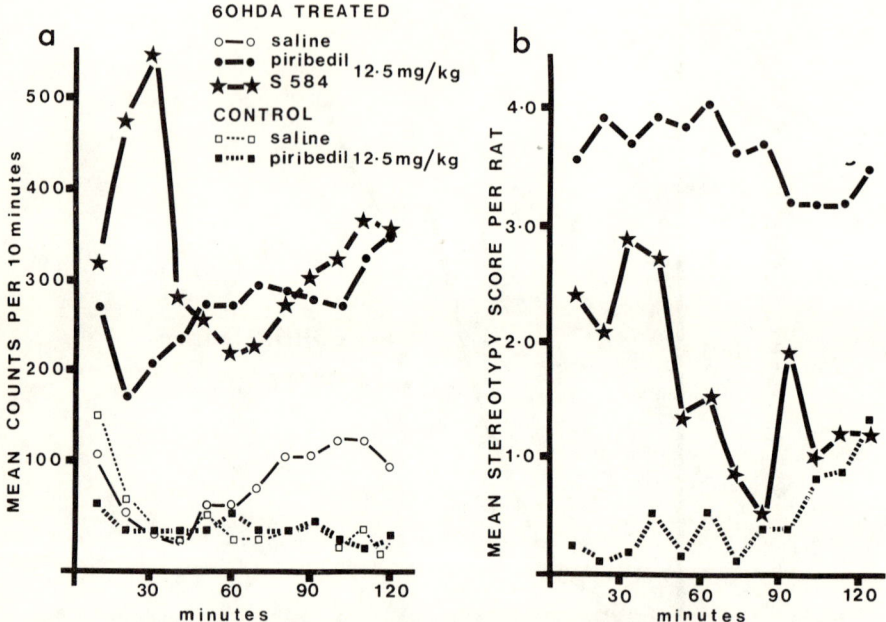

Fig. 7. a: Activity response to piribedil (12.5 mg/kg) and saline for adult 6-hydroxydopamine neonate lesioned rats and controls. The locomotor response of the 6-hydroxydopamine lesioned rats to S584 (12.5 mg/kg) is also shown. b: Stereotypy response to piribedil (12.5 mg/kg) for adult 6-hydroxydopamine lesioned rats and controls and to S584 (12.5 mg/kg) for the 6-hydroxydopamine lesioned rats. The 6-hydroxydopamine lesioned rats (98% striatal tyrosine hydroxylase depletion) showed an enhanced behavioural response to these dopamine agonists.

the free concentration of dopamine formed from the L-DOPA to interact with the receptors. However, such a mechanism would not explain the behavioural supersensitivity to apomorphine; apomorphine is not a competitive inhibitor of dopamine uptake [34] and is thus not normally taken up by presynaptic terminals. Moreover, we investigated the time course of the development of the enhanced behavioural response to apomorphine [14] and found that it continued to increase for at least 48 days following substantia nigra lesion (Figure 8). Ungerstedt [18] reported a similar time course for the increased rotational behaviour to apomorphine seen in unilaterally substantia nigra lesioned rats. The slow and continued rise in apomorphine sensitivity would be consonant with a postsynaptic mechanism.

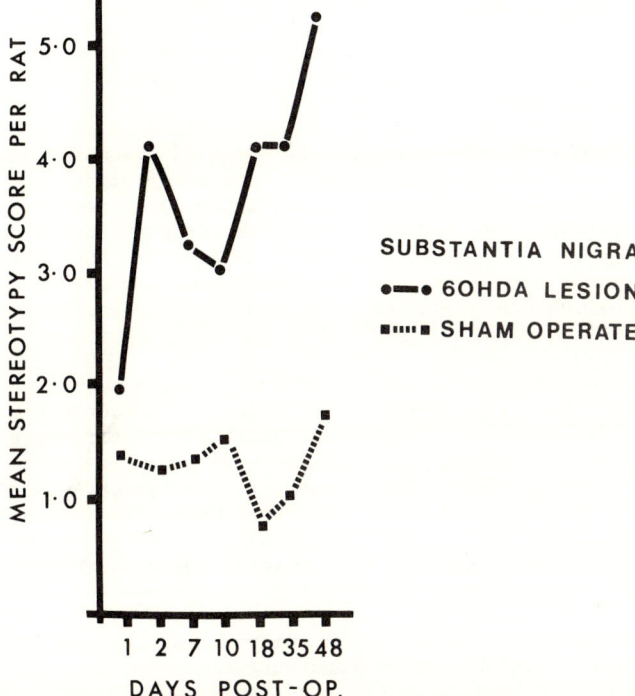

Fig. 8. Mean stereotypy response to 1 mg/kg apomorphine for bilateral substantia nigra 6-hydroxydopamine lesioned rats and sham operate controls. The response was measured for 1 hr after drug injection on the post-operative days listed. The substantia nigra lesioned rats (over 99% striatal tyrosine hydroxylase depletion) showed a significantly enhanced and increasing response compared to the sham operate controls.

Elegant studies by Stricker, Zigmond and Friedman [35] have also illuminated this point. They found that whereas a wide range of dopamine depletions were followed by a correlated increase in responsiveness to L-DOPA, an increase in sensitivity to apomorphine only occurred when at least an 80% dopamine depletion had been achieved. They interpreted this as indicating that each dopamine receptor in the striatum has, what amounts to, a functional multiple synaptic innervation. Hence the removal of a few dopamine terminals, while reducing the number of dopamine uptake sites and increasing the effectiveness of a given dose of L-DOPA, does not necessarily denervate receptors from dopamine stimulation. They hypothesize that sufficient dopamine is released from a dopamine terminal to stimulate not only its own receptor across the synapse, but "spill over" to activate other receptors in the vicinity. This continued stimulation of the denervated receptors prevents the development of postsynaptic supersensitivity. Thus it is only when almost all the dopamine terminals are removed and receptors become truly denervated from stimulation by dopamine that supersensitivity at the receptor level is instigated and an enhanced behavioural response to apomorphine occurs.

Such a mechanism would explain the enhanced locomotor stimulant effects of a low dose of amphetamine in substantia nigra lesioned rats with an 85-90% dopamine depletion (Figure 3). These rats would have both supersensitive receptors in certain denervated areas as well as functional dopamine terminals elsewhere. Amphetamine would augment the normal release of dopamine which would spread to the supersensitive receptors and result in the enhanced behavioural response.

Although we found no evidence for the primary involvement of noradrenaline in the amphetamine stimulation of locomotor activity [14], Segal, McAllister and Geyer have shown that the intraventricular infusion of noradrenaline can result in an increase in spontaneous activity [36]. Pretreatment with 6-hydroxydopamine enhances this effect and since a noradrenaline uptake inhibitor, DMI, did not affect the response in normal rats, they interpret the increased responsiveness of the 6-hydroxydopamine treated rats as indicating a postsynaptic noradrenergic supersensitivity.

Interruption of synaptic transmission in the central nervous system by pharmacological rather than surgical means can also give rise to an enhanced behavioural response to amine agonists. Dominic and Moore [37] showed that the chronic treatment of mice with α-methyl-p-tyrosine, which inhibits amine synthesis, enhanced the stimulant action of amphetamine when the treatment was discontinued. Ungerstedt [18] found that reserpine treatment, which depleted the striatal nerve terminals of their dopamine content, increased the sensitivity of rats with unilateral lesion of the striatum to apomorphine. In an extensive series of experiments, Tarsy and Baldessarini [38,39] have shown that an enhanced responsiveness to apomorphine not only follows these presynaptic manipulations of amine availability, but can occur if the postsynaptic dopamine receptors are chronically blocked with chlorpromazine or haloperidol. Klawans and McKendall [40] have suggested that such a mechanism is responsible for the appearance of tardive dyskinesia seen in humans following the prolonged treatment with neuroleptic drugs. From these experiments it seems probable that the lack of dopamine reaching the postsynaptic cells is, in itself, able to induce an increase in the sensitivity to apomorphine.

Is the development of supersensitivity of functional significance? Lesions to the substantia nigra generally give rise to aphagia and adipsia [41,42]. The greater the extent of the lesion the more severe and prolonged is the impairment of food and water intake. Zigmond and Stricker [43] have found that almost all aspects of normal regulation do recover if the lesion to the nigro-striatal pathway is not complete. However, the full syndrome can be reinstated by treating the rats with subthreshold doses, for normal rats, of α-methyl-p-tyrosine. This indicates that the catecholamine neuronal systems were maintaining these recovered functions rather than compensatory mechanisms in other systems. A similar enhanced behavioural depressant effect of α-methyl-p-tyrosine or reserpine has been found on the performance of a number of operant tasks following 6-hydroxydopamine treatment [44]. Consistent with this is the finding that an initial pretreatment with α-methyl-p-tyrosine [45] or haloperidol [46] which might be expected to induce supersensitivity prior to lesion can reduce the time needed to recover from lateral hypothalamic and nigro-striatal damage. The increased sensitivity of patients with Parkinson's disease may indicate that supersensitivity of dopamine receptors has occurred in response to the degeneration of the nigro-striatal pathway in an attempt to maintain normal function.

However, postsynaptic supersensitivity is a pharmacological concept referring to specific biochemical changes at the receptor level itself. All the previous data reported have used behavioural responses as a possible correlate of such receptor changes. But many unknown steps lie between the combination of a neurotransmitter with its receptor and the generation of an overt behavioural response. We must be careful not to be misled and interpret changes in behavioural sensitivity as necessarily implying changes in the number or sensitivity of the receptor sites. We already know that decreases in central cholinergic activity can enhance the behavioural effects of apomorphine [47]. Weight loss, whether caused by deprivation per se [48] or treatment with some of the aminergic drugs [49] used in the above studies, can be sufficient in itself to enhance the stimulant effects of amphetamine or apomorphine [50]. It is possible that such indirect mechanisms may have been responsible for the observed enhanced behavioural responses to dopamine agonists.

In order to determine, with certainty, that a postsynaptic supersensitivity has occurred, observations need to be made at the neuronal level, or better still, at the receptor site itself. Electrophysiological recording of single unit activity in the caudate nucleus following 6-hydroxydopamine treatments has demonstrated that changes do, in fact, occur in the sensitivity of neurones to the depressant effects of iontophoretically applied dopamine [51,52]. Since the depressant effects of apomorphine also have a lower threshold [52], a postsynaptic supersensitivity appears indicated.

Recent studies [28-30] have indicated the presence of a dopamine sensitive adenyl cyclase in the rat striatum. That many dopamine antagonists block the stimulatory effects of dopamine on this enzyme in proportion to their behavioural effects has led to the suggestion that this enzyme system may well be the dopamine receptor itself. Cyclic AMP so considered would be a "second messenger". Interestingly, the electrophysiological data indicate that cells which are depressed by dopamine and apomorphine are also depressed by cyclic AMP [52]. In keeping with the second messenger hypothesis, 6-hydroxydopamine does not alter their responsiveness to cyclic AMP while concurrently enhancing the effects of dopamine and apomorphine [52]. Postsynaptic supersensitivity in this system would be manifested by an increase in the production of cyclic AMP for a given amount of dopamine. This could be achieved either by a change in the kinetic parameters of the enzyme system, or an increase in the total number of receptor-enzyme sites.

A number of studies have investigated the dopamine sensitive adenyl cyclase in 6-hydroxydopamine lesioned rats. Mishra et al. [53] found that dopamine or S584, the behaviourally active metabolite of piribedil, caused a seven fold increase in striatal cyclic AMP production on the denervated side following a unilateral substantia nigra lesion. The contralateral, control striatum showed only a two to three fold stimulation of cyclic AMP production under the same conditions. There was also a moderate increase in the maximal stimulation of cyclic AMP production by dopamine in the denervated striatum. These findings are consistent with the behavioural data previously presented. Other researchers have not found a similar increase in cyclic AMP production following 6-hydroxydopamine treatment [54] which may be due to methodological differences. However, it is important that adequate controls are used in these experiments as nerve terminals are rich in phosphodiesterase activity and by destroying presynaptic elements with 6-hydroxydopamine the decrease in phosphodiesterase activity may spare cyclic AMP from catabolism and thus apparently increase the cyclic AMP response to dopamine without any changes occurring in the receptor-enzyme complex. A noradrenergic stimulation of cyclic AMP production has also been described in the central nervous system and the pineal gland. Intraventricular 6-hydroxydopamine treatment [55-57] or denervation of the pineal [58,59] increase the cyclic AMP production following noradrenaline stimulation. This phenomenon appears to be a common feature of catecholaminergic denervation. At the present time it appears probable that the dopamine sensitive adenyl cyclase in the striatum may well be part of the dopamine receptor, and that changes in cyclic AMP production do occur in the behaviourally supersensitive animal.

In the peripheral nervous system cholinergic denervation at the neuromuscular junction is well known to produce both an increase in the number and a spread of receptor sites [60]. This has been elegantly demonstrated by combining electrophysiological techniques with the autoradiography of the binding of radioactively labeled α-bungarotoxin which binds to the acetylcholine receptor [61]. Such binding studies with labeled dopamine agonists or antagonists should, in theory, be capable of determining whether or not there are increases in the number of dopamine receptor sites in the behaviourally supersensitive animal.

At the present time the most parsimonious explanation of the numerous experimental results reported here is that both pre- and post-synaptic mechanisms are responsible for the observed changes in reactivity to dopamine agonists seen following the interruption of dopaminergic activity in these varied systems. However, a post-synaptic supersensitivity analagous to that occurring in the peripheral cholinergic system remains to be demonstrated directly at the receptor level.

REFERENCES

[1]. N. -E. Andén, A. Carlsson, A. Dahlström, K. Fuxe, N. -A. Hillarp and K. Larsson, Life Sci., 3, 1964, 523-530.

[2]. U. Ungerstedt, Acta physiol. scand., suppl. 367, 1971, 1-48.

[3]. U. Ungerstedt, Eur. J. Pharmac., 5, 1968, 107-110.

[4]. U. Ungerstedt, in 6-Hydroxydopamine and Catecholamine Neurones (T. Malmfors and H. Thoenen, eds.), North-Holland, Amsterdam and London, 1971, pp. 101-127.

[5]. T. Hökfelt and U. Ungerstedt, Brain Res., 60, 1973, 269-297.

[6]. Y. Agid, F. Javoy, J. Glowinski, D. Bouvet and C. Sotelo, Brain Res., 58, 1973, 291-301.

[7]. C. Sotelo, F. Javoy, Y. Agid and J. Glowinski, Brain Res., 58, 1973, 269-290.

[8]. N. J. Uretsky and L. L. Iversen, J. Neurochem., 17, 1970, 269-278.

] 9]. K. D. Evetts, N. J. Uretsky, L. L. Iversen and S. D. Iversen, Nature, 225, 1970, 961-962.

[10]. R. Laverty and K. M. Taylor, Br. J. Pharmac., 40, 1970, 836-846.

[11]. K. M. Taylor and R. Laverty, Eur. J. Pharmac., 17, 1972, 16-24.

[12]. I. Creese and S. D. Iversen, Nature New Biol., 238, 1972, 247-248.

[13]. I. Creese and S. D. Iversen, Brain Res., 55, 1973, 369-382.

[14]. I. Creese and S. D. Iversen, Brain Res., 1974, (in press).

[15]. I. Creese and S. D. Iversen, Psychopharmacologia, 1974,(in press).

[16]. I. Creese, Eur. J. Pharmac., 28, 1974, 55-58.

[17]. Y. Agid, F. Javoy and J. Glowinski, Nature New Biol., 245, 1973, 150-151.

[18]. U. Ungerstedt, Acta physiol. scand., suppl. 367, 1971, 69-93.

[19]. A. M. Ernst, Psychopharmacologia, 7, 1965, 391-395.

[20]. N. -E. Andén, A. Rubenson, K. Fuxe and T. Hökfelt, J. Pharm. Pharmac., 19, 1967, 627.

[21]. R. Schoenfeld and N. Uretsky, Eur. J. Pharmac., 19, 1972, 115-118.

[22]. N. J. Uretsky and R. I. Schoenfeld, Nature New Biol., 234, 1971, 157-159.

[23]. H. Corrodi, L. Farnebo, K. Fuxe, B. Hamberger and U. Ungerstedt, Eur. J. Pharmac., 20, 1972, 195-204.

[24]. M. Goldstein, B. Anagnoste and C. Shirran, J. Pharm. Pharmacol., 25, 1973, 348-351.

[25]. H. Corrodi, K. Fuxe and U. Ungerstedt, J. Pharm. Pharmacol., 23, 1971, 989-991.

[26]. B. Costall and R. J. Naylor, Nauyn-Schmiedebergs Arch. Pharmacol., 278, 1973, 117-133.

[27]. R. J. Miller and L. L. Iversen, Nauyn-Schmiedebergs Arch. Pharmacol., 282, 1974, 213-216.

[28]. R. K. Mishra and M. H. Makman, Pharmacologist, 16, 1974, 287.

[29]. J. W. Kebabian, G. L. Petzold and P. Greengard, Proc. Nat. Acad. Sci. USA, 69, 1972, 2145-2149.

[30]. R. J. Miller, A. S. Horn and L. L. Iversen, Molecular Pharmacology, 10, 1974, 759-766.

[31]. U. Trendelenburg, Pharmacol. Rev., 15, 1963, 225-276.

[32]. U. Trendelenburg, Pharmacol. Rev., 18, 1966, 629-640.

[33]. S. Z. Langer, P. R. Draskóczy and U. Trendelenburg, J. Pharmacol. Exp. Ther., 157, 1967, 255-273.

[34]. S. Symchowicz, C. A. Korduba and J. Veals, Life Sci., 10, 1971, 35-42.

[35]. E. M. Stricker, M. J. Zigmond and M. I. Friedman, "Recovery of Function Following Damage to Central Catecholamine-Containing Neurons", presented at Fourth Annual Meeting of the Society for Neuroscience, St. Louis, Missouri, 1974.

[36]. D. S. Segal, C. McAllister and M. A. Geyer, Pharmacol. Biochem. and Behav., 2, 1974, 79-86.

[37]. J. A. Dominic and K. E. Moore, Psychopharmacologia, 15, 1969, 96-101.

[38]. D. Tarsy and R. J. Baldessarini, Nature New Biol., 245, 1973, 262-263.

[39]. D. Tarsy and R. J. Baldessarini, Neuropharmacology, 1974, (in press).

[40]. H. L. Klawans Jr. and R. R. McKendall, J. neurol. Sci., 14, 1971, 189-192.

[41]. U. Ungerstedt, Acta physiol. scand., suppl. 367, 1971, 95-122.

[42]. S. D. Iversen, in The Neurosciences Third Study Program (F. O. Schmitt and F. G. Worden, eds.) M. I. T. Press, Cambridge, Mass., 1974, pp. 705-711.

[43]. M. J. Zigmond and E. M. Stricker, in Neuropsychopharmacology of Monoamines and their Regulatory Enzymes (E. Usdin, ed.) Raven Press, N.Y., 1974, pp. 385-402.

[44]. B. R. Cooper, G. R. Breese, J. L. Howard and L. D. Grant, Psychopharmacologia, 27, 1972, 99-110.

[45]. S. D. Glick, S. Greenstein and B. Zimmerberg, Science, 117, 1972, 534-535.

[46]. M. D. Hynes, H. Lal and C. D. Anderson, Proc. 81st Annual Convention, APA, 1973, 1047-1048.

[47]. J. Scheel-Kruger, Acta pharmac. tox., 28, 1970, 1-16.

[48]. B. A. Campbell and H. C. Fibiger, Nature, 233, 1971, 424-425.

[49]. H. C. Fibiger, C. Trimbach and B. A. Campbell, Neuropharmacology, 11, 1972, 57-67.

[50]. B. J. Sahakian and T. Robbins, Neuropharmacology, 1975, (in press).

[51]. P. Feltz and J. De Champlain, Brain Res., 43, 1972, 601-605.

[52]. G. R. Siggins, B. J. Hoffer and U. Ungerstedt, Life Sci., 15, 1974, 779-792.

[53]. R. K. Mishra, E. L. Gardner, R. Katzman and M. H. Makman, Proc. Nat. Acad. Sci. USA, 71, 1974, 3883-3887.

[54]. P. F. Von Voigtlander, S. J. Boukma and G. A. Johnson, Neuropharmacology, 12, 1973, 1081-1086.

[55]. G. C. Palmer, Neuropharmacology, 11, 1972, 145-149.

[56]. A. Kalisker, C. O. Rutledge and J. P. Perkins, Molecular Pharmacology, 9, 1973, 619-629.

[57]. M. Huang, A. K. S. Ho and J. W. Daly, Molecular Pharmacology, 9, 1973, 711-717.

[58]. B. Weiss, J. Pharmacol. Exp. Ther., 168, 1969, 146-168.

[59]. T. Deguchi and J. Axelrod, Molecular Pharmacology, 9, 1973, 612-618.

[60]. R. Miledi and L. T. Potter, Nature, 233, 1971, 599-603.

[61]. H. C. Hartzell and D. M. Fambrough, J. General Physiol., 60, 1972, 248-262.

DISCUSSION

Dr. Smith wondered if the increased motor activity in the 70-80% lesioned animals could be explained via a beta noradrenergic mechanism. Dr. Creese felt that this was improbable since when control lesions in rats in the dorsal and ventral noradrenaline pathways were produced with 6-hydroxydopamine, resulting in very similar depletion of noradrenaline, such animals showed no change in their amphetamine response.

Dr. Snyder thought that the data might indicate more of a supersensitivity effect with DOPA than with apomorphine; he wondered if this might indicate something about the relative significance of the reuptake inactivation. Dr. Creese felt that reuptake was not very important here. As far as quantitation of supersensitivity was concerned, he felt this was difficult to measure in absolute terms, particularly since maximal stimulation is observed at incredibly low dosages.

Dr. Hornykiewicz suggested that Dr. Creese did not destroy the noradrenaline pathways projecting caudally to the medulla and the spinal cord. Dr. Creese said that he did not measure this, that the lesions were made in the dorsoventral pathway, not in the suborbital regions. He agreed with Dr. Hornykiewicz that noradrenaline is involved in locomotor activity. Infusion of noradrenaline resulted in increased spontaneous activity, particularly in 6-hydroxydopamine-lesioned animals. Dr. Creese stated that what he had been trying to demonstrate was the lack of primary involvement of the noradrenaline forebrain systems in the amphetamine stimulation of locomotor activity, not involvement of noradrenaline in movement per se.

Dr. Moore discussed the relative importance of reuptake versus postsynaptic sensitivity. He felt that there would be a rather rapid destruction of presynaptic terminals and therefore if this were the operative mechanism it should occur quite rapidly. In fact, he found as Dr. Fuxe had suggested that there was a continued progression of increased responsiveness for well over thirty days. Dr. Creese felt that there may well be presynaptic uptake component.

Dr. Gessa disagreed with the statement that apomorphine does not block the uptake of dopamine. He has found that apomorphine is very potent, blocking the uptake of dopamine (in caudate nucleus homogenates) via a competitive mechanism. Apomorphine was taken up by cells in these homogenates; the uptake was blocked by dopamine. Some of the supersensitivity to apomorphine could be explained by this reduced uptake. Dr. Creese explained that he had reported not his own data but that of Symchowicz et al. If apomorphine is taken up into presynaptic terminals, then the conclusions of those who have considered that apomorphine is simply postsynaptic in action are invalidated.

Dr. Gessa stated that he has also shown that apomorphine blocks monoamine oxidase, that it actually blocks dopamine in vivo. Dr. Creese suggested that the strongest argument for postsynaptic supersensitivity would be finding that the response increased past

48 days since if it were simply a presynaptic phenomenon, degeneration should be complete long before then. Thus, even if apomorphine is finally demonstrated to be taken up presynaptically, there is still good evidence that there is a postsynaptic supersensitivity in the dopamine system.

Dr. Adler was surprised by the return at about 33 days to the control level, with regard to sensitivity. Dr. Creese admitted that he did not have a complete explanation for this. He felt that the system exhibits a great deal of flux and if 20% of the dopamine terminals are still intact, it is conceivable that there might be sprouting onto those denervation receptors which initially were supersensitive. As this occurred, as they became reinnervated, they would lose their supersensitivity and a plateauing would result and response would return to normal.

BIOCHEMICAL IDENTIFICATION OF THE POSTSYNAPTIC SEROTONIN RECEPTOR
IN MAMMALIAN BRAIN

Solomon H. Snyder and James P. Bennett, Jr.
Departments of Pharmacology and Experimental Therapeutics
and
Psychiatry and Behavioral Sciences
The Johns Hopkins University School of Medicine
Baltimore, Maryland 21205

Modern psychopharmacology owes a great debt to biochemical studies of neurotransmitters in the brain. The bulk of this biochemical information characterizes presynaptic properties such as synthesis, release and reuptake of neurotransmitters and the influence of psychotropic drugs on these processes. Only recently has it been possible to identify biochemically postsynaptic receptor sites for central nervous neurotransmitters. For glycine [1] and the muscarinic acetylcholine receptor [2], binding of antagonists has provided the most efficient labeling technique, while for γ-aminobutyric acid (GABA), binding of the transmitter itself has been effective [3].

Very little is known of the pharmacology of postsynaptic serotonin receptors in the brain. Besides postsynaptic receptors, there appear to be presynaptic receptors for serotonin which can be identified neurophysiologically by measuring the influence of iontophoretically injected serotonin upon the firing rate of raphe cells, which represent the major cell bodies of all serotonin neurons in the forebrain [4,5,6]. Iontophoretic administration of serotonin to areas of the brain enriched in serotonin terminals provides a means of studying the postsynaptic serotonin receptor

[7]. The properties of presynaptic and postsynaptic serotonin receptors differ somewhat. d-Lysergic acid diethylamide (LSD) potently mimics the effects of serotonin on raphe cells, that is upon the presynaptic serotonin receptor, while d-LSD only weakly mimics serotonin at postsynaptic receptor sites. Other psychedelic drugs such as dimethyltryptamine also mimic serotonin at presynaptic receptors and more weakly at postsynaptic receptors. Indeed, since maximal neurophysiologic responses cannot be obtained with dimethyltryptamine at postsynaptic sites, it is possible that dimethyltryptamine is a partial agonist at these loci. Moreover, while local anesthetic effects preclude the administration of high concentrations of LSD to postsynaptic sites, available evidence is consistent with the possibility that LSD itself may only be a partial agonist at the postsynaptic serotonin receptors, hence may be both agonist and antagonist at these sites (G. Aghajanian, personal commnnication).

The psychedelic actions of LSD are thought to derive from the potent effects of this drug upon presynaptic serotonin receptors, inhibiting raphe cell firing, which would be consistent with the great psychotropic potency of LSD and the fact that 2-bromo-LSD, which is much weaker in its psychotropic effects than LSD, is also considerably weaker in its influence on raphe cell firing [5,6,7].

Using equilibrium dialysis, Farrow and Von Vunakis [8,9] observed stereospecific binding of LSD to particulate fractions of the cerebral cortex, but could detect no binding in other brain regions even though serotonin terminals occur more prominently in areas other than the cerebral cortex. With a more sensitive filtration technique, Bennett and Aghajanian observed stereospecific binding of LSD to membrane fractions throughout the brain [10,11]. Since destruction of serotonin neurons by raphe lesions failed to affect the binding it was concluded that the binding did not involve the presynaptic receptors for serotonin but may have involved postsynaptic receptors. In this study, we describe LSD and serotonin binding to membrane fractions of the brain which appear to involve the postsynaptic serotonin receptor [12].

SUBCELLULAR LOCALIZATION

As observed previously for other neurotransmitter receptors in the brain, the greatest amount of specific LSD binding occurs in the crude mitochondrial (P_2) and low speed microsomal fraction (Table 1). Similar to findings of Bennett and Aghajanian [11] the microsomal fraction contains highest specific activity of LSD binding, (P_3) almost three times greater than the next highest subcellular fractions. Although the highest specific activities for opiate, muscarinic and GABA binding also occur in the P_3 fraction, their enrichment is proportionately less than for LSD. Since LSD binding to intact or lysed P_3 fractions is the same [12], we presume that binding takes place to membrane surfaces and does not involve transport into intact particles. In our studies a lysed P_3 fraction is used routinely for binding assays.

REGIONAL DISTRIBUTION OF RECEPTOR BINDING AND THE EFFECT OF RAPHE LESIONS

If LSD binding involves serotonin receptors, one anticipates some correlation between binding and the density of serotonin nerve terminals. In a detailed study with monkey brain [12] highest ^{3}H-LSD binding occurred in several regions of the cerebral cortex with values for the frontal cortex more than 10 times those of areas enriched in white matter [10,11]. Confirming the observations of Bennett and Aghajanian, binding in the cerebellar cortex of the monkey was only about 1/8th that of the frontal cortex and similar differences between cerebral cortex and cerebellum are evident in rat brain (Table 2). Except for the cerebral cortex, highest LSD binding occurred in the hippocampus, caudate and putamen of the monkey with several diencephalic areas

TABLE 1

Subcellular Distribution of Specific d-[^{3}H]LSD Binding in Rat Cerebral Cortex

Fraction	Specific d-[^{3}H]LSD Binding		
	Percent of Total	fmoles/100 mg wet weight	fmoles/mg protein
Crude Nuclear (P_1)	7	50.4±1.1	61.5±1.4
Mitochondrial (P_2)	32	239±6	58.2±1.5
Low Speed Microsomal	35	257±3	103±2
Microsomal (P_3)	26	196±4	317±6

Rat cerebral cortex was homogenized in 15 vol of cold 0.32 M sucrose and centrifuged at 900 x g for 10 min to yield P_1 which was washed with 2-10 ml portions of 0.32 sucrose. The combined supernatants were centrifuged at 11,500 x g for 20 min with one sucrose wash to yield P_2. The combined supernatants were then centrifuged at 20,000 x g for 30 min to yield the low speed microsomal pellet and the supernatant at 100,000 x g for 60 min to yield P_3. All fractions were then disrupted in 20 vol of cold water with the Polytron and centrifuged at 50,000 x g for 20 min. The membrane pellets were then resuspended in 20 vol (based on original tissue wet weight) of 50 mM Tris HCl buffer with 0.1% ascorbic acid. Two ml aliquots were incubated with 3 nM d-[^{3}H]-LSD with and without 1 µM unlabeled d-LSD for 10 min at 37°C. The samples were filtered and washed as described in METHODS. Specific binding is defined as total d-[^{3}H]LSD binding minus binding in the presence of 1 µM unlabeled d-LSD. Each sample is the mean ± SEM of four determinations.

TABLE 2

Regional Distribution of [^{3}H]Serotonin and [^{3}H]LSD
Specific Binding in Rat Brain

Region	[^{3}H]-LSD	[^{3}H]-Serotonin
Cerebral cortex	3.19	1.01
Corpus striatum	4.52	1.24
Hippocampus	1.52	--
Thalamus-hypothalamus	1.19	--
Midbrain	1.63	--
Brainstem	1.13	--
Cerebellum	0.70	0.21

Rat brain P_3 membranes from each region were incubated with [^{3}H]-LSD (4 nM) or [^{3}H]-serotonin (8 nM). After filtration and washing, specific binding was calculated by subtracting from total binding the nonspecific binding occurring in the presence of excess unlabeled serotonin (10 µM) or d-LSD (1 µM). Values are given in terms of picomoles bound per gram original tissue wet weight.

containing somewhat less binding. In general the monkey brain regions clostered into 3 groups with highest binding in the cerebellum and intermediate values in the diencephalic regions. In the rat the corpus striatum has higher LSD binding than the cerebral cortex (Table 2).

This distribution differs from that of serotonin uptake in the monkey, which was highest in the hypothalamus and inferior and superior colliculi as well as substantia nigra and amygdala [12], all of which contain high levels of endogenous serotonin [13,14]. By contrast cerebral cortical areas were relatively low in serotonin uptake. Interestingly, high affinity serotonin uptake which presumably labels serotonin nerve terminals, did not itself correlate closely with endogenous serotonin. The superior colliculus contains 5 times as much endogenous serotonin as the inferior colliculus [14] yet had about the same amount of serotonin uptake. If one omits the cerebral cortex from consideration, there was a statistically significant correlation between LSD binding and serotonin uptake in various brain regions [12].

As anticipated from other evidence that serotonin and LSD binding involve the same sites, we do find similar regional variations in serotonin as in LSD binding in rat brain with corpus striatum highest, somewhat greater than cerebral cortex, and cerebellum 5-6 times lower (Table 2).

If LSD and serotonin bind to the postsynaptic serotonin receptor how do we explain the discrepancies between the regional distribution of endogenous serotonin and presumed receptor binding sites? Receptor site concentration is presumably determined by the proportion of cells in a given brain region which receive input from a transmitter. If the majority of cells in the cerebral cortex each receives one serotonin nerve terminal, while a minority of cells in the hypothalamus each receives 100 serotonin terminals, one would anticipate higher endogenous serotonin levels and uptake of serotonin in the hypothalamus than in the cerebral cortex but a greater density of serotonin receptors in the cerebral cortex. Kuhar et al. [13] discuss histochemical evidence that the faint but diffuse serotonin fluorescence in the cerebral cortex represents serotonergic innervation of a major portion of cerebral cortex cells, possibly more extensive than in the hypothalamus. Thus the density of postsynaptic receptors need not correlate with endogenous levels of a neurotransmitter.

There is some precedent for this conclusion derived from other neurotransmitter receptors. The relative density of muscarinic cholinergic receptors in various brain regions shows only a limited correlation with levels of endogenous acetylcholine [15]. Norepinephrine sensitive cyclic AMP accumulating systems, presumably associated with norepinephrine receptor sites, are most enriched in the cerebellum which contains the lowest levels of endogenous norepinephrine in the brain [16,17]. Receptor binding sites for thyrotropin releasing hormone (TRH) throughout the brain do not correlate with endogenous levels of TRH [18]. In addition, receptor binding for GABA (γ-aminobutyric acid) in various brain areas of the rat does not correlate well with endogenous GABA concentration [3].

BINDING OF LSD IN VIVO COMPETES WITH ENDOGENOUS SEROTONIN

Without an extensive series of compounds evaluated neurophysiologically and by binding for serotonin-like postsynaptic effects, one has difficulty in establishing unequivocally that LSD and serotonin binding do involve the postsynaptic serotonin receptor. Definitive evidence has been obtained by measuring LSD binding in vivo (Bennett, Szabo and Snyder, in preparation). When small doses of ^{3}H-LSD are injected intravenously, the regional distribution of membrane bound radioactivity in rat brain closely parallels that of ^{3}H-LSD binding in vitro. LSD binding in vivo is saturable such that 40 µg/kg of unlabeled LSD inhibits the binding of ^{3}H-LSD by 50%.

If LSD binds to the postsynaptic serotonin receptor, then changes in levels of endogenous serotonin might be expected to alter LSD binding. Depleting serotonin in the brain and presumably in the synaptic cleft as well should lessen competition for the receptor and enhance LSD binding, while elevation of brain serotonin should lower receptor binding of LSD. We did find that reserpine elevates LSD binding in vivo.

SATURATION OF LSD BINDING

We examined the saturation of LSD binding in two ways. In one experiment increasing amounts of ^{3}H-LSD were added while in another, the ability of nonradioactive LSD to inhibit ^{3}H-LSD binding was measured (Fig. 1,2). LSD binding is fully saturated

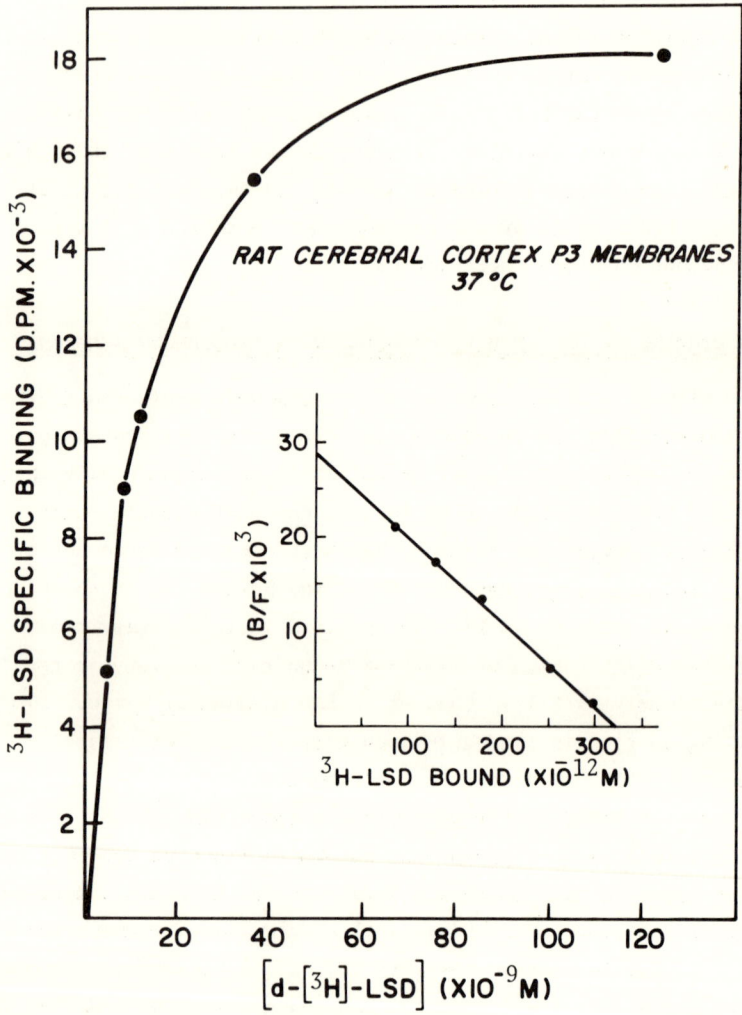

Fig. 1. d-[³H]LSD binding as a function of increasing concentration of d-[³H]LSD. Aliquots of rat cerebral cortex P3 membranes equivalent to 100 mg original tissue wet weight were incubated with various concentrations of d-[³H]LSD for 10 min at 37°C in 50 mM Tris-HCl buffer with 0.1 % ascorbic acid (pH 6.7 at 37°). Total d-[³H]LSD binding and nonspecific d-[³H]LSD binding occurring in the presence of 1 µM unlabeled d-LSD were assayed as described in METHODS. Each point is the mean of quadruplicate samples whose standard error was less than 5%.

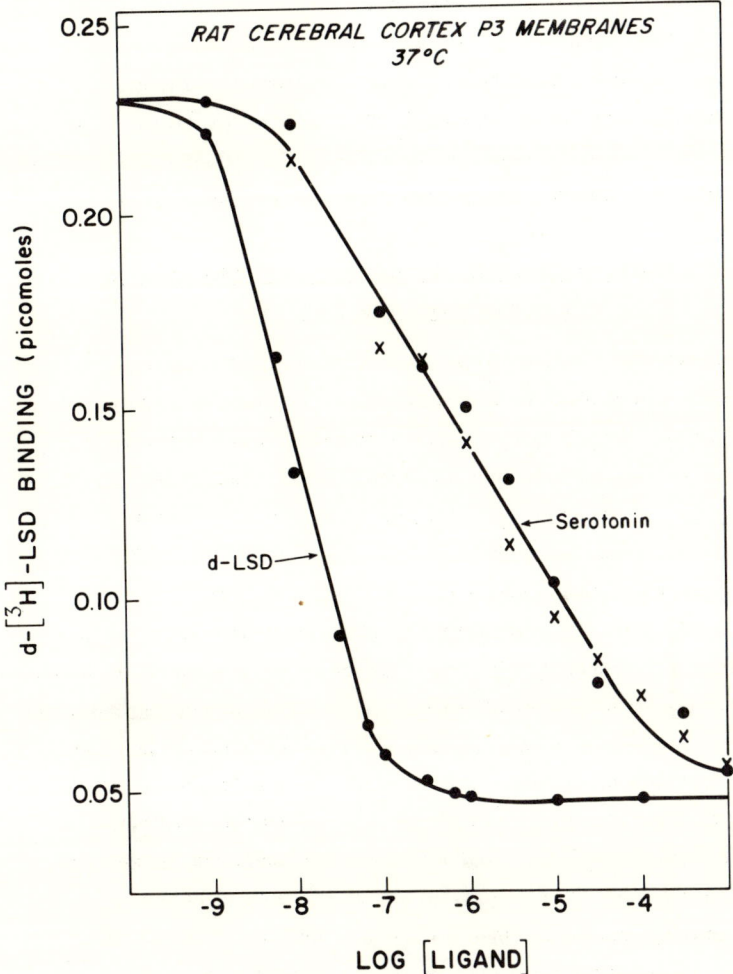

Fig. 2. Total d-[^{3}H]LSD binding displaced by unlabeled d-LSD and serotonin. Aliquots of cerebral cortex P$_3$ membranes equivalent to 100 mg original tissue wet weight were incubated with 3 nM d-[^{3}H]LSD and various concentrations of unlabeled d-LSD or serotonin for 10 min at 37°C. The incubation medium was 50 nM Tris-HCl with 0.1% ascorbic acid and 10 μM pargyline (pH 6.7 at 37°C). d-[^{3}H]LSD binding was assayed as described in METHODS. The displacement by serotonin was performed both with (X--X) and without (●—●) a 10 min preincubation (37°C) of the tissue with serotonin before the d-[^{3}H]LSD was added. Each point represents the mean of quadruplicate samples whose standard errors were less than 5%.

at about 200 nM and half-maximal saturation occurs at 10 nM, similar to the findings of Bennett and Aghajanian [10,11]. Scatchard analysis indicates a single saturable site with a dissociation constant of about 11 nM. A plot of these data according to the Hill equation reveals a Hill coefficient of 1.0 indicating the absence of cooperative interactions [12].

RELATIVE AFFINITY OF DRUGS AND NEUROTRANSMITTERS FOR LSD AND SEROTONIN BINDING SITES

Identity of ligand binding with the opiate, glycine, muscarinic acetylcholine and GABA receptors was demonstrated by showing close correlations between pharmacologic and binding potencies for a variety of neurotransmitter analogues [1,2,3,19]. In the case of glycine and GABA the pharmacologic potency values were obtained from neurophysiologic studies of the ability of amino acids to mimic glycine or GABA respectively in their synaptic effects. To determine if LSD binds directly to the postsynaptic serotonin receptor, it would be desirable to compare the affinity of a series of serotonin analogues for LSD binding sites and neurophysiologic serotonin-like effects at postsynaptic sites. Unfortunately very little data is available regarding the serotonin-like activities of drugs and serotonin analogues at postsynaptic receptors. Another approach would be to measure serotonin binding directly. If serotonin binding were to evince characteristics essentially the same as that of LSD binding, we could assume that they involve the same or similar sites and that the LSD binding was associated with true serotonin receptors.

We can demonstrate directly the binding of serotonin to membrane preparations of rat brain. Since this binding possesses a similar regional distribution and substrate specificity to that of LSD binding, we conclude that LSD and serotonin bind to the same or closely related sites. The high affinity of serotonin for its binding sites, when assayed directly (K_D of

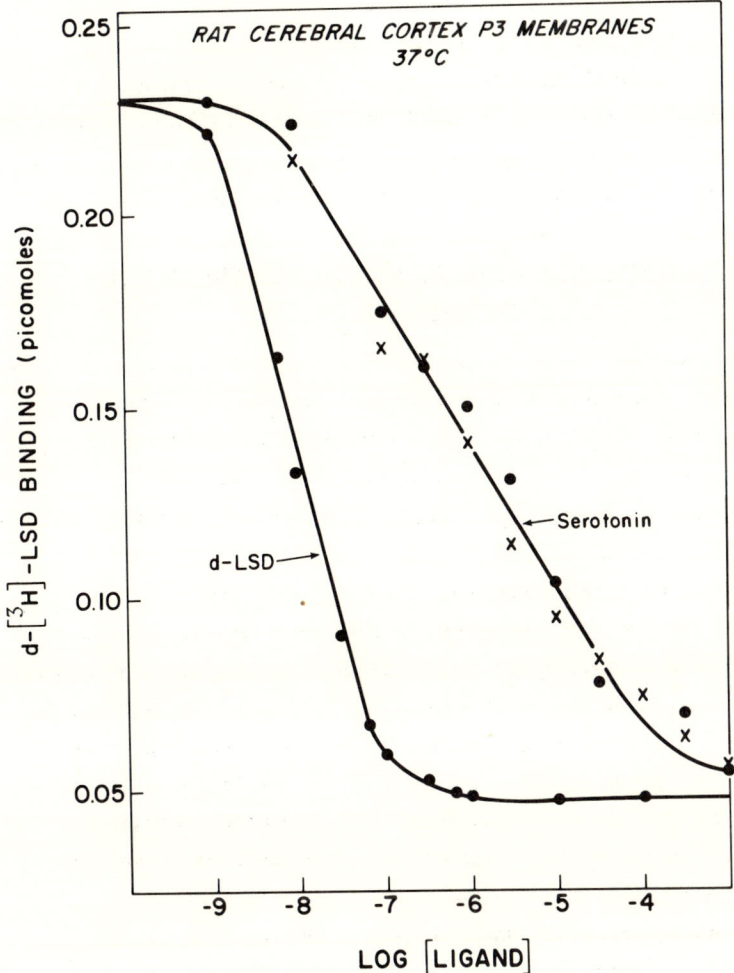

Fig. 2. Total d-[³H]LSD binding displaced by unlabeled d-LSD and serotonin. Aliquots of cerebral cortex P_3 membranes equivalent to 100 mg original tissue wet weight were incubated with 3 nM d-[³H]LSD and various concentrations of unlabeled d-LSD or serotonin for 10 min at 37°C. The incubation medium was 50 nM Tris-HCl with 0.1% ascorbic acid and 10 μM pargyline (pH 6.7 at 37°C). d-[³H]LSD binding was assayed as described in METHODS. The displacement by serotonin was performed both with (X--X) and without (●—●) a 10 min preincubation (37°C) of the tissue with serotonin before the d-[³H]LSD was added. Each point represents the mean of quadruplicate samples whose standard errors were less than 5%.

at about 200 nM and half-maximal saturation occurs at 10 nM, similar to the findings of Bennett and Aghajanian [10,11]. Scatchard analysis indicates a single saturable site with a dissociation constant of about 11 nM. A plot of these data according to the Hill equation reveals a Hill coefficient of 1.0 indicating the absence of cooperative interactions [12].

RELATIVE AFFINITY OF DRUGS AND NEUROTRANSMITTERS FOR LSD AND SEROTONIN BINDING SITES

Identity of ligand binding with the opiate, glycine, muscarinic acetylcholine and GABA receptors was demonstrated by showing close correlations between pharmacologic and binding potencies for a variety of neurotransmitter analogues [1,2,3,19]. In the case of glycine and GABA the pharmacologic potency values were obtained from neurophysiologic studies of the ability of amino acids to mimic glycine or GABA respectively in their synaptic effects. To determine if LSD binds directly to the postsynaptic serotonin receptor, it would be desirable to compare the affinity of a series of serotonin analogues for LSD binding sites and neurophysiologic serotonin-like effects at postsynaptic sites. Unfortunately very little data is available regarding the serotonin-like activities of drugs and serotonin analogues at postsynaptic receptors. Another approach would be to measure serotonin binding directly. If serotonin binding were to evince characteristics essentially the same as that of LSD binding, we could assume that they involve the same or similar sites and that the LSD binding was associated with true serotonin receptors.

We can demonstrate directly the binding of serotonin to membrane preparations of rat brain. Since this binding possesses a similar regional distribution and substrate specificity to that of LSD binding, we conclude that LSD and serotonin bind to the same or closely related sites. The high affinity of serotonin for its binding sites, when assayed directly (K_D of about 30 nM) is consistent with direct binding to serotonin receptor sites. This provides valuable additional evidence that the binding sites for serotonin and LSD do represent the postsynaptic receptor.

d-LSD is the most potent displacer of ^{3}H-LSD and ^{3}H-serotonin, reducing binding by 50% at 10 nM (Table 3). LSD binding is markedly stereospecific, since d-LSD is more than 1000 times as potent as l-LSD, which corresponds to the stereospecificity of psychedelic effects. However, 2-bromo-LSD, whose psychotropic effects are very weak, is just as potent a displacer of serotonin and LSD binding as d-LSD. In marked contrast, 2-bromo-LSD is much weaker than d-LSD at presynaptic receptors involved in slowing raphe neuron firing [5] which supports the supposition that psychedelic effects of d-LSD are exerted via presynaptic and not postsynaptic receptors. Methysergide and d-isolysergic acid amide are both less than a tenth and d-lysergic acid 0.1% as potent as d-LSD in inhibiting both LSD and serotonin binding.

There are discrepancies between the affinities of tryptamine analogues for serotonin and LSD binding sites (Table 3). Serotonin itself has 100 times greater affinity for serotonin than LSD binding sites and the discrepancy in the same direction is between 20 and 200 fold for other tryptamines. These disparities might indicate that serotonin and LSD do not bind to the same receptor at all. However, the close similarity of regional distribution and the affinities of LSD derivatives indicates that they must bind to intimately related sites. We propose that serotonin and LSD bind to two distinct conformations of the same postsynaptic serotonin receptor.

A MODEL FOR CONFORMATIONAL ALTERATIONS OF THE POSTSYNAPTIC SEROTONIN RECEPTOR

Neurotransmitter receptors may exist in "agonist" and "antagonist" conformations. Drugs which have a high affinity for the agonist conformation effect neurotransmission since the

TABLE 3

Displacement of Specifically Bound [^{3}H]Serotonin and [^{3}H]LSD by LSD Analogues and Tryptamines

		ED$_{50}$	
		[^{3}H]Serotonin	[^{3}H]LSD
I.	**LSD Analogues**		
	d-LSD	10 nM	9.5 nM
	2-bromo-LSD	30 nM	7.0 nM
	d-isolysergic acid amide	100 nM	200 nM
	methysergide	300 nM	100 nM
	d-lysergic acid	3 µM	10 µM
	l-LSD	100 µM	20 µM
II.	**Tryptamines**		
	serotonin	30 nM	3000 nM
	bufotenine	60 nM	530 nM
	N,N-dimethyltryptamine	100 nM	2400 nM
	5-methoxytryptamine	10 nM	2000 nM
	tryptamine	60 nM	5000 nM

Rat cerebral cortex P$_3$ membranes were incubated with [^{3}H]serotonin (8 nM) or d-[^{3}H]LSD (4 nM) in the presence of several concentrations of drugs. After filtration and washing, specific binding was calculated by subtracting nonspecific binding occurring in the presence of excess unlabeled serotonin (10 µM) or d-LSD (1 µM) from total binding.

"second messenger", ionic conductance change or cyclic nucleotide alteration, occurs only when an agent binds to the agonist conformation of the receptor. Drugs which bind to the antagonist conformation make fewer agonist sites available for the neurotransmitter and thus block synaptic transmission. In receptor binding studies antagonists and agonists, though clearly binding to the same receptor, may exhibit different affinities depending on whether they are competing for binding of a radiolabeled agonist or antagonist respectively. Pure antagonists may compete better for the binding of a radiolabeled antagonist than for the binding of a radiolabeled agonist. The situation is reversed for agonists and, of course, is intermediate for mixed agonist-antagonists, also known as partial agonists. This model of synaptic transmission has been postulated for the nicotinic cholinergic receptor [20,21] and has been demonstrated for the opiate [19] and glycine [22] receptors.

If LSD and serotonin bind to different conformations of the same receptor, one might predict cooperative interactions in their mutual displacement, though this need not be obligatory. Interestingly, the slope for displacement of LSD binding by serotonin differs markedly from that of LSD displacement by LSD (Fig. 2). Hill coefficients calculated from this experiment are 1.0 for LSD and 0.57 for serotonin suggesting the existence of negative cooperativity between serotonin and LSD [12].

According to this model of synaptic function, our data with serotonin and LSD suggest that while serotonin is the agonist, LSD is the antagonist or at least a partial agonist. In the limited iontophoretic studies which have been performed at postsynaptic serotonin receptors in the brain [7], LSD weakly mimics serotonin as might be expected for a partial agonist. Partial agonists generally cannot produce "maximal" effects, because their antagonist properties hinder full expression of their agonist actions. LSD has not been demonstrated to produce maximal serotonin-like effects at postsynaptic brain receptors because of its local anesthetic effects [7]. Thus we do not know whether it is merely a weak agonist or a mixed agonist-antagonist. In the absence of local anesthetic effects, dimethyltryptamine appears to be only a partial agonist [7]. Segal [23,24] has directly demonstrated blockade of postsynaptic serotonin actions in the brain by LSD at identified serotonin synapses and at unidentified synapses Boakes et al. [25] have also observed blockade of serotonin effects by LSD

Though the situation is by no means clear, we postulate that the postsynaptic serotonin receptor can exist in two conformations and that serotonin binds with major affinity to the agonist conformation while LSD binds with partial affinities to both agonist and antagonist conformations and is itself a partial agonist.

In summary, the saturable binding of LSD and serotonin to membranes of brain tissue appears to reflect an interaction with the postsynaptic serotonin receptor. Mutual displacements between serotonin and LSD suggest that the serotonin receptor exists in two conformations, with serotonin binding to the agonist conformation and LSD binding to both agonist and antagonist conformation.

REFERENCES

[1]. A.B. Young and S.H. Snyder, Proc. Nat. Acad. Sci. USA 7, 1973, 2832.

[2]. H.I. Yamamura and S.H. Snyder, Proc. Nat. Acad. Sci. USA 71, 1974, 1725.

[3]. S.R. Zukin, A.B. Young, and S.H. Snyder, Proc. Nat. Acad. Sci. USA, in press.

[4]. G.K. Aghajanian, W.E. Foote, and M.H. Sheard, Science 161, 1968, 706.

[5]. G.K. Aghajanian, W.E. Foote, and M.H. Sheard, J. Pharmacol. Expt. Ther. 171, 1970, 178.

[6]. G.K. Aghajanian, H.J. Haigler, and F.E. Bloom, Life Sci. Part I, Physiol. Pharmacol. 11, 1972, 615.

[7]. H.J. Haigler, and G.K. Aghajanian, J. Pharmacol. Expt. Ther. 188, 1974, 688.

[8]. J.T. Farrow, and H. Van Vunakis, Nature 237, 1972, 164.

[9]. J.T. Farrow, and H. Van Vunakis, Biochem. Pharmacol. 22, 1973, 1103.

[10]. J.L. Bennett, and G.K. Aghajanian, Fed. Proc. 33, 1974, 256.

[11]. J.L. Bennett, and G.K. Aghajanian, Life Sci., in press.

[12]. J.P. Bennett and S.H. Snyder, Brain Res., submitted for publication.

[13]. M.J. Kuhar, G.K. Aghajanian and R.H. Roth, Brain Res. 44, 1972, 165.

[14]. M. Palkovits, M. Brownstein, and J.M. Saavedra, Brain Res. 80, 1974, 237.

[15]. H.I. Yamamura, M.J. Kuhar, D. Greenberg and S.H. Snyder, Brain Res. 66, 1974, 541.

[16]. M. Chasin, I. Rivkin, F. Mamrak, S.G. Samaniego, and S.M. Hess, J. Biol. Chem. 246, 1971, 3037.

[17]. B. Weiss, and E. Costa, Biochem. Pharmacol. 17, 1968, 2107.

[18]. D.R. Burt and S.H. Snyder, Brain Res., submitted for publication.

[19]. C.B. Pert and S.H. Snyder, Mol. Pharmacol. 10, 1974, 868.

[20]. A. Karlin, J. Theor. Biol. 56, 1967, 306.

[21]. J.-P. Changeux, Mol. Pharmacol. 2, 1966, 369.

[22]. A.B. Young and S.H. Snyder, Proc. Nat. Acad. Sci. USA 71, 1974, 4002.

[23]. M. Segal, Brain Res., in press.

[24]. M. Segal, J. Pharmacol. Expt. Ther., in press.

[25]. R.J. Boakes, P.B. Bradley, I. Briggs and A. Dray, Brain Res. 15, 1969, 529.

DISCUSSION

Dr. Spector requested that Dr. Snyder describe which fractions he had used in his studies, how pure they were, etc. Dr. Snyder replied that for the GABA receptor, for the glycine receptor and for the serotonin receptor, crude synaptic membrane preparation (à la de Robertis) had been used; for the opiate receptor, a whole brain membrane preparation had been used. He went on to aver that the specificity of receptor binding is not a function of the purity of the preparation, but rather is a function of the specificity of the assay method.

Dr. Weiner wondered if the same effects occurred with sodium, but Dr. Snyder thought this unlikely since Dr. Loh had reported no effects when he had tried sodium. Dr. Snyder stated that cerebroside sulfate is not the opiate receptor since this compound is a lipid and the opiate receptor is definitely primarily proteinaceous: it is very sensitive to trypsin (0.1 mg/ml will eliminate opiate receptor binding), to chymotrypsin, and to phospholipase A. The cerebroside binding may be a component or somehow contribute to receptor binding, but the cerebrosides certainly are not the opiate receptor: Whereas cerebrosides are almost ubiquitous (located all over the body, down to the big toe), recent autoradiographic localization studies by Kuhar show that the opiate receptor has extreme specificity in location.

STRUCTURE-ACTIVITY RELATIONSHIPS FOR AGONIST,
AND ANTAGONIST DRUGS, AT PRE- AND POST-
SYNAPTIC DOPAMINE RECEPTOR SITES IN RAT BRAIN

L.L. Iversen, A.S. Horn and R.J. Miller

Medical Research Council Neurochemical Pharmacology Unit,
Department of Pharmacology,
University of Cambridge, Cambridge, England.

I. INTRODUCTION

The hypothesis that antipsychotic drugs act by blocking dopamine receptors in the central nervous system is widely accepted. Many of the effects of such drugs on dopamine metabolism in brain can be explained in this way (1-3). Studies of the pharmacological properties of dopamine receptors in CNS have proved difficult, owing to the absence of any simple model for such receptor sites in the peripheral nervous system. Recently however, two useful model system have emerged. One is based on the remarkable similarity between the CNS effects of dopaminergic drugs and their effects on the renal artery, a system which responds to dopamine and related agonists by vasodilatation (4-5). This has proved to be a valuable peripheral model for studies of dopaminergic agonists and antagonists. The second model arose from the finding that low concentrations of dopamine stimulate the formation of cyclic AMP in bovine superior cervical ganglia (6), rat and bovine retina (7-8) and cell-free homogenates of rat basal ganglia (9) and other dopamine-rich areas of brain such as olfactory tubercle and nucleus accumbens (10-11). The effects of dopamine in some of these systems are antagonized by neuroleptic drugs such as chlorpromazine and haloperidol, and are mimicked by apomorphine (8-9). The dopamine-sensitive adenylate cyclase is absent from brain regions, such as cerebellum, which lack dopamine-containing nerve terminals, and it is not potently affected by classical α- or β-adrenoceptor agonists or antagonists. The enzyme appears to be located predominantly on post-synaptic cells in the striatum, since the dopamine-stimulated activity persists unchanged or is even increased after destruction of the nigro-striatal dopaminergic terminals (12-13). The existence of a dopamine-sensitive adenylate cyclase is consistent with the hypothesis that many of the post-synaptic actions of catecholamines are mediated by cyclic AMP production in adrenergically innervated cells (6-14-15). In our own work we have used the dopamine-sensitive adenylate cyclase of the rat striatum as a biochemical model in an attempt to define some of the structural requirements for dopamine receptor agonists and antagonists (16-20).

II. ACTIONS OF AGONIST DRUGS ON CYCLIC AMP FORMATION
A. Methods

The method was as described by Kebabian et al. (9). Rat striata or other brain regions were dissected according to the procedure described by Glowinski and Iversen (21), and homogenized with a motor-driven teflon-glass homogenizer in approximately 25 volumes of 2mM tris-maleate pH 7.4 containing 2mM EGTA. Aliquots of this homogenate were transferred to a solution containing 80 mM tris-maleate buffer pH 7.4 with 2mM magnesium sulphate, 0.2mM EGTA and 10mM theophylline, and various drugs. The incubation tubes were kept at $0^{\circ}C$ while ATP was added to a final concentration of 0.5mM and they were then incubated at $30^{\circ}C$ for 2.5 min. The reaction was stopped by heating at $100^{\circ}C$ and the contents of the tubes were then assayed for cyclic AMP using the protein binding method of Brown et al (22).

B. Effects of dopamine and related β-phenylethylamines

Addition of dopamine to rat striatal homogenates increased cyclic AMP production by approximately 100% during a brief incubation in vitro (Fig.1). Half-maximum stimulation was produced by about 3µM dopamine. Of the sixteen other phenylethylamines tested (Table 1), the only one that was as potent as dopamine was the N-methyl analogue, epinine. The N-dimethyl and N-trimethyl analogues were weaker agonists. Compounds with 1,3 or 4 carbon side chains, instead of the two carbon chain of dopamine, were completely inactive, as were non-catecholamines, such as m-tyramine, p-tyramine, amphetamine and O-methoxylated dopamine metabolites (Table 1). (±)-α-Methyldopamine was about 50 times less potent than the parent compound, and l-norepinephrine was 20 times less potent. d-Norepinephrine was inactive at concentrations up to 1mM, as was L-DOPA.

C. Naphthalene and tetrahydro-isoquinoline derivatives

The compound 2-amino-6,7-dihydroxy-1,2,3,4-tetrahydronaphthalene (ADTN), in which the side chain of dopamine is incorporated into a second ring system in the fully extended form, was equipotent with dopamine. The non-catechol analogue, however, was completely inactive (Table 2). When the dopamine side chain was

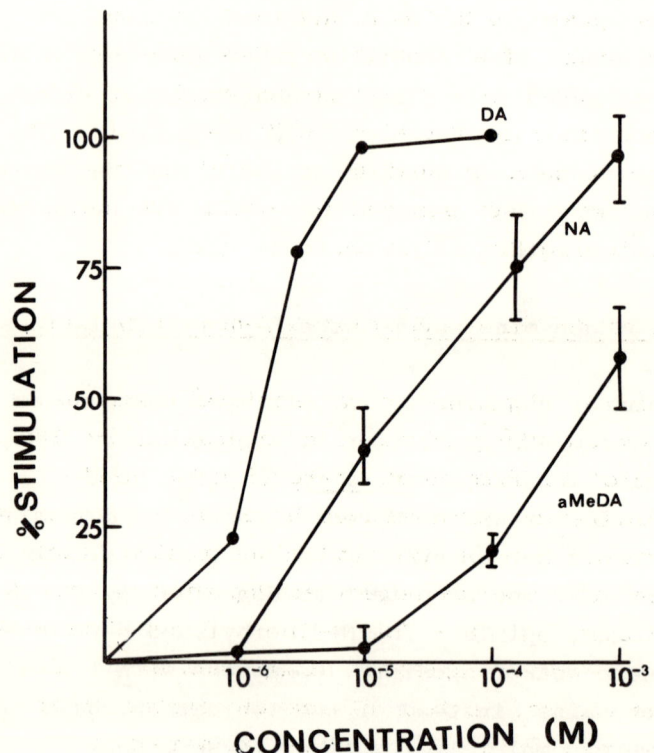

Fig.1. Stimulation of cyclic AMP formation in rat striatal homogenates by dopamine (DA),l-norepinephrine (NA) and (±)-α-methyldopamine (aMeDA). The amount of cyclic AMP formed during a 2.5 min incubation increased from 31.8 ± 0.96 pmol per assay tube (2mg tissue) to 66.9 ± 3.69 pmol per tube in the presence of a maximally stimulating concentration of dopamine (100μM), (means ± S.E., n = 9). Results are means ± S.E.M. of 4-10 separate incubations.

incorporated into a ring system in its non-extended form, as in 6,7-dihydroxy-tetrahydroisoquinoline, the compound was much less active than ADTN (19). Tetrahydropapaveroline and emetine were completely inactive at concentrations up to 1mM.

TABLE 1
Stimulation of cyclicAMP Formation by β-Phenylethylamines

Compound	Maximum stimulation % of dopamine*	EC50-μMolar**
Dopamine (DA)	100	2.0
Epinine	100	1.5
N-dimethylDA	48	1000.0
N-trimethylDA	30	>1000.0
l-Norepinephrine	97	40.0
(±)-α-MethylDA	58	850.0

Compounds inactive at 10^{-3}M: m-Tyramine; p-Tyramine; 3,4-Dihydroxyphenylbutylamine; 3,4-Dihydroxyphenylpropylamine; 3,4-Dihydroxyphenylbenzylamine; d-Norepinephrine; 3-Methoxy, 4-hydroxyphenylethylamine; 3-Hydroxy, 4-methoxyphenylethylamine; L-DOPA; (±)-Amphetamine; Amantadine.

*Maximum stimulation above basal cyclic AMP production is expressed as a percentage of that obtained with 100μM dopamine, with 1mM drug concentration.

**EC50 is the drug concentration needed to produce 50% of the maximum effect observed with 100μM dopamine.

D. Piribedil and its metabolite S584

Piribedil is a non-catechol analogue of dopamine, and was found to be inactive in stimulating cyclic AMP formation in concentrations up to 0.1 mM. The catechol metabolite of this drug, however, S-584, was highly effective in the test system, and was approximately

TABLE 2

EFFECT OF β-NAPHTHYLAMINE ANALOGUES ON
RAT STRIATAL CYCLIC AMP PRODUCTION

Compound	Maximum stimulation % of dopamine	EC50-μMolar
2-amino-6,7-dihydroxy-(1,2,3,4) tetrahydronaphthalene	115	4.0
2-amino-1,2,3,4-tetrahydronaphthalene	–	–

equipotent with dopamine (17). This finding suggests
that the long-lasting dopamine-like effects of piribedil
observed *in vivo* may be mediated through the production
of active catechol metabolites such as S-584, which is
known to be an important urinary metabolite of the
parent drug in man and rat (23-24). The simpler analogue
of S584, 1-(3,4-dihydroxyphenyl)-piperazine was also
active, with a potency comparable to that of dopamine in
stimulating cyclic-AMP formation.

E. (-)-Apomorphine and related compounds

(-)-Apomorphine stimulates striatal adenylate
cyclase at low concentrations but is inhibitory at
higher concentrations (9,19). It has been found that (+)-
apomorphine possesses only inhibitory effects (25).
Of various other aporphines tested only (±)-N-n-propyl-
norapomorphine possessed any stimulatory activity
(Miller, Kelly and Neumeyer - unpublished). Lal et al.,
(26) have shown that both apocodeine and 10,11-

methylenedioxy-apomorphine have some ability to elicit stereotyped behaviour in rats. It is possible that the in vivo activity of these compounds is due to metabolic conversion to apomorphine in a similar manner to that suggested above for ET 495 and its metabolite S584. Several aporphines when tested at 10^{-5}M had some ability to inhibit the stimulation produced by dopamine. (+)-Bulbocapnine was the most potent in this respect; it acted as a competitive inhibitor with a Ki of 1.6×10^{-7}M. The dopamine blocking effects of bulbocapnine found in these experiments agree with the known ability of the alkaloid to produce catalepsy in animals either when given peripherally (27) or when injected directly into the striatum (28). The Ki value of 1.6×10^{-7}M indicates that bulbocapnine is not as potent a dopaminergic antagonist as some of the conventional neuroleptics, and in accordance with this it is somewhat less potent than chlorpromazine as a neuroleptic agent (27).

F. Topography of the dopamine receptor

Sheppard and Burghardt (25,29) have also tested a number of dopamine analogues on the striatal adenylate cyclase and have reported findings similar to those described here. It is of interest that in two other dopamine sensitive preparations a similar spectrum of agonist activity has also been observed, namely in the renal artery of the dog, (4) and in neurones of the snail Helix aspersa (30). In all of these systems the structure activity relations for agonists are quite distinct from those of classical α- or β-adrenoceptors. In each case epinine was found to be equipotent with dopamine. For agonists there is an absolute requirement for a catechol grouping and a two carbon side chain attached to an amino group. Among rigid analogues of dopamine, in which the side chain is incorporated into a second ring system, the compounds with the greatest potency are those in which the dopamine side chain is in the fully extended form, as in ADTN and apomorphine. This suggests the fully extended _trans_ form of the dopamine side chain is the preferred conformation of the molecule on interaction with the dopamine-sensitive adenylate cyclase (19,25,29, 31,32). This suggestion also supports the hypothesis of Horn and Snyder (33) that the preferred conformation of dopamine at its receptor site is the fully extended _trans_ form, which can be superimposed on the X-ray crystallographic structure of chlorpromazine, hence accounting possibly for the receptor blocking activity of the latter compound

III. NEUROLEPTIC DRUGS AS ANTAGONISTS OF DOPAMINE-SENSITIVE CYCLIC-AMP FORMATION IN STRIATAL HOMOGENATES

A number of neuroleptics and other drugs have been examined as antagonists of the dopamine-stimulated adenylate cyclase in rat striatal homogenates (Table 3). In these studies a constant concentration of 100µM dopamine was used to ensure maximum stimulation. Assuming competitive antagonism as the prevalent mode of inhibition (11,18) it was possible to calculate Ki values for each compound from the graphically determined IC50 values (drug concentration producing 50% inhibition of dopamine-stimulated cyclic-AMP formation) as described by Clement-Cormier et al., (11). The results reported by Clement-Cormier et al., (11) (see also accompanying chapter by Greengard), by Brown and Makman (9) and by Karobath and Leitich (34) from similar experiments are largely in accordance with our own.

STRUCTURE-ACTIVITY RELATIONSHIPS

A. Phenothiazines

Among the phenothiazines tested there was good agreement between the potency of drugs as inhibitors of the dopamine-stimulated adenylate cyclase and their known <u>in vivo</u> potencies as neuroleptics. Thus for example, among the phenothiazines (Fig.2,3) the potent neuroleptics fluphenazine and trifluoperazine were the most active, while promazine and promethazine, which have only very weak neuroleptic activity were several orders of magnitude less potent as antagonists of the dopamine-sensitive adenylate cyclase (Table 3). The 7-hydroxy and N-desmethyl metabolites of chlorpromazine retained substantial inhibitory activity in the cyclase test system, while the N-oxide and sulphoxide were inactive (Table 4) (16). These findings are in agreement with the activity of these compounds in accelerating dopamine turnover in the intact brain (3)

B. Thioxanthenes

The thioxanthenes are an interesting group of neuroleptic drugs in which a double bond connects the side chain to the heterocyclic nucleus (Fig.2). Because of the presence of a 2-substituent they exhibit geometric cis/trans isomerism. The relative effects of the different isomeric forms of flupenthixol, clopenthixol and chlorprothixene are shown in Fig.4. In each case the α-isomer was considerably more potent than the β-isomer in antagonising the effects of dopamine on adenylate cyclase activity. This was particularly marked with α- and β-flupenthixol. The activity of flupenthixol in the mixed αβ-form used clinically appears to be entirely due to a α-isomer. These findings agree well with the

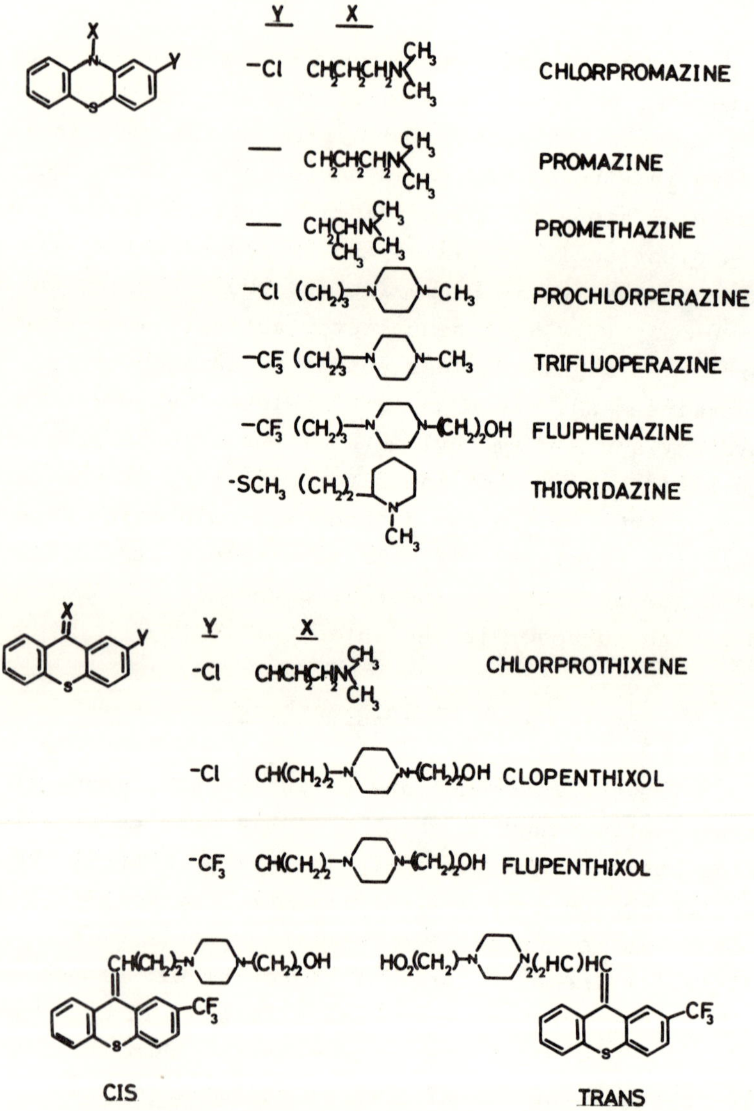

Fig. 2. Structures of some neuroleptic drugs.

reported neuropharmacological properties of these drugs Moller-Nielsen et al (35) showed that α-flupenthixol was very considerably more potent than β-flupenthixol in

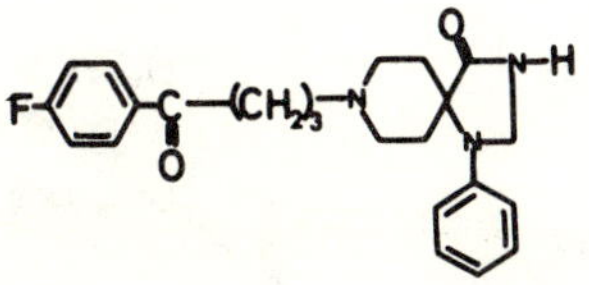

STRUCTURE-ACTIVITY RELATIONSHIPS

SPIROPERIDOL

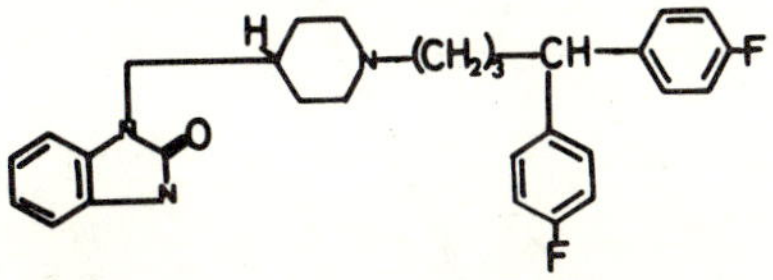

PIMOZIDE

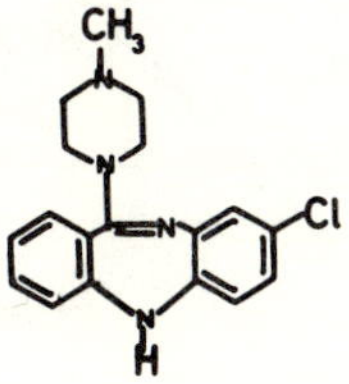

CLOZAPINE

Fig. 2. (continued).

various animal tests for neuroleptic activity, and more potent than clopenthixol and chlorprothixene. It is known from X-ray and n.m.r. analysis (36-39) that the pharmacologically more active α-isomers of the thioxanthenes have the cis configuration; i.e. the 2-substituent and the amine side chain are on the same side of the double bond linking the side chain to the ring system (Fig.2).

The results obtained with the biochemical test system are consistent with the known structure-activity rules for neuroleptic activity in both phenothiazines and thioxanthenes, (40,41). A 2-substituent is of critical importance (Fig.2), and the most potent compounds (fluphenazine, trifluoperazine and flupenthixol) are those having a CF_3 substituent in this position. The highest potency both in in vivo tests and in the present system was also found in compounds having a β-hydroxyethylpiperazinyl side chain (fluphenazine, flupenthixol).

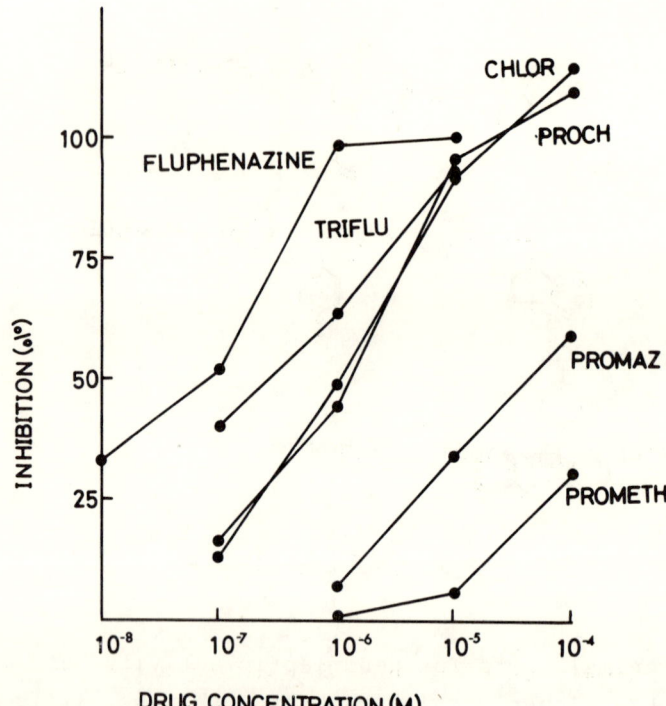

Fig.3. Effect of phenothiazines on dopamine stimulated cyclic AMP production in striatal homogenates. Basal level of cyclic AMP production was 45.5 ± 3.6 pmol per sample (2mg wet weight) and stimulated (100μM dopamine) was 88.7 ± 9.1 pmol per sample. (Means $\pm$ S.E. for 6 experiments). Each point is the mean of at least five separate incubations; standard errors were less than $\pm$ 10% of means. At 10^{-4}M some drugs inhibited basal cyclic AMP production, this is represented as an inhibition of more than 100%.

It was of interest that the tricyclic antidepressant chlorimipramine, which differs from chlorpromazine only in having a dimethylene bridge instead of a sulphur atom in the heterocyclic ring, had about one tenth of the

TABLE 3
Inhibition of Dopamine-Stimulated Adenylate Cyclase by Neuroleptic Drugs

Drug	Inhibition Constant Ki - nM*
α-Flupenthixol	1.0
αβ-Flupenthixol	3.5
Fluphenazine	4.3
(+)-Butaclamol	8.8
α-Clopenthixol	16.0
Trifluoperazine	19.0
α-Chlorprothixene	37.0
Chlorpromazine	48.0
Spiroperidol	95.0
Prochlorperazine	100.0
Thioridazine	130.0
Pimozide	140.0
(+)-Bulbocapnine	160.0
Chlorimipramine	420.0
β-Chlorprothixene	950.0

Compounds lacking neuroleptic activity and with Ki values > 1000 nM:-** Promazine, β-Clopenthixol, Morphine, β-Flupenthixol, (-)-Butaclamol, Promethazine, Benztropine, Desipramine, Ethopropazine, Diethazine, Mezapine, Fenethazine, Chlorpromazine sulphoxide, Pyrathiazine, Diphenhydramine, Methdilazine, Pentolamine, Propranolol, Prostaglandin E_1, dl-Amphetamine, Amantadine.

*Ki values calculated from IC50 values determined graphically as in Figure 3. Values from (18).
**Data from references (8) (11) (18) and (34).

TABLE 4

Inhibition of Dopamine Sensitive Adenylate
Cyclase by Metabolites of Chlorpromazine

Metabolite	Ki nM
Chlorpromazine	48
Desmethyl Chlorpromazine	270
Bisdesmethylchlorpromazine	510
7-Hydroxy Chlorpromazine	600
Chlorpromazine Nitroxide	2220
Chlorpromazine Sulphoxide	7500

potency of chlorpromazine. Phenothiazines which lack neuroleptic activity, and various other drugs such as benztropine, morphine and desipramine are relatively ineffective as inhibitors of the dopamine-sensitive adenylate cyclase (Table 3).

C. Butyrophenones

Neuroleptic drugs of the butyrophenone class, such as spiroperidol and pimozide were active in the present test system, although their potencies in the biochemical experiments were low in view of the very high potencies reported for these compounds as dopaminergic antagonists in whole animal experiments and clinically. Thus pimozide and spiroperidol, which are many times more potent than chlorpromazine in vivo, were 2-3 times less active than chlorpromazine in the in vitro tests. This appears to be the most serious discrepancy at the moment between results obtained using the dopamine-sensitive adenylate cyclase and those obtained from in vivo studies.

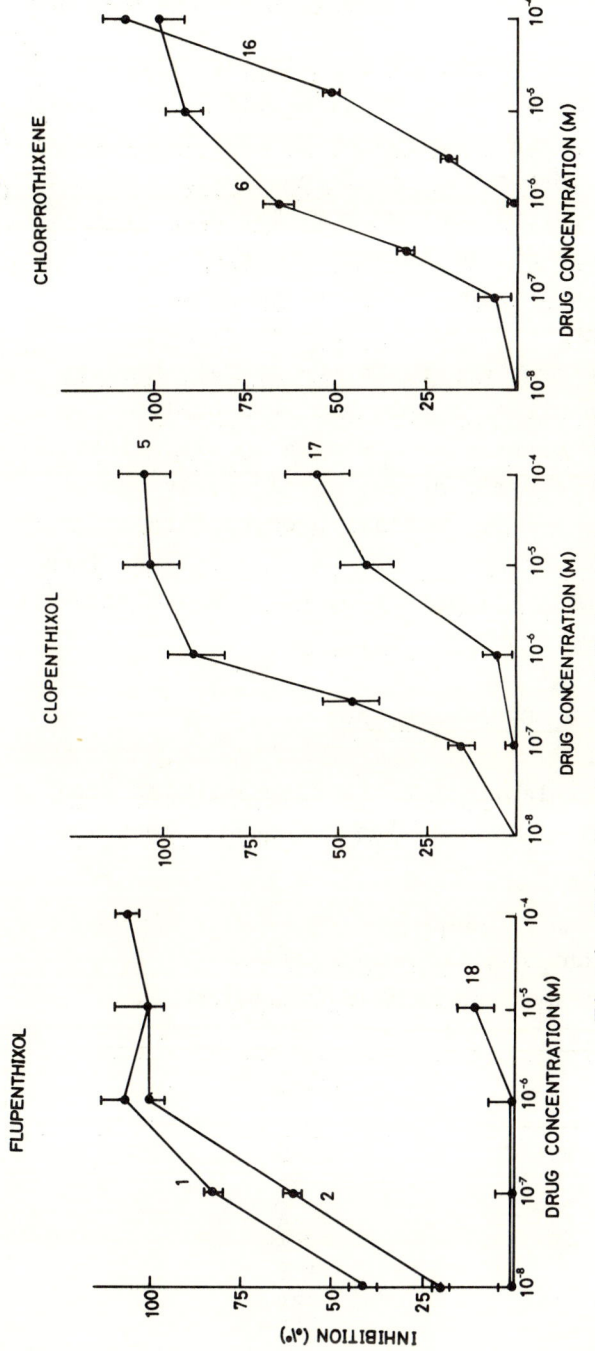

Fig.4. Effect of α- and β-isomers of thioxanthenes on dopamine stimulated cyclic AMP production in striatal homogenates. Basal levels of cyclic AMP were 33.0 pmol per sample (2mg wet weight) and stimulated levels (100μM DA) 69.0 pmol per sample. Each point is the mean ± S.E.M. for at least five separate incubations

This discrepancy cannot be explained, although there are various possible reasons for it which should be carefully examined before rejecting the hypothesis that neuroleptic potency correlates closely with anti-dopaminergic potency as measured by the present test system. The high in vivo potency of these drugs may be related to their differential distribution in the CNS after in vivo administration. In the case of pimozide a selective concentration of the drug occurs in the caudate nucleus after systemic administration (42) and this could account for the high potency of the drug in vivo. The possibility that neuroleptic drugs, particularly those of the butyrophenone series, may act presynaptically by blocking impulse conduction and transmitter release from dopaminergic terminals, however, remains as an alternative explanation for these findings (43-45).

D. Dibenzazepines

A series of neuroleptics of the dibenzazepine class has also been tested (Table 5). The compounds clozapine,

TABLE 5

Inhibition of Dopamine Sensitive Adenylate Cyclase by Dibenzazepines

Compound	K_i - nM
HF 2046 (cis analogue CLZ)	18
Clothiapine	25
Loxapine	45
Clozapine	170
Perlapine	480

clothiapine, and loxapine are of known anti-psychotic efficacy, and were effective as inhibitors of the dopamine-stimulated adenylate cyclase. The drug clozapine proved to be a competitive inhibitor (Fig.5), although its potency was less than that of chlorpromazine. The substance HF 2046, which is equivalent to the "cis" analogue of clozapine, in that the basic substituent and the halogen are oriented to the same side of the molecule, was almost ten times more potent than clozapine. Perlapine, which is an analogue lacking the halogen substituent and with no detectable anti-psychotic effects, was only weakly active as an inhibitor. The failure of clozapine to react positively in several whole animal tests for anti-dopaminergic properties (46) is thus not in agreement with our in vitro findings, which suggest that this drug is a dopamine antagonist, albeit with only modest potency. The reasons for the negative findings in whole animal experiments are discussed further below.

E. Butaclamol

That the effects of drugs as inhibitors of the dopamine-sensitive adenylate cyclase do have predictive value in assessing neuroleptic activity, however, is shown by our more recent findings with a newly described neuroleptic drug, butaclamol (47-48). This compound is unique among the neuroleptics in possessing assymetric carbon atoms, and thus exhibiting stereoisomersim (Fig.6). In animal tests only the (+) enantiomer possesses neuroleptic activity, and when the enantiomers were tested at concentrations up to 10μM only the (+) enantiomer was active as an inhibitor of the dopamine-stimulated formation of cyclic AMP (Fig.6) (49). The

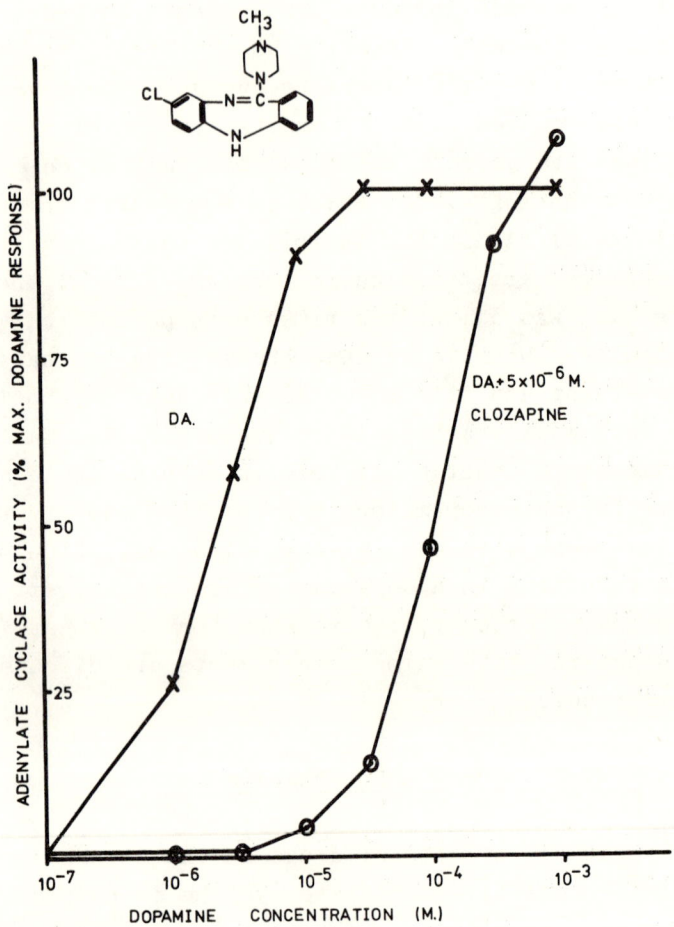

Fig.5. Stimulation of adenylate cyclase in rat striatal homogenates by dopamine in the presence and absence of clozapine (5×10^{-6}M). Each point is the mean of four separate incubations. Mean basal levels were 31.3 pmol cyclic AMP (2mg wet weight) and maximally stimulated levels 58.8 pmol cyclic AMP (2mg wet weight). The parallel shift to the right of the dose response curve induced by clozapine indicates a competitive mode of inhibition by this drug.

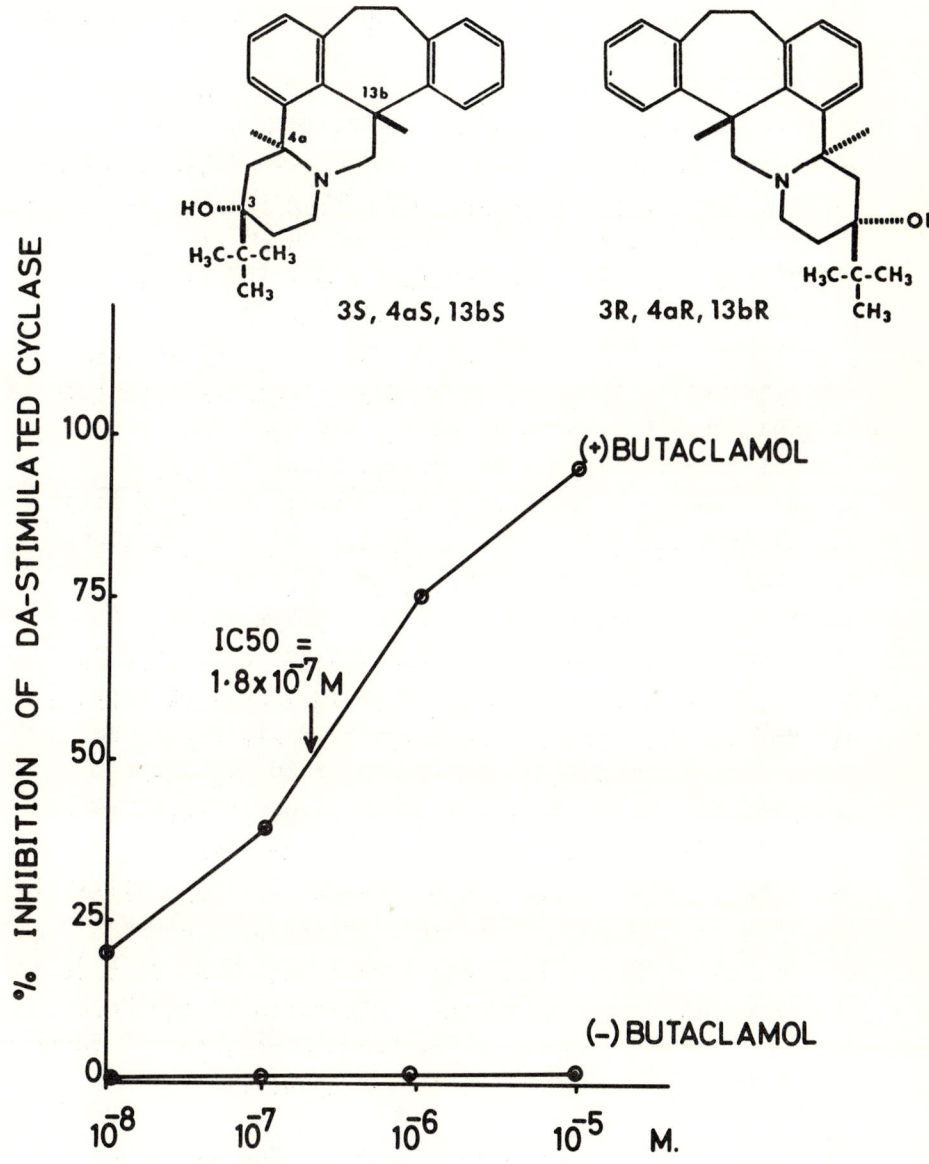

Fig.6. The inhibition by various concentrations of (+)- and (-) enantiomers of butaclamol of the stimulation of striatal adenylate cyclase by 10^{-4}M dopamine. Each point is the mean of five separate incubations.

(+)-enantiomer proved to be an effective competitive inhibitor, with a Ki value of approximately 10^{-8}M, making it one of the four most potent compounds examined so far. Similar findings have been reported for the effects of (+) and (-) butaclamol on the dopamine-stimulated adenylate cyclase in homogenates of rat olfactory tubercle (48). The active and inactive enantiomers of butaclamol are clearly of considerable pharmacological interest as research tools for studies of dopaminergic systems in brain. The compounds are also of interest from a structural point of view in several respects. Chemically butaclamol resembles more closely the tricyclic antidepressants than conventional neuroleptic drugs. Butaclamol also lacks the 2-substituent characteristic of most other active neuroleptics. Unlike other neuroleptics, the nitrogen containing portion of the molecule is locked in a rigid system, and the presence of three asymmetric carbons gives rise to optical isomerism. As in other potent neuroleptics, however, there is a hydroxyl "tail" to the molecule. On the basis of our studies of other neuroleptic drug structures we suggest that the critical distance in butaclamol for dopamine receptor blockade may be that from the nitrogen atom to the most distant benzene ring, since molecular model building indicates that the distance to the other benzene ring is too short to be compatible with effective antagonism.

IV. EFFECTS OF NEUROLEPTIC DRUGS ON OTHER TRANSMITTER AND HORMONE RECEPTORS

In addition to their effects as dopamine antagonists various neuroleptic drugs also inhibit a variety of other transmitter and hormone-sensitive cyclases, although there is little evidence that such effects correlate with neuroleptic activity (50-51). The α-adrenoceptor blocking actions of chlorpromazine and related drugs are well known. We have found that chlorpromazine antagonizes the stimulating actions of l-norepinephrine on adenylate cyclase activity in cell membrane fragments from rat adipose cells, a response mediated by β-adrenoceptors (52) The inhibition caused by chlorpromazine proved to be competitive with norepinephrine, indicating that chlorpromazine probably has some affinity for binding to β-adrenoceptors, although the affinity is far less than that for the dopamine-sensitive adenylate cyclase in brain. In addition the effects of norepinephrine in adipocytes could be weakly inhibited by haloperidol and by α and β-flupenthixol. The α- and β-isomers of flupenthixol were approximately equipotent in this test system, in contrast to their widely different neuroleptic potencies. Chlorpromazine also partially antagonized the activation of adenylate cyclase by glucagon in a rat liver plasma membrane preparation (53). To antagonize the effects of glucagon in this preparation, however, relatively high concentrations of chlorpromazine were required (IC50 10^{-4}M). In contrast to the effects of chlorpromazine on catecholamine-sensitive adenylate cyclase, the effects of chlorpromazine on the glucagon activated system proved to be non-competitive with respect to the peptide hormone. It has been shown that certain detergents can destroy the gluacagon sensitivity of adenylate cyclase in liver membranes (54) without affecting basal enzyme activity. The effects of chlorpromazine reported here may be of similar origin.

The effects of certain neuroleptic drugs as antagonists at muscarinic cholinergic receptors are extremely potent, and may contribute importantly to the neuropharmacological profiles of such drugs (55-58). Miller and Hiley (59) and Snyder et al., (60) tested various neuroleptic drugs as muscarinic antagonists, using recently developed in vitro assays which depend on measurements of the binding of radioactively labelled muscarinic receptors ligands. Miller and Hiley measured the atropine-sensitive component of the binding of ^{3}H-N-propyl-benzilylcholine mustard to membrane fragments in homogenates of rat cerebral cortex as the test system (61). The results with neuroleptic drugs and related substances (Table 6) showed that neuroleptics exhibit a wide range of antimuscarinic potencies. Very similar results were reported by Snyder et al., (60). The most potent anticholinergic compounds were thioridazine and clozapine, followed by chlorpromazine, whereas flupenthixol, trifluoperazine, pimozide and spiroperidol were relatively weak anticholinergics. If one expresses the results in terms of the ratio of anticholinergic to anti-dopaminergic potencies, the neuroleptics span a wide range from those such as thioridazine and clozapine which are considerably more potent as anti-cholinergics than as anti-dopaminergics, to flupenthixol and spiroperidol which show the converse properties (Table 6). We believe that these results may have an important bearing on the neuropharmacological properties of individual neuroleptic drugs. In particular the low incidence of Parkinson-like side effects seen with drugs such as clozapine and thioridazine (62-64) could be related to the fact that such compounds carry a built in anti-cholinergic activity, which may prevent them from manifesting extrapyramidal side effects as a consequence of their anti-dopamine effects (55). On the other hand potent anti-dopamine agents which are weak anti-

STRUCTURE-ACTIVITY RELATIONSHIPS

TABLE 6

Relative Potencies of Drugs as Muscarinic or Dopamine Antagonists

Compound	Dissociation Constant for binding to receptor sites-nM		Ratio of Cholinergic: Dopaminergic Potency
	Muscarinic	Dopaminergic	
Atropine	0.5	–	
Benztropine	1.3	–	
Ethopropazine	10.0	–	
Thioridazine	25.0	130	5.2
Clozapine	55.0	170	3.1
Pimozide	160.0	140	0.87
Chlorpromazine	350.0	48	0.14
α-Flupenthixol	2200.0	1	0.0005
Trifluoperazine	4000.0	19	0.005
Spiroperidol	12000.0	95	0.008

cholinergics, such as spiroperidol, haloperidol, flupenthixol and fluphenazine are known to induce extrapyramidal side effects much more frequently. The anticholinergic properties of clozapine and thioridazine may also obscure the effects of these compounds as dopamine antagonists in many of the animal behavioural and biochemical tests used to assess neuroleptic agents. For example, thioridazine and clozapine do not antagonize the behavioural effects of amphetamine, either in intact animals or in animals with unilateral lesions of the nigro-striatal pathway. This has led some authors to suggest that these drugs lack dopamine-antagonist properties, and that they are thus exceptions to the "dopamine antagonist" hypothesis of neuroleptic activity (46,65,66). Miller and Sahakian (67), however, were able to show that clozapine and thioridazine can act as antagonists of the locomotor stimulation induced by amphetamine if tested in 11 day old rats; in such animals the cholinergic systems of the basal ganglia are not fully developed (68), so that the anticholinergic properties of the drugs do not obscure their anti-dopamine properties. Thioridazine and clozapine clearly do have anti-dopamine properties on the dopamine adenylate cyclase system and it seems more parsimonious to propose that their anomalous behaviour in standard tests for anti-dopaminergic properties points to weaknesses in the design of such whole animal tests, rather than to any weakness in the hypothesis concerning their mode of action as neuroleptics.

V. PRESYNAPTIC ACTIONS OF DOPAMINERGIC DRUGS

It is well known that dopaminergic agonists cause a slowing of dopamine turnover in the nigrostriatal pathway <u>in vivo</u>, and that dopaminergic antagonist drugs cause an acceleration (3). At least part of these effects persist after impulse traffic in the nigrostriatal neurones is abolished, either by acute lesions, or after administration of γ-hydroxybutyric acid (69,70), suggesting that these actions may be mediated in part by drug interactions locally at the presynaptic dopamine-containing nerve terminals. We have recently examined the model described by Christiansen and Squires (71-72). They described an inhibitory effect of apomorphine on the rate of hydroxylation of ^{3}H-L-tyrosine by intact synaptosomes from rat striatum (73-74). We were able to repeat these findings, and found that apomorphine is indeed a potent inhibitor of tyrosine hydroxylation in intact synaptosomes (Fig.7). In this system the rate of conversion of ^{3}H-tyrosine to tritiated catechoalmines is measured in a crude synaptosome preparation from rat

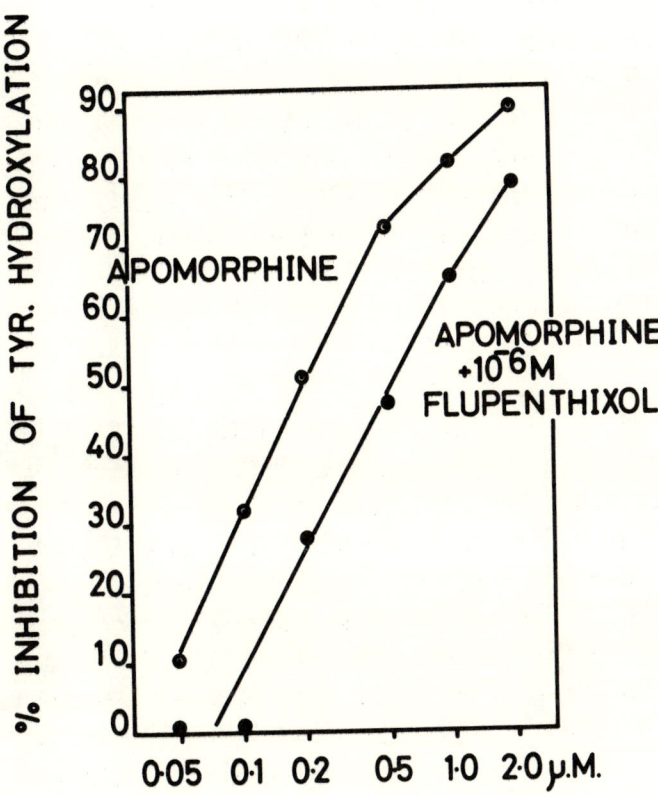

Fig.7. Inhibition of tyrosine hydroxylation in intact synaptosomes from rat striatum by apomorphine in the presence or absence of 1μM α-flupenthixol. Resuspended crude mitochondrial fraction was incubated for 10 min with L-^{3}H-tyrosine (5μM) and ^{3}H-catechols were isolated by absorption on alumina. Each point is the mean of 3-6 determinations.

striatum incubated in Krebs-Ringer phosphate medium with no added pteridine cofactor. Under these conditions apomorphine inhibited the reaction with an IC50 of 0.2μM. If the synaptosomes were lysed, and free tyrosine hydroxylase assayed in the presence of added biopterin cofactor, apomorphine again inhibited the reaction but much higher concentrations were required (IC50 approximately 10μM). The inhibitory effects of apomorphine on tyrosine hydroxylation in intact synaptosomes do not seem to be related to an uptake and accumulation of this catechol substance by the particles, since its inhibitory effects were unaffected by the presence of an inhibitor of dopamine uptake sites, benztropine (2μM). This suggests that the inhibition of tyrosine hydroxylation in intact synaptosomes particles by apomorphine may reflect an action on presynaptic dopamine receptors. Further support for this notion is derived from the finding that the inhibitory effects of apomorphine in this system can be partly reversed by neuroleptic drugs (71-72). Like these authors, however, we found that a maximum reversal of the apomorphine effect of only about 50% was attainable under the present experimental conditions, making it difficult to assess quantitatively the relative potencies of different neuroleptic drugs in this test system. However, preliminary results indicate that α-flupenthixol was considerably more potent than β-flupenthixol and that spiroperidol and haloperidol were potent inhibitors. These findings are particularly interesting in view of the results reported by Seeman and his colleagues (43,45) who found that various neuroleptic drugs had potent effects on presynaptic sites in dopaminergic nerve terminals. Certainly the existence of such pharmacological mechanisms should make us hesitant at this stage to ascribe all the actions of neuroleptic

STRUCTURE-ACTIVITY RELATIONSHIPS

drugs to a single post-synaptic mechanism, such as the dopamine-sensitive adenylate cyclase system. It may be that the "anti-dopamine" actions of neuroleptic drugs are achieved by various combinations of post-synaptic and pre-synaptic effects, and the relative importance of these effects may vary from one neuroleptic, or class of neuroleptics, to another.

VI. EFFECTS OF INTRACEREBRAL INJECTION OF CHOLERA TOXIN

The enterotoxin from <u>Vibro cholerae</u> (choleragen) has been shown to have the property of activating the enzyme adenylate cyclase in all cell systems in which it has been tested, and in consequence it has been shown to activate cyclic AMP mediated processes in all these systems (75). Progress has been made in identifying the receptor for the toxin, which is probably the GM_1 gangliosides on the cell surface (76). After binding of the toxin to the cell surface there is a characteristic lag period lasting several hours before adenylate cyclase activation occurs. In order to examine the hypothesis that dopaminergic transmission in the CNS is mediated by cyclic AMP we have attempted to mimic some behavioural effects of dopamine receptor stimulation with cholera toxin.

It is known that bilateral injections of dopamine into the nucleus accumbens area in the rat brain causes a transient stimulation of locomotor activity (77). We injected choleragen (1µg) bilaterally into the nucleus accumbens of rat and observed its effect on locomotor activity. During the first two hours after the injection rats treated with vehicle or toxin showed no difference in their locomotor activity. During the third and fourth hour the toxin treated animals showed increased locomotor

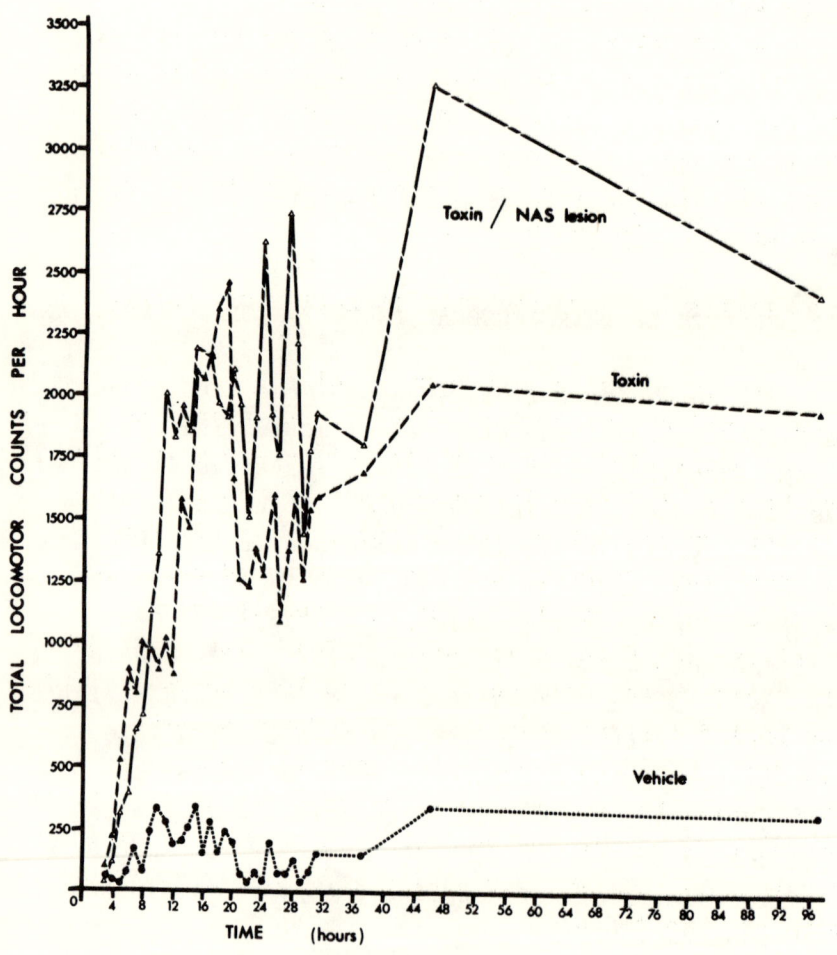

Fig.8. Effect of choleragen on locomotor activity in rats. Rats were prepared with cannullae bilaterally in the nucleus accumbens. Some animals had previously had the dopamine terminals in the nucleus accumbens destroyed by injection of 6-OH dopamine. Rats (n = 6) received either vehicle (1µl), toxin (1µg/1µl), or toxin (1µg/1µl) after 6-OH DA treatment (NAS lesion). (R.J. Miller and P. Kelly - unpublished).

activity. This stimulation became even more pronounced over the subsequent time period, and at twelve hours toxin treated animals showed an approximately 10-fold increase in locomotor activity. This is comparable to the stimulation seen on injecting dopamine into the same area (77). However, in contrast to the effects of dopamine the effects of choleragen were very long lasting. Increased locomotor activity was still observed in the toxin treated animals up to twelve days after the injection. Assay of the adenylate cyclase activity in the nucleus accumbens area of toxin treated rats showed that there was also a lag period before this became activated. There was no significant activation at 90 min but there was an approximately 4-fold increase after 5 hours. The enzyme was even further increased at 22 and 48 hours.

In view of recent reports that cyclic AMP can activate tyrosine hydroxylase in pre-synaptic dopamine terminals (78), we also injected toxin into rats where these terminals had been destroyed in the nucleus accumbens by previous injection of 6-hydroxydopamine. The behavioural response to toxin in these animals was the same as that in animals not pretreated with 6-hydroxydopamine. These preliminary findings suggest that choleragen may be a useful tool for investigation of cyclic AMP mediated processes in the central nervous system.

REFERENCES

(1). S. Matthysse, Fed. Proc., $\underline{32}$,1970, 200-205.

(2). S.H. Snyder, S.P. Banarjee, H.I. Yamamura and D. Greenberg, Science, $\underline{184}$, 1974a, 1243-1253.

(3). G. Sedvall, Receptor feedback and dopamine turnover in the central nervous system. In Handbook of Psychopharmacology, Ed. L. Iversen, S. Iversen and S. Snyder, Plenum Publishing Corp. New York (in press).

(4). L.I. Goldberg, P.F. Sonneville and J.I. McNay, Pharmac. exp. Ther., 163, 1968, 188-197.

(5). L.I. Goldberg, Advances in Neurology, 9, Ed. D.B. Calne, Raven Press, New York (in press).

(6). P. Greengard, D.A. McAfee and J.W. Kebabian, In Advances in cyclic nucleotide research, Vol. 1, Ed. P. Greengard and G.A. Robinson, Raven Press, New York 337-357, 1972.

(7). J.H. Brown and M.H. Makman, Proc. Nat. Acad. Sci. US. 69, 1972, 539-543.

(8). J.H. Brown and M.H. Makman, J. Neurochem. 21, 1973, 477-479.

(9). J.W. Kebabian, G.L. Petzold and P. Greengard, Proc. Nat. Acad. Sci. US, 68, 1972, 2145-2149.

(10). A.S. Horn, A.C. Cuello and R.J. Miller, J. Neurochem. 22, 1974, 265-270.

(11). Y.C. Clement-Cormier, H.W. Kebabian, G.L. Petzold and P. Greengard, Proc. Nat. Acad. Sci. US. 71, 1974, 1113-1117.

(12). P.F. Von Voigtlander, S.J. Boukma and G.A. Johnson, Neuropharmacology, 12, 1973, 1081-1086.

(13). R.K. Mishra, E.L. Gardner, R. Katzman and M.H. Makman, Proc. Nat. Acad. Sci. US. 71, 1974, 3883-3887.

(14). B. Weiss and E. Costa, J.Pharmac. exp. Ther. 161, 1968, 310-319.

(15). B.J. Hoffer, G.R. Siggins, A.P. Oliver, and F.E. Bloom, In "Advances in cyclic nucleotide research" Vol.1, Ed. by P. Greengard and G.A. Robinson, Raven Press, New York 411-432, 1972.

(16). R.J. Miller and L.L. Iversen, J. Pharm. Pharmac., 26, 1974, 142-144.

(17). R.J. Miller and L.L. Iversen, N.S. Archiv. Pharmac. 282, 1974, 213-216.

(18). R.J. Miller, A.S. Horn and L.L. Iversen, Molec. Pharmac., 10, 1974, 759-766.

(19). R.J. Miller, A.S. Horn, L.L. Iversen and R.M. Pinder, Nature, 250, 1974, 238-240.

(20). R.J. Miller, A.S. Horn and L.L. Iversen, In Brain c-AMP and drugs acting on the CNS, Ed. E. Costa, Proceedings of IX Congress Collegium Internationale Neuropharmacologicum, Excerpta Medica Congress Series (in press).

(21). J. Glowinski and L.L. Iversen, J. Neurochem. 13, 1966, 655-669.

(22). B.L. Brown, R.D. Ekins and J.D.M. Albano, In "Advances in cyclic nucleotide research", Vol. 2 Ed. P. Greengard and G.A. Robinson, Raven Press, New York 25-40, 1972.

(23). P. Jenner, A.R. Taylor and D.B. Campbell, J. Pharm. Pharmac., 25, 1973, 749-750.

(24). D.B. Campbell, P. Jenner and A.R. Taylor, In "Advances in Neurology", Vol. 3 Ed. D.B. Calne, Raven Press, New York, 199-213, 1974.

(25). H. Sheppard, In Brain c-AMP and drugs acting on the CNS, Ed. E. Costa, Proceedings of IX Congress Collegium Internationale Neuropshychopharmacologicum, Excerpta Medica Congress Series (in press).

(26). S. Lal, T. Soukes, K. Missala and G. Belendick, Eur. J. Pharmac., 20, 1972, 71-79.

(27). B. Costall and R.J. Naylor, Psychopharmacology, 32, 1973, 161-170.

(28). F. Tseng, E. Wei and H. Loh, Eur. J. Pharmac, 22, 263-366.

(29). H. Sheppard and C.R. Burghardt, Res. Commun. Chem. Path. Pharmac., 8, 1974, 527-534.

(30). G.N. Woodruff and R.J. Walker, Int. J. Neuropharmac. 8, 1969, 279-286.

(31). R.F. Recker, D.J.C. Engel and G.G. Nys, J. Pharm. Pharmac., 24, 1973, 589-591.

(32). J.G. Cannon, In "Advances in Neurology, 9, Ed. D.B. Calne, Raven Press, New York (in press).

(33). A.S. Horn and S.H. Snyder, Proc. Nat. Acad. Sci. US. 68, 1971, 2325-2328.

(34). M. Karobath and H. Leitich, Proc. Nat. Acad. Sci. US. 71, 1974, 2915-2918.

(35). I. Moller-Nielsen, V. Pedersen, M. Nymak, K.F. Franc, U. Boek, B. Fjallan and A.V. Christiansen, Acta Pharmac. Toxicol. 33, 1973, 353-362.

(36). J.D. Dunitz, H. Eser and P. Strickler, Helv. Chim. Acta, 47, 1964, 1897-1902.

(37). J.P. Schaefer, Chem. Comm. 1967, 743-744.

(38). M.L. Post, O. Kennard and A.S. Horn, Acta Cryst. B. 30, 1974, 1644-1646.

(39). C. Kaiser, R.J. Warren and C.L. Zirkle, J. Med. Chem. 17, 1974, 131-133.

(40). C.L. Zirkle and C. Kaiser, In "Medicinal Chemistry" Vol. II, pp. 1420-1469, Ed. A. Burger, Wiley Interscience, New York, 1970.

(41). P.V. Petersen and I. Moller-Nielsen, In " Psychopharmacological Agents", Vol. 1 pp.301-324, Ed. M. Gordon, Academic Press, New York, 1964.

(42). W. Soudijn and I. van Wijngaarden, J. Pharm. Pharmac. 24, 1972, 773-780.

(43). P. Seeman, Pharmac. Rev., 24, 1972, 583-655.

(44). P. Seeman and T. Lee, J. Pharmac. exp. Ther. 190, 1974, 131-140.

(45). P. Seeman and T. Lee, In "Antipsychotic drugs, pharmacodynamics and pharmacokinetics", Ed. G. Sedvall, Wenner-Gren International Center Symposia, Pergamon Press, Oxford (in press).

(46). G. Stille and H. Hippius, Neuropsychopharmacol., 4, 1971, 182-191.

(47). L.G. Humber and F. Bruderlein, In American Chemical Society 167th ACS National Meeting, Division of Medicinal Chemistry, Abstract No.5, 1974.

(48). W. Lippman, T. Pugsley and J. Merker, Life Sci. (in press).

(49). R.J. Miller, A.S. Horn and L.L. Iversen, submitted for publication.

(50). J. Wolff and A.B. Jones, Proc. Nat. Acad. Sci. US. 65, 1970, 454-459.

(51). C.A. Free, V.S. Park and J.D. Shada, In The Phenothiazines and Related Drugs, Ed. O.S. Forrest, C.J. Carr and E. Usdin, Raven Press, New York, pp. 739-748, 1974.

(52). L. Birnbaumer and M. Rodbell, J. Biol. Chem. 244, 1969, 3477-3482.

(53). S.L. Pohl, L. Birnbaumer and M. Rodbell, J. Biol. Chem., 246, 1971, 1849-1856.

(54). P. Cuatrecasas, Ann. Rev. Biochem., 43, 1974, 169-214.

(55). E.L. Schelkunov, Activit. nerv. sup. 9, 1967, 207-217.

(56). N.E. Anden, J. Pharm. Pharmac. 24, 1972, 905-906.

(57). N.E. Anden, J. Pharm. Pharmac. 25, 1973, 346-348.

(58). N.E. Anden and P. Bedard, J. Pharm. Pharmac. 23, 1971, 460-462.

(59). R.J. Miller and C.R. Hiley, Nature 248, 1974, 596-577.

(60). S.H. Snyder, D. Greenberg and H. Yamamura, Archiv. Gen. Psychiat. 31, 1974, 58-61.

(61). A.S.V. Burgen and J.M. Young, Brit. J. Pharmac., 51, 1974, 279-285.

(62). J.O. Cole and D.J. Clyde, Rev. Canad. de Biol. 10, 1961, 565-574.

(63). R.I. Shader and A. Di Mascio, Psychotropic drug side effects, Williams and Wilkins Co., Baltimore, 1970.

(64). J. Angst, D. Bente, P. Berner, H. Heiman, H. Helmchen and H. Hippius, Pharmakopsychiat. 4, 1971, 201-211.

(65). T.J. Crow and C. Gillbe, Nature, 245, 1973, 27-28.

(66). A.C. Sayers, H.R. Burki, W. Ruch and H. Asper, Psychopharmac., (in press).

(67). R.J. Miller and B. Sahakian, Brain Res., 81, 1974, 387-392.

(68). E.G. McGeer, H.C. Fibiger and V. Wickson, Brain Res., 32, 1971, 433-440.

(69). W. Kehr, A. Carlsson, M. Lindqvist, T. Magnusson and C. Atack, J. Pharm. Pharmac. 24, 1972, 744-747.

(70). J.R. Walters, B.S. Bunney and R.H. Roth, In " Advances in Neurology", 9, Ed. D.B. Calne, Raven Press, New York (in press).

(71). J. Christiansen and R.F. Squires, J. Pharm. Pharmac., 26, 1974, 367-369.

(72). J. Christiansen and R.F. Squires, In "Antipsychotic drugs, pharmacodynamics and pharmacokinetics", Ed. G. Sedvall, Wenner-Gren International Center Symposia, Pergamon Press, Oxford, (in press).

(73). M. Karobath, Proc. Nat. Acad. Sci. US. 68, 1971, 2370-2373.

(74). R.L. Patrick and J.D. Barchas, J. Neurochem. 23, 1974, 7-15.

(75). R.A. Finkelstein, CRC Critical Reviews in Microbiology, 2, 1973, 553-623.

(76). P. Cuatrecasas, Biochemistry, 12, 1973, 3547-3558.

(77). A.J.J. Pijnenburg and J.M. Rossum, J. Pharm. Pharmac., 25, 1973, 1003-1005.

(78). J.E. Harris, V.H. Morgenroth III, R.H. Roth and R. J. Baldessarini, Nature, 252, 1974, 156-158.

DISCUSSION

Dr. Lovenberg inquired whether neuroleptics had any effect in preventing the action of cholera toxin. Dr. Iversen replied that he would predict that the neuroleptics would not be effective but that the experiment has not yet been performed.

Dr. Mandel was interested in the action of neuroleptics in blocking various adenyl cyclases. Dr Iversen stated that at concentrations of 10^{-5}M and higher chlorpromazine shows a slight inhibition of basal adenylate cyclase activity in striatal homogenates; this activity is not at all marked and not very potent. Dr. Miller has assessed some of the neuroleptic drugs against a norepinephrine response in fat cell ghosts which have an adenylate cyclase that responds to norepinephrine; this seems a classical beta type of response. Here the neuroleptics are very weakly active in blocking this response: chlorpromazine and the alpha and beta isomers of flupenthixol, all require about 10^{-4}M. Thus, no correlation is seen here between neuroleptic activity and the ability to block.

Dr. Hornykiewicz proposed that there might be some similarity between the formulas of butaclamol and reserpine. He wondered if anybody had tried reserpine on the adenyl cyclase system. Dr. Iversen said that Dr. Janssen had recently pointed out the similarity in Stockholm recently. Dr. Iversen emphasized that butaclamol does not resemble chemically any of the traditional neuroleptic classes.

Dr. Everett inquired whether any studies had been done on the adenyl cyclase system in the chronic administration of drugs. Dr. Iversen said that this was an intriguing possibility since behavioral data suggest that chronic treatment with neuroleptics can lead to some type of behavioral supersensitivity, e. g., exaggerated responses of CNS dopamine receptors. However, two attempts to

STRUCTURE-ACTIVITY RELATIONSHIPS

observe a change in dopamine-sensitive adenylate cyclase activity in striatal homogenates after treating rats chronically for 1 or 2 weeks with chlorpromazine (or haloperidol or pimozide) have been unsuccessful.

Dr. Hornykiewicz added that recently some Basle workers have reported that chronic treatment with neuroleptics does make adenylate cyclase more sensitive to dopamine.

CRITERIA FOR AND PITFALLS IN THE IDENTIFICATION OF RECEPTORS

Pedro Cuatrecasas

Department of Pharmacology and Experimental Therapeutics
and
Department of Medicine
The Johns Hopkins University School of Medicine
Baltimore, Maryland

I. INTRODUCTION

Considerable progress has been made in the identification and study of cell membrane receptors for such peptide hormones as insulin, glucagon, adrenocorticotropin, thyrotropin, angiotensin, calcitonin, growth hormone, prolactin, follicle stimulating hormone, leutinizing hormone, chorionic gonadotropin, oxytocin and vasopressin, as well as nonpeptide hormones and drugs such as catecholamines, prostaglandins, acetylcholine and opiates (reviewed in Ref. 1). The general approach in these studies has been to measure the interaction (binding) of a radioactively labelled hormone with intact target cells or with isolated membrane preparations derived from such cells. The binding is surmised to reflect "specific" receptor interactions if it demonstrates a) strict structural and steric specificity; b) saturability, which indicates a finite and limited number of binding sites; c) tissue specificity in accord with biological target cell sensitivity; d) high affinity, in harmony with the physiological concentrations of the hormone; and e) reversibility which is kinetically consistent with the reversal of the physiological effects observed upon removal of the hormone from the medium. In addition, it is of considerable help if specific chemical or enzymatic perturbations of the cells or

of the hormone result in changes in the biological activity which
parallel closely similar changes in binding.

The term "receptor" in all these studies is a general term which
is used for convenience, and its use implies a lack of knowledge of
the discrete or unique chemical structures involved in the interactions. As the history of the study of drugs has shown, the use of
the term "receptor" is in effect a reflection of ignorance of the
molecular locus of action of the drug; when this locus is known (e.g.,
whether a specific enzyme such as a kinase for cyclic AMP, or hemaglobin or a vitamin for certain drugs), we no longer refer to it as
the receptor but rather refer to it by its chemical nature. "Receptor" in the context used currently in hormonal studies is defined
operationally as those molecules which specifically <u>recognize</u> and
bind the hormone, and which as a consequence of this recognition can
lead to other changes (or series of changes) which ultimately result
in the biological response. This is done in analogy with classical
enzyme-substrate systems, in which substrate binding and catalysis
are separate and discrete but sequential processes which can be studied independently. As in the case of competitive inhibitors of
enzymes, hormone analogs (e.g., as known for glucagon, ACTH, angiotensin and oxytocin) may in certain cases bind to "receptors" but
fail to trigger biological responses, thus serving as relative or
absolute inhibitors depending on the quantitative comparison of their
intrinsic activity relative to their binding affinity.

II. PROBLEMS AND PITFALLS IN THE STUDY OF HORMONE RECEPTORS

A number of problems and pitfalls can be encountered in the
kinds of studies described above [1, 2] and considerable caution must
be exercised in the interpretation of data, especially when detailed
mechanistic inferences are made or when extrapolating to complex <u>in
vivo</u> biological systems or disease states. Some examples of such
actual or potential problems relating to different aspects of hormone-binding studies will be presented here.

A. The Problem of "Nonspecific" Binding

Because physiological membrane receptors are present in extremely small quantity in membranes, the hormone must if possible be labeled to very high specific activity (e.g., with ^{125}I or ^{131}I at 1 to 2 Ci/μmole) without destroying the biological activity of the hormone. Since virtually all chemical compounds used as binding ligands (hormones) exhibit some nonspecific adsorptive or binding properties to a variety of inert as well as nonreceptor biological materials, since such "binding" may be of extremely high affinity, and since the number ("infinite", by definition) of such nonspecific binding sites may greatly exceed that of specific receptors, great difficulties may be encountered in <u>detecting</u> such specific receptors. The 'background binding' of labeled hormone to a filter or apparatus used to separate membrane-bound from free hormone, or to the tissue material itself, may contribute very significantly to the total amount of hormone bound.

Of particular importance is the fact that such nonspecific binding can appear as 'specific' by many criteria such as saturability, specificity, reversibility, etc. which are generally used to define receptors. We have observed many instances where this has been a troublesome complication. For instance, it has been observed that in the absence of cellular material vigorous shaking in glass but not plastic tubes of ^{125}I-insulin solutions in Hank's or Krebs-Ringer-bicarbonate buffers in the presence and absence of native insulin yields large quantities of spurious 'displaceable counts' which are trapped on Millipore filters [3].

Furthermore, binding of ^{125}I-insulin in a manner competitively displaceable by native insulin can be demonstrated and studied in various nonreceptor systems consisting of inorganic substances such as talc, alumina powder, and microsilica [3]. In addition, 'specific' binding can be shown to occur to certain organic molecules in model systems such as agarose beads containing thyroglobulin and fetuin but not albumin. Since in all hormone binding studies nonspecific or nonreceptor interactions occur and must therefore be understood as much as possible, some of the above simple systems may be useful models for the study of such phenomena. As a result of such studies some initially surprising and instructive general observations have been made. For example, the "saturable" binding of ^{125}I-insulin to talc can be shown to exhibit some specificity with respect to the nature of the hormone [3]. A variety of peptide hormones are less effective than insulin, and insulin at low concentrations is more effective than proinsulin, in analogy with biological receptor interactions. However, it is notable that growth hormone can compete as effectively as insulin at high concentrations. The binding of insulin to talc, which is also a time-dependent process, can be shown under certain conditions to exhibit irregular kinetic behavior suggestive of "positive cooperativity".

Another striking example of a very simple, controlled case where binding can feign as "receptor" binding is illustrated by studies of the binding of ^{125}I-labeled glucagon. The hormone can be shown to bind very well to certain lots of cellulose acetate (EG or EH) Millipore filters in the absence of tissue, and this binding shows very nice 'displacement' by native glucagon; the apparent affinity for glucagon in this system is about 5×10^{-7} M [2]. Numerous other hormones (FSH, LH, prolactin, secretin, oxytocin, ACTH, TSH and insulin) at high concentration (100 µg per ml) did not inhibit the binding significantly. Growth hormone, however, demonstrated specificity, although with a 10-fold lower affinity. The only other hormone tested which could inhibit binding was vasopressin, which inhibited binding by 50% at 50 µg per ml. This system therefore shows saturability and remarkable specificity with respect to hormone binding. In this and the various other artifactual "receptor" binding systems studied in this laboratory the apparent affinity constant for the hormone usually does not exceed 10^8 M. This does not, however, exclude the existence of higher affinity nonspecific binding systems for particular hormones in biological tissues, since these are chemically extremely heterogeneous and complex compared to the simple model systems described above.

Other examples exist of moderately high affinity and highly specific binding which are biological "accidents" rather than meaningful recognition phenomena. It is well known that albumin can bind D-trytophan but not the L-isomer [4]. ^{3}H-Naloxone has also been shown to bind stereospecifically to glass filters [5]. Opiate drugs have been shown to bind to cerebroside sulfate stereospecifically and with an order of potency which is remarkably similar to the biological in vivo potency of these drugs [6].

Perhaps it should not be surprising to find such specificity of binding in "nonspecific" chemical interactions. Regardless of the chemical basis (nature of bonds) of such adsorptive binding, the overall interaction and its affinity must depend on and be dictated by the chemical composition and structure of the interacting components, and these will change drastically with alterations in steric properties as well as in the primary, secondary and tertiary structure of the polypeptides involved. This can be expected to be particularly true for any high-affinity system in which a complex composite of different bonds must be coordinated to achieve such high affinity. Therefore, demonstration that binding of hormone is lost or altered by changes in its structure is not by itself sufficient proof of "receptor" specificity. Thus, the chemical properties which govern receptor recognition may in whole or in part also determine nonreceptor adsorptive properties.

These considerations should prove cautionary for the interpretation of receptor binding studies. For example, even when a given interaction at low hormone concentrations may clearly result from a specific receptor, more complicated processes and 'nonspecific', saturable binding may be encountered at higher concentrations of the hormone. Since the latter are much more likely to be observed in these conditions, great care should be exercised in attaching significance to "second binding" sites of low affinity and high capacity. In view of the ubiquity with which nonreceptor but "specific" binding of moderate affinity (apparent K_m, 10^{-6} to 10^{-8} M) can be demonstrated in a variety of simple nontissue containing systems, it would indeed be surprising if complex biological tissues did not also exhibit such properties. In this respect it is pertinent that virtually all hormones of peptide and other (e.g., catecholamine, acetylcholine, steroid) composition can be demonstrated under proper circumstances to exhibit a "second" low affinity and high capacity binding component when analyzed by Scatchard plots. Unfortunately, it is most difficult to study these functions properly in complex tissues. However, special care should be exercised in interpreting this second component as a single, unique binding structure or class of receptors rather than as the sum of a complex mixture of components unrelated to receptors.

B. Some Other Problems Related to Methodology

In addition to the problems discussed above, numerous others related to methodology and interpretation exist. For example, labeling of a hormone may result in lowered or even enhanced [7] affinity and potency for biological activity. Considerable variability in the "quality" of various lots of Na ^{125}I used for peptide iodination exist which can result in altered properties of the hormone. Many peptide hormones undergo facile degradation by ubiquitous or specific proteases, glass surfaces or even spontaneously. Troublesome deiodination and transpeptidation reactions can be catalyzed by enzymes or chemical components in membranes, especially when these are performed at elevated temperatures for protracted periods. Some of these reactions may occur with greater facility in crude, solubilized preparations of membranes. When binding to intact cells is studied, attention must be paid to the possibility of ligand internalization (e.g., by pinocytosis), especially if elevated temperatures are utilized. Considerable variability may exist between different cell types with respect to such pinocytotic behavior.

C. Ligand Self-Aggregation and "Negative Cooperativity"

The existence of negatively cooperative interactions between insulin receptors in liver membranes has been proposed [8] on the

IDENTIFICATION OF RECEPTORS 251

basis of the fact that the spontaneous rate of dissociation of the ^{125}I-insulin-membrane complex is accelerated by the addition of native insulin to the incubation medium. Using human placenta membranes, which bind much greater quantities of insulin and thus greatly facilitate accurate measurements, we have confirmed these observations (Fig. 1). The major effect of adding native insulin occurs very rapidly (first few minutes), depending on the concentration of native insulin which is used. If very early times in the course of dissociation are examined, significant differences can be seen between various concentrations of insulin which are all supersaturating with respect to receptor binding.

Effects similar to those described above for the enhancement by native insulin of the dissociation of the insulin-placenta membrane complex can be reproduced with insulin-talc complexes (Fig. 2). Although in this system the spontaneous rate of dissociation is slower, profound effects are observed with concentrations of native insulin comparable to those used with placenta membranes. Similar results have also been observed with other kinds of nonreceptor insulin complexes [3]. Analogous results have been described for the interaction of epidermal growth factor (EGF) [3] and nerve growth factor (NGF) [9] to membrane preparations.

Since the above effects can be reproduced in nonreceptor systems, the data cannot be interpreted to reflect "negatively cooperative" interactions between receptors. The observed effects are most likely the results of interactions between the ligand molecules [3]. It is well known that insulin forms dimers and higher aggregates. The dissociation constant for dimer formation (at neutral pH) has been reported to be 7×10^{-7} M [10].

Relatively low affinity constants of dimerization may permit rapid "exchange" and thus "dissociation" of the labeled receptor-bound hormone by even relatively low concentrations of the unlabeled hormone, provided the total quantity of the unlabeled hormone exceeds that of the labeled. This is because in such binding studies only the behavior of the ^{125}I-labeled material is examined and the rates

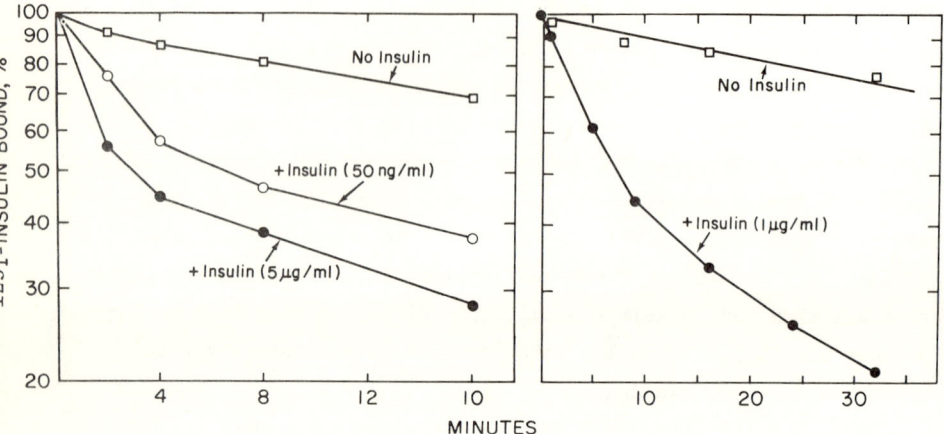

Fig. 1. Native insulin enhances the rate of dissociation of the ^{125}I-insulin-placenta membrane complex, as measured by two very different methods (left and right).

Left: Nine ml of Krebs-Ringer-bicarbonate buffer containing 0.1% albumin and 2.5 mg of placenta membrane protein were incubated for 30 min at 24° with ^{125}I-insulin (8 x 10^4 cpm per ml, 1.4 Ci per mmole). The suspension was cooled in ice, centrifuged at 40,000 rpm, and the pellet was washed three times with ice-cold buffer. The pellet was suspended in 8 ml of ice-cold buffer and divided in 0.4 ml portions for assay. Native insulin (50 ng or 5 µg per ml) was added to some samples, and some were immediately (within 2 min) filtered on EG Millipore filters for determination of the zero time values. The samples were then placed in a 24° water bath and assayed for binding at various times. The zero time values (100%) correspond to about 22,000 cpm.

Right: Spontaneous dissociation of ^{125}I-insulin in the absence of native insulin was determined after first collecting and washing the samples on filters (EGWP) with buffer at 4° and then percolating buffer at 24° for timed intervals. Results are corrected for non-specific binding (1 µg per ml of native insulin added before ^{125}I-insulin). The 100% value corresponds to about 35,000 cpm. Data from Ref. 3.

of diffusion and dimer formation are extremely fast; thus, rapid exchange can occur when the proportion of the total ligand present in the dimer form is very small (Fig. 3). In this interpretation it is also implicit that the receptor-bound monomer can still participate in dimerization, and that this alters its conformation such that its affinity for the receptor is greatly reduced. Dimerization must

IDENTIFICATION OF RECEPTORS

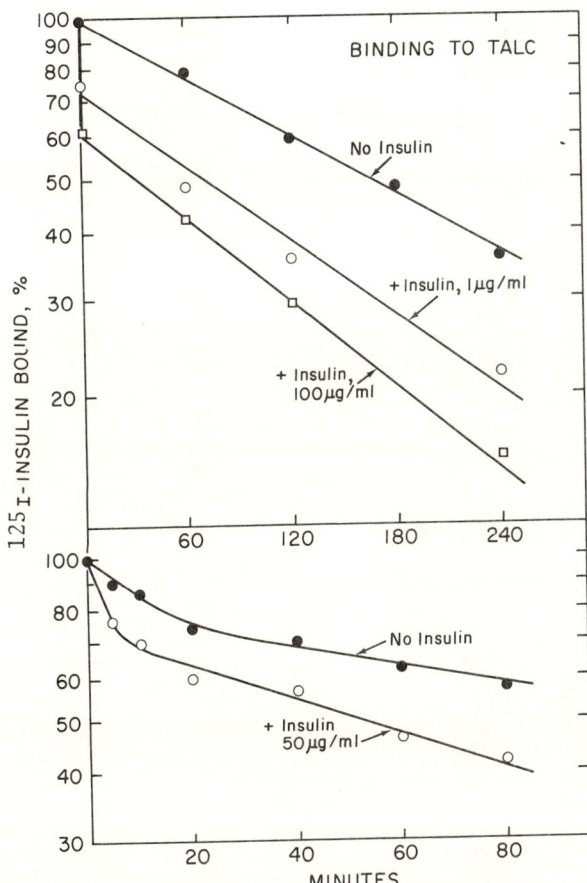

Fig. 2. Enhancement of dissociation of ^{125}I-labeled insulin-talc complex by native insulin. A suspension of talc (0.25 mg per ml) in Hank's buffer - 0.1% albumin was incubated for 40 min at 37° with ^{125}I-insulin (2.5 x 10^5 cpm per ml, 1.7 Ci per mmole). The suspension was cooled in ice and washed two times with ice-cold buffer to remove all the unbound ^{125}I-insulin. The talc was suspended (30 µg of talc per ml) in ice-cold buffer and native insulin was added to some samples. Samples without (100% value) and with insulin were filtered at once (EG Millipore filters) to determine zero time values. The suspensions were then incubated at 37° and samples were filtered periodically to determine insulin binding. Data from Ref. 3.

change the monomer structure sufficiently to alter its binding to receptors as well as its adsorptive properties to talc and other materials.

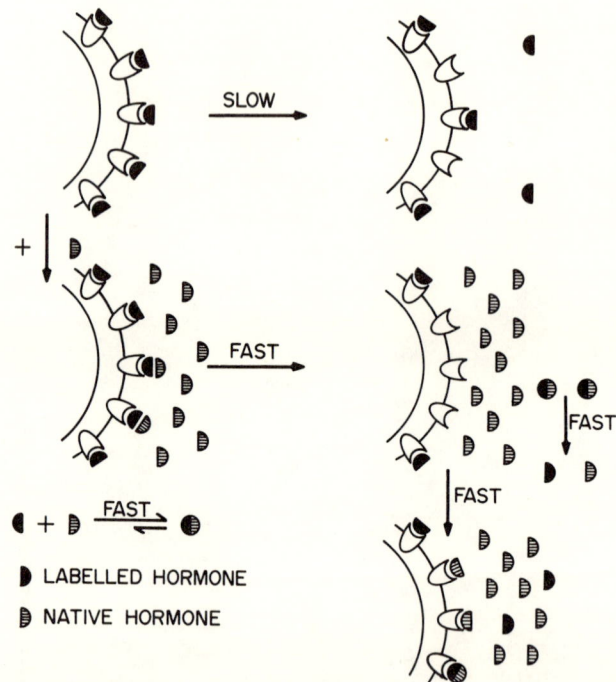

Fig. 3. Process by which ligand (hormone) dimerization can cause rapid dissociation of receptor-bound labeled hormone, giving the appearance of "negative cooperativity". By this mechanism relatively low concentrations (far below K_D of dimerization) of unlabeled hormone can accelerate dissociation even with weak stability constants for dimer formation.

Since numerous other ligands and hormones are known to isomerize or polymerize in a concentration-dependent manner, it is predictable that if studied by the methodology described here, the "apparent" behavior of "negative cooperativity" may be detected in other systems provided a) that the formation of these associated ligand states is not precluded by binding of the monomer to the receptor and b) that the altered ligand state has a decreased affinity for the receptor. Enhanced receptor binding of the self-associated ligand state would of course result in "positively cooperative" behavior. Self-interactions are well known and have been well studied for several kinds of ligands such as proteins, nucleosides, chlorophylls, pyrimidines, purines, cholesterol, and organic dyes.

IDENTIFICATION OF RECEPTORS

Self-aggregation of the type suggested here for insulin, NGF and EGF will obviously also introduce curvatures in Scatchard plots of binding data, especially if the data are obtained from competition-displacement curves measured over a wide range of native hormone concentration. It is notable that in many studies where Scatchard analysis and kinetic interpretations have been made from the competition of labeled-ligand binding by varying the concentration of unlabeled ligand, the plots have been nonlinear and suggestive of additional "low affinity, high capacity" binding sites. Such data could be explained at least in part by the aggregation effects discussed here.

D. Receptor Concentration, "Displacement" Curves and Scatchard Plots

A serious problem which has seldom been appreciated in the analysis of high-affinity receptor systems relates to the aberrant data that is obtained for such dissociable systems if the concentration of receptor used in the assay is greater than the dissociation constant under study. In analogy with enzyme systems, such conditions will not result in normal "Zone A" behavior [11]; under such circumstances affinity constants will be underestimated, and bizarre properties may be unjustifiably invoked for the system. These conditions will often prevail in the study of biological receptors because the affinities of such systems are very high, the quantities of receptors in tissue samples are small and the specific radioactivity of the ligands used is not sufficiently high. Thus, to <u>detect</u> receptors by direct binding it is necessary to use very high concentrations (exceeding K_m) of tissue material.

The effect of receptor concentration on binding is illustrated in Fig. 4 for the binding of ^{125}I-labeled EGF to placenta membranes. It is evident immediately that estimates of the apparent affinity of complex formation simply from the concentration of native hormone required to achieve half-maximal displacement may lead to grossly erroneous results. It is of interest in this respect that where estimates of hormone-receptor affinity have been made on the basis of the ratio (k_{-1}/k_1) of the rates of dissociation (k_{-1}) and association (k_1) of complex formation, the dissociation constants have been lower than those estimated by competition data [3]. Rate constant measurements have the advantages that they can be done with the labeled hormone alone and with very low concentrations of the hormone.

Under certain conditions in very high affinity systems (e.g., Fig. 4) the binding of the ligand appears to be directly proportional to the ligand concentration, at least over the low range of hormone concentration. Such data result in a horizontal line in a Scatchard plot (Fig. 5), superficially or falsely indicating the existence of an infinite number of such receptor sites (e.g., "nonspecific" binding).

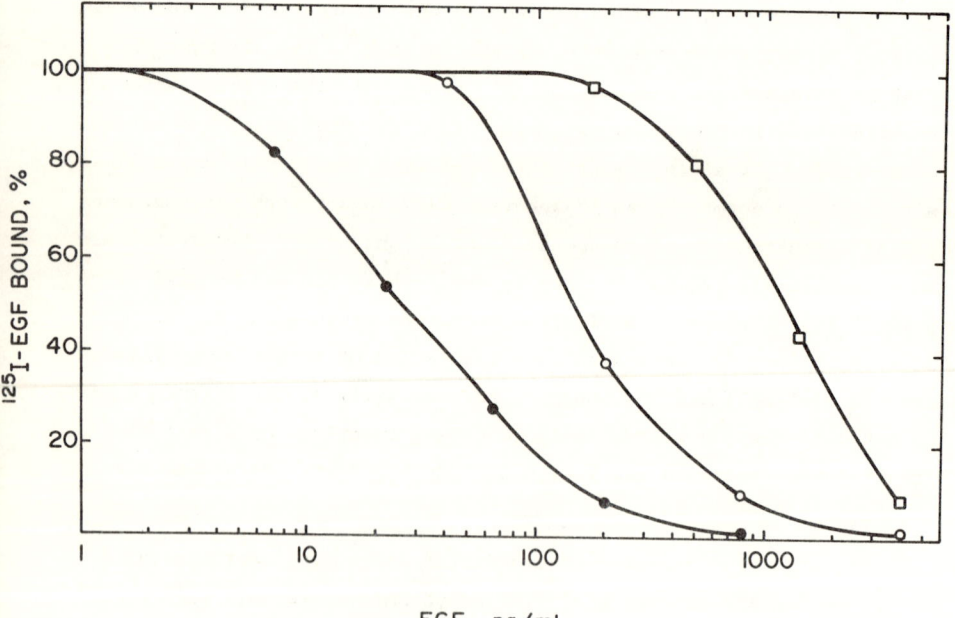

Fig. 4. Effect of varying the receptor (membrane) concentration on the ability of native epidermal growth factor (EGF) to compete for the binding of ^{125}I-labeled EGF. Samples containing 9.3×10^4 cpm of ^{125}I-labeled EGF (260 µCi/µg) were incubated in 0.2 ml of Krebs-Ringer bicarbonate, 0.1% albumin, for 20 min at 24° with 10 µg (●), 50 µg (○) or 300 µg (□) of placenta membrane protein and varying amounts of unlabeled EGF. The latter was added 5 min before the labeled hormone. Binding was determined by Millipore membrane filtration.

IDENTIFICATION OF RECEPTORS

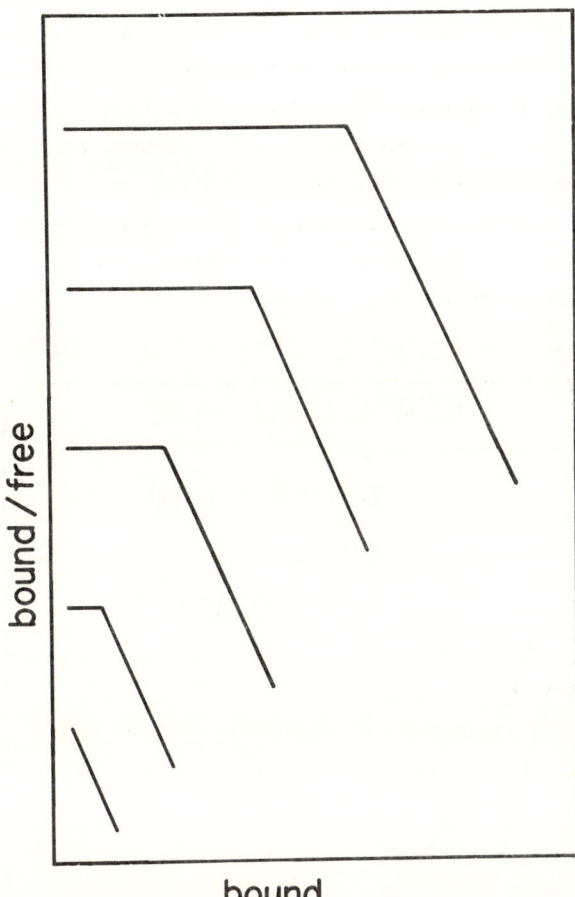

Fig. 5. Scatchard plots obtained from binding data of very high affinity systems where the concentration of receptor (e.g., membranes) is higher than the dissociation constant of the complex, as illustrated in Fig. 4. Each curve represents a different receptor concentration in the same assay; the length of the horizontal portion decreases as the receptor concentration is decreased, but the slopes of the remaining curves are unchanged.

Since Scatchard plots visually describe both extremities of the binding curve, even minor nonspecific interactions of the type described earlier (whether saturable or not) will grossly distort the curves giving the impression of a "second class" of binding sites of low affinity and high capacity (Fig. 6). It is most difficult if not impossible to distinguish between multiple not saturable, nonspecific sites differing in affinity and various or single saturable nonspecific binding sites. In systems such as this, perhaps the best information is obtained from the low saturation points, which describe the highest affinity processes occurring as far as possible from the low affinity and possibly nonspecific sites. Other possible causes for such concave upward inflections in Scatchard plots include a) negative

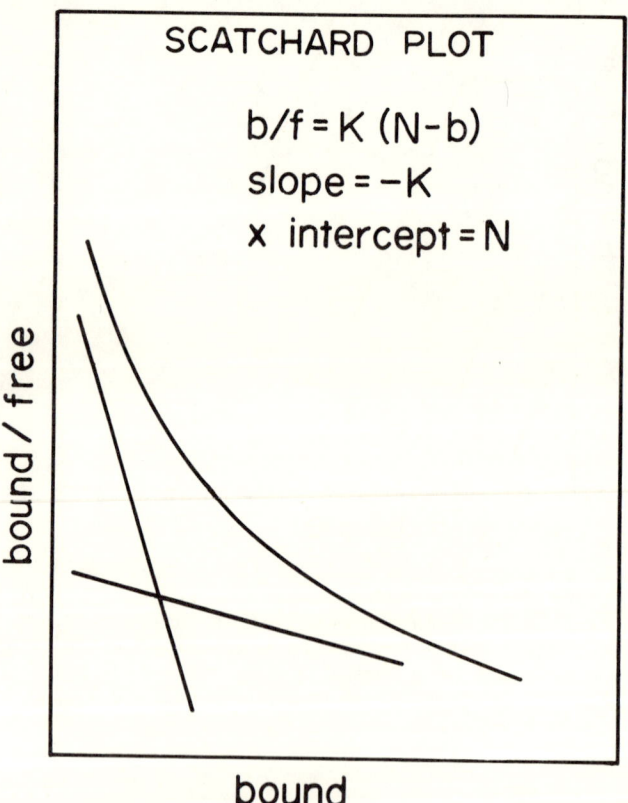

Fig. 6. Scatchard plot of binding data showing two hypothetical binding components differing in affinity and quantity. The curvature at the lower values of B/F, which is often interpreted as suggesting a "second order" of binding sites, is found frequently and has many other possible explanations, as described in the text.

cooperativity between receptors, b) self association (as described earlier) of the ligand, and c) a higher affinity of the labeled ligand compared to the unlabeled species.

E. Cross-Reactivity in Hormone-Receptor Systems

Even in cases where considerable evidence points to the specific nature of an interaction between a hormone and a tissue preparation, the possibility must be considered that the hormone under study may not be the normal or natural ligand which ordinarily triggers that system under physiological conditions. This should be especially important in cases where the affinity of the system is particularly low.

Several examples now exist which demonstrate that different but probably structurally related hormones can interact with each other's receptors, but with different affinities. Fat cell membrane sites which bind secretin and which were originally thought to represent the physiologic receptor for this hormone have in fact a much higher (2 orders of magnitude) affinity for vasoactive intestinal polypeptide (VIP), and both hormones appear to affect adenylate cyclase through a common receptor [12, 13]. In liver, on the other hand, both hormones have separate receptors, but the hormones can cross-react and stimulate both receptors at appropriately high concentrations. Other examples of peptides with overlapping receptor specificity may be found with vasopressin and oxytocin [14, 15] and human growth hormone, human placental lactogen and prolactin [16]. A similar situation may exist for the binding and biological activity of insulin in lymphocytes and fibroblast cells in tissue culture since the binding and biological activities reflect unphysiologically high binding affinities.

F. Heterogeneity of Cell Populations

Serious problems can arise in interpreting quantitative data obtained on mixed cell populations since the assumption is frequently made that all of the cells present are contributing equally to the binding process. Cases are known, however, where only a very small fraction of the cells under study possess the specific receptors being studied [2]. Such situations are particularly dangerous if comparisons are made between one tissue and another, between species or between one clinical state and another. The erroneous conclusion can be made, for example, that fewer receptors per cell exist in a given clinical state when in actuality the change is in the relative composition of the cells under study. Similar considerations apply to studies of cell membranes isolated from tissues of heterogeneous cell composition.

G. Correlation of Apparent Affinity for Binding and for Biological Activity

An important criterion for evaluating the validity of hormone binding studies is correlation of the affinity observed in these binding studies with the affinity of the hormone for the biological response. A reasonable approximation of the apparent K_m for the biological response can be estimated by careful measurements of the fasting (or under other appropriate conditions) concentration of the hormone in the blood. However, detailed and more rigorous studies and correlations are generally required. Unfortunately, in some cases (e.g., growth hormone) no simple _in vitro_ systems are available, while in others (e.g., insulin) stable, reproducible or sufficiently large effects cannot be measured in broken cell preparations to permit precise kinetic correlations with binding studies.

Even in cases where large effects can be observed in simple, intact systems _in vitro_, and even in simpler broken-cell systems, important problems and ambiguities are often encountered. For example, the apparent affinity of ACTH or catecholamines for stimulating lipolysis in isolated fat cells can be manipulated within rather large ranges (4-fold) by the addition of very low concentrations of theophylline, which alone are virtually without effect (Fig. 7). In addition, "sigmoidal" curves suggestive of cooperative interactions become hyperbolic by such treatment. It is apparent that in cases

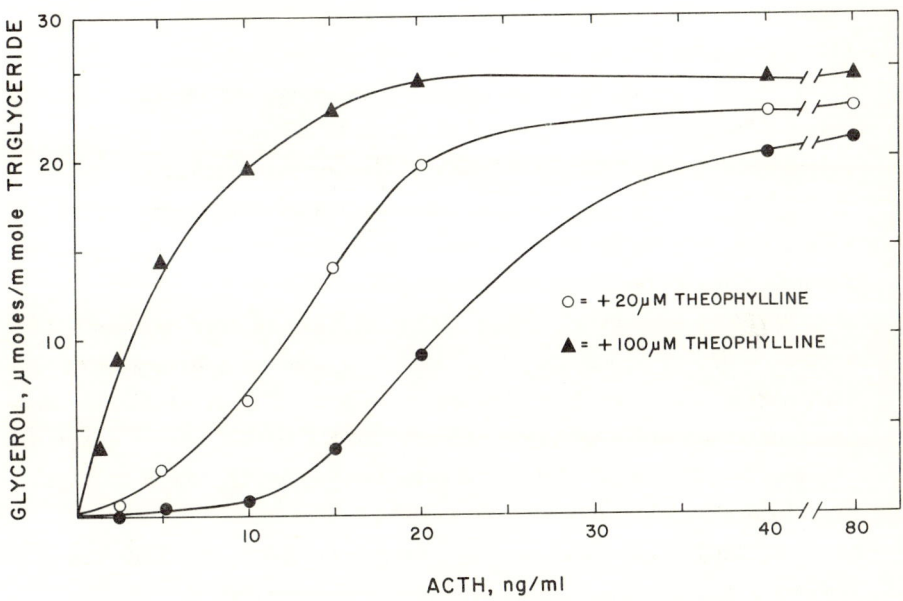

Fig. 7. Effect of low concentrations of theophylline on the concentration dependence of ACTH for lipolysis in isolated fat cells. Fat cells were incubated for 60 min at 37° in Krebs-Ringer-bicarbonate buffer containing 3% albumin. Very similar results are observed if lipolysis is measured with epinephrine instead of ACTH.

where a distant metabolic effect is measured (e.g., lipolysis) estimates of hormone affinity are hazardous, regardless of the explanation for these interesting results. Similarly, it is not possible to use biological assays of this type to examine the combined effect of different hormones to determine whether such hormones may operate through the same adenylate cyclase molecules.

Equally important, studies of responses in such simple, intact systems (e.g., lipolysis, glycogen synthesis, protein synthesis, etc.) cannot be used to judge uncritically the possible existence of "spare receptors". For example, the data in Fig. 6 would suggest that in the presence of 100 μM theophylline fewer hormone receptors must be occupied to achieve the same response. Although in this narrow context "spare receptors" exist, the term has little real chemical meaning since these receptors are only "spare" with respect to the specific biological response being measured under those specific conditions. For example, if a hormone acts on a variety of separate intracellular processes through cyclic AMP, all of these end responses may in principle exhibit different sensitivity to the nucleotide. Thus, hormone dose-response relationships may differ widely for each of these responses, and receptors which appear to be "spare" for one response may not be for another.

Valid assessment of "spare receptors" can be made only in situations where an immediate one-to-one correspondence between hormone binding and the initial or primary biochemical effect of the hormone-receptor interaction can be measured. Such a situation may exist for hormones which stimulate adenylate cyclase activity, where it is in principle possible to relate in subcellular systems the number of binding sites which exist to the number required to activate the enzyme. In such studies of lysine-vasopressin binding, Bockaert et al., [15] found rather close but not entirely simple correspondence between receptor occupancy and adenylate cyclase activation.

ACKNOWLEDGMENT

Reported studies from this laboratory were supported by NIH, ACS and The Kroc Foundation.

REFERENCES

[1]. P. Cuatrecasas, Ann. Rev. Biochem., 43, 1974, 169-214.

[2]. P. Cuatrecasas, M. D. Hollenberg, K.-J. Chang, and V. Bennett, Recent Progress in Hormone Research, Vol. 31, Academic Press, New York 1975, in press.

[3]. P. Cuatrecasas and M. D. Hollenberg, Biochem. Biophys. Res. Commun., 1975, in press.

[4]. K. K. Stewart and R. F. Doherty, Proc. Nat. Acad. Sci. USA, 70, 1973, 2850-2852.

[5]. S. H. Snyder, C. B. Pert, and G. W. Pasternak, Handbook of Psychopharmacology, (eds.) L. I. Iversen, S. Iversen, and S. H. Snyder, Plenum Press, New York, in press.

[6]. H. H. Loh, T. M. Cho, Y.-C. Wu, and E. L. Way, Life Sciences, 14, 1974, 2231-2245.

[7]. W. W. Bromer, M. E. Boucher, and J. M. Patterson, Biochem. Biophys. Res. Commun., 53, 1973, 134-139.

[8]. P. De Meyts, J. Roth, D. M. Neville Jr., J. R. Gavin III, and M. A. Lesniak, Biochem. Biophys. Res. Commun., 55, 1973, 154-161.

[9]. W. A. Frazier, L. F. Boyd, and R. A. Bradshaw, J. Biol. Chem. 249, 1974, 5513.

[10]. A. H. Parker and B. H. Frank, Biochemistry, 11, 1972, 4013.

[11]. A. Goldstein, L. Aronow, and S. M. Kalman, Principles of Drug Action, John Wiley & Sons, New York, 1974.

[12]. B. Desbuquois, M. H. Laudat, and P. H. Laudat, Biochem. Biophys. Res. Commun., 53, 1973, 1187-1194.

[13]. B. Desbuquois, Eur. J. Biochem., 46, 1974, 439-450.

[14]. M. Soloff, T. Swartz, M. Morrison, and M. Saffran, Endocrinology, 92, 1973, 104-107.

[15]. J. Bockaert, C. Roy, R. Rajerison, and S. Jard, J. Biol. Chem., 248, 1973, 5922-5931.

[16]. R. P. C. Shiu, P. A. Kelly, and H. G. Friesen, Science, 180, 1973, 968-971.

DISCUSSION

Dr. Snyder asked for an explanation of the three zones described by Dr. Goldstein. Dr. Cuatrecasas said that this could best be done by mathematical derivation. He pointed out that it is very easy to demonstrate the binding of tritiated catecholamines (e. g., norepinephrine) to cells or to particulate fractions (e. g., microsomes). A number of investigators have described such binding studies and thought specific receptor interactions were involved since superficially they appear to be of fairly high affinity and more or less consistent with the biological effects of the catecholamines. Not only is the binding of fairly high affinity, it is saturable, etc. However, when the binding is examined in more detail, it is found to be totally lacking in stereospecificity - the sole specificity is for catechols. Thus, e. g., pyrocatechol or dihydroxymandelic acid, compounds without effect on biological activity, will displace and compete as well as norepinephrine. Since these compounds which have no biological activity even when their concentrations are raised by five orders of magnitude will displace the observed binding, such binding cannot reflect a true biological receptor.

Dr. Clark asked if this meant that, in general, all binding studies had to be correlated with pharmacological activity. Dr. Cuatrecasas agreed; he emphasized this point by mentioning that there are frequently two or three orders of magnitude greater numbers of catecholamine binding sites than receptors. There may be 100,000 sites and only 2,000 of these are true β-adrenergic receptors. A major problem is how to detect the true receptors among the multitude of binding sites.

PINEAL BETA-ADRENERGIC RECEPTOR:
REGULATION OF SENSITIVITY

Jorge A. Romero
Julius Axelrod
Laboratory of Clinical Science
National Institute of Health
Bethesda, Maryland

1. INTRODUCTION

In the rat pineal gland, enviornmental lighting markedly influences the metabolism of indoleamines and the synthesis of the hormone melatonin. The first specific step in the synthesis of melatonin is the acetylation of serotonin by the enzyme serotonin N-acetyltransferase (NAT) to form N-acetylserotonin (NAS) (1). NAS is then methylated by hydroxyindole-O-methyltransferase (HIOMT) to yield melatonin (2). In rats kept under diurnal lighting conditions (alternating 12-hour periods of light and dark), the activities of NAT (3,4) and HIOMT (5) are much higher during the night than during the day. The circadian rhythm in the activity of these enzymes is in phase with similar cycles in the levels of NAS (6, 7) and melatonin (8) in the pineal gland. Serotonin levels, however, show a reciprocal relationship to the above cycles, the highest levels of serotonin occurring during the day (9). If animals are kept in constant light, serotonin levels rise, while the activities of NAT and HIOMT, and the levels of NAS and melatonin remain at their lowest levels. This reciprocal relationship between serotonin and the enzymes and intermediates of the pathway for melatonin synthesis suggests that a single basic mechanism drives these rhythms. A stimulus which increases the activity of NAT (and HIOMT) would increase the production of melatonin and accelerate the utilization of serotonin, thus generating the above relationships.

The external signal that synchronizes these cycles is environmental lighting. Information about lighting conditions is relayed to the pineal gland via postganglionic sympathetic fibers with cell bodies in the superior cervical ganglion (10). Denervation of the pineal gland by bilateral superior cervical ganglionectomy abolishes these cycles (11). The rate of firing of the postganglionic sympathetic fibers innervating the pineal gland reflects changes in environmental lighting (12); electrical activity recorded at the pineal gland with extracellular electrodes is inhibited by exposure of the rats to light. In addition, the turnover of the neurotransmitter noradrenaline (NA) in the pineal gland is reduced by daylight (13).

At the cellular level, there is compelling evidence that activation of the β-adrenergic receptor regulates the cycles in indole metabolism in the pineal gland. The β-adrenergic receptor is activated by norepinephrine released from the sympathetic terminals innervating the gland. We will describe in this report the relationship of the β-adrenergic receptor to NAT, and present evidence indicating that exposure of the receptor to its agonist not only induces NAT activity, but also modifies the capacity of the gland to respond to further stimulation.

2. CONTROL OF N-ACETYLTRANSFERASE ACTIVITY

The activity of NAT in the pineal gland is controlled by a β-adrenergic receptor mechanism (14, 15). Administration of l-propranolol, a potent β-adrenergic blocker, prevents the physiologic rise in enzyme activity at night; if propranolol is injected into rats after NAT activity is already increased, the drug causes a precipitous fall in enzyme activity with a half-life of less than 10 minutes (16). Similar rapid inactivation of the

enzyme occurs when sympathetic nerve activity is
sharply reduced by exposing the rats to light at night
(16, 17). During the day, when enzyme activity is
low, administration of catecholamines in vivo, or
incubation of the glands in organ explant culture in
the presence of catecholamines, will cause 50-100 fold
increases in enzyme activity. This action of catecholamines is antagonized by β-adrenergic blocking agents,
both in vivo and in vitro (15).

It is very likely that the β-adrenergic receptor
acts intracellularly via an adenylate cyclase coupled
system (14, 15). Catecholamines cause a sharp peak
in cyclic AMP levels within 5 to 10 minutes, which
can be prevented by l-propranolol. This increase in
cyclic AMP precedes the induction of NAT (15).
Dibutyryl cyclic AMP mimics the effects of catecholamines in inducing NAT activity in cultured rat
pineals (14). The action of dibutyryl cyclic AMP
by-passes the membrane receptor, and is unaffected
by propranolol (18).

Cycloheximide, an inhibitor of protein synthesis,
prevents the nighttime rise in NAT activity (16),
and also the induction of NAT by catecholamines
in vivo and in vitro (14, 15). Furthermore,
cycloheximide blocks the induction of NAT activity
by dibutytyl cyclic AMP (14).

These findings indicate that NAT activity is controlled by a β-adrenergic receptor coupled to adenylate cyclase. Intracellularly, cyclic AMP acts as a second messenger and increases NAT activity by a process which requires new protein synthesis.

3. RECEPTOR SUPER AND SUBSENSITIVITY

And study of super- and subsensitivity of a receptor to its agonist must consider a variety of possible mechanisms which can cause changes in sensitivity. Specifically, in the pineal gland, denervation supersensitivity could be either pre-synaptic or postsynaptic in character.

Presynaptic sensitivity changes imply the interference with, or the elimination of, presynaptic mechanisms for the removal of neurotransmitter from the vicinity of the receptor in the postsynaptic membrane (19). This is one of the early effects of denervation supersensitivity, and does not include any alteration in end-organ responsiveness (19). Changes in sensitivity of the end-organ proper, independent of any presynaptic changes, are classified as postsynaptic (20) or postjunctional. Several mechanisms may account for postjunctional sensitivity in the pineal gland: a) a change in the number of receptors available, b) changes in receptor affinity for its agonist, c) changes in the coupling of the receptor to adenylate cyclase, and d) intracellular phenomena such as feedback inhibition, substrate activation, depletion of intermediates, and other similar mechanisms affecting end-organ responsiveness.

A. **Denervation Supersensitivity in the Pineal Gland**

In studying the effects of catecholamines on the pineal gland, it was noted that denervated animals showed an enhanced induction of NAT, in response to catecholamines (21). Superinduction of NAT was evident as early as 24 hours after denervation of the pineal gland by superior cervical ganglionectomy (21). This superinduction of NAT in denervated glands was found to be a manifestation of the postsynaptic supersensitivity. The dose response curve for induction of NAT by NE and isoproterenol in denervated glands of N-acetyltransferase by catecholamines was markedly shifted to the left as compared to that in intact glands (21). By using isoproterenol, a β-adrenergic agonist which is not subject to presynaptic reuptake mechanisms (22), it was established that these changes in sensitivity were of the postjunctional type. No increase in the sensitivity of NAT to induction by dibutyryl cyclic

AMP was found, and therefore the changes in sensitivity were proximal to the site of action of cyclic AMP (23).

Other manipulations which decrease the availability of neurotransmitter at the receptor sites also produce supersensitivity (23). Treatment with reserpine or 6-hydroxydopamine causes supersensitivity of NAT to induction by catecholamines (23). Of particular significance is the fact that prolonged exposure to light, which reduces sympathetic nerve activity, also causes supersensitivity (23).

The sensitivity of adenylate cyclase to stimulation by norepinephrine in pineal homogenates is enhanced after chronic denervation or prolonged exposure to light (24). In contrast to these reported changes in adenylate cyclase responsiveness, which require 4 weeks to develop, the changes in the sensitivity of NAT to induction by catecholamines are present as early as 24 hours after denervation or reserpinization (23). However, enhanced elevation of cyclic AMP by isoproterenol after denervation develops by the sixth or seventh postoperative day (23). At the present time there is no satisfactory explanation for this apparent discrepancy in the time required for development of supersensitivity of adenylate cyclase and cyclic AMP in response to catecholamines.

Repeated administration of isoproterenol to rats with denervated pineal glands suppresses the supersensitivity caused by denervation. If intact animals are treated similarly, subsensitivity of NAT to induction by isoproterenol develops (25).

Thus, surgical or pharmacological manipulations which decrease the availability of neurotransmitter at the receptor sites cause supersensitivity of pineal NAT to induction by catecholamines. Repeated stimulation with exogenous catecholamines produces subsensitivity and abolishes surgically or pharmacologically produced supersensitivity. Prolonged exposure to light, which reduces the activity of the nerves innervating the pineal gland, also causes supersensitivity.

B. <u>Physiologic Cycles in Sensitivity to β-Adrenergic Stimulation</u>

The highest levels of NAT activity during the normal cycle occur 6 to 8 hours after the onset of darkness. After reaching a peak, enzyme levels return to baseline prior to the onset of light (4). Attempts to induce NAT activity by exposure of rats to darkness during the normal light period have shown that the enzyme is refractory to induction by darkness during the first 6 hours of the normal light period (16, 26).

It has been shown that this refractoriness to induction by darkness in the early hours of the light period is a manifestation of subsensitivity of the β-adrenergic receptor to activation by catecholamines (4). Furthermore, since repeated attempts to demonstrate changes in NA turnover during the night have been unsuccessful, the nighttime fall in NAT activity may also be a manifestation of subsensitivity (4).

A physiologic, diurnal variation in the sensitivity of the pineal gland to catecholamines has been shown by utilizing rats kept in alternating light-dark cycles of 12 hours duration (4). In pineal explant culture, higher concentrations of isoproterenol are required to produce equi-effective responses in glands from rats killed at the end of the dark period as compared to rats killed at the end of the light period (4). With increasing duration of exposure to light, there is a shift to the left of the dose response curve of NAT to induction by isoproterenol (4). In addition, there is an increase in the maximum response attainable (4).

Thus, during the latter half of the night, NAT activity falls and subsensitivity develops. As a pharmacologic stimulus, isoproterenol is able to override this subsensitivity which nevertheless remains evident as a shift to the right in the dose response curve.

If rats are made supersensitive by exposure to light overnight, and then injected with isoproterenol repeatedly at 2 hour intervals, NAT activity rises and then falls following a very similar time course to the normal physiologic cycle (28).

C. Time Course of NAT Induction

A single dose of isoproterenol given to rats at noon or later during the daylight hours induces NAT activity after a lag of about 1 hour. Peak activity of NAT occurs 3 hours after the injection, and enzyme activity returns to baseline within 5 hours. If the animals are challenged with a second dose of isoproterenol, the corresponding rise in NAT activity is smaller, and the time course of the induction is accelerated: the lag is clearly less than 1 hour, while peak activity is attained between 1 and 2 hours. Three hours after the second injection, NAT activity has returned to baseline (29).

Increasing the duration of exposure to light, in addition to causing supersensitivity, also increases the lag for induction of NAT by isoproterenol (28). In the afternoon (1800 hrs), after

12 hours of exposure to light, isoproterenol induces NAT in vivo with a lag period greater than 1 hour. Peak activity of NAT occurs between 3 and 4 hours after the injection. In contrast, in the morning (0630 hrs), the lag for induction of NAT is shorter, and peak activity occurs earlier (28). The extreme case is illustrated by rats which are exposed to light for 20 minutes at midnight, thereby causing enzyme activity to fall to baseline. In these animals, NAT levels rise immediately after isoproterenol injection and peak activity occurs within 1 hour (16, 29).

This variation in the lag period for induction of NAT by isoproterenol suggests that there is a precursor present in rats that have been recently stimulated either by darkness or by exogenous catecholamines. During the day, this precursor decays, thus explaining the increasing lag period. The rapid reinduction of NAT at midnight after exposure to light indicates that such a precursor is available at this time. Since inhibition of protein synthesis with cycloheximide completely blocks stimulation by isoproterenol, even at midnight, the rapid reinduction of NAT probably does not represent the reactivation of an inactive form of the enzyme.

Actinomycin D, which inhibits RNA synthesis, blocks the induction of NAT in rats injected with isoproterenol at the end of the light period by 80 to 90 percent. Actinomycin D does not block the reinduction of NAT by isoproterenol at midnight after exposure to light for 20 minutes. At 0600 hrs, induction by isoproterenol is partially blocked (50 to 80 percent) by actinomycin D. Thus, the sensitivity to actinomycin D correlates with the length of the lag period for induction of NAT, suggesting that the lag period is due to the requirement for new RNA synthesis (30).

The above experiments with actinomycin D and cycloheximide strongly suggest that activation of the β-adrenergic receptor by isoproterenol results in stimulation of both transcription and translation. At midnight, stimulation of translation is sufficient to reinduce enzyme activity since reinduction occurs even in the presence of 90-95 percent inhibition of RNA synthesis by actinomycin D (30). However, the inhibition of the action of isoproterenol by actinomycin D at 1800 hrs implies that in these animals both transcription and translation are necessary for induction of NAT activity (30).

Similar results obtained using dibutyryl cAMP to induce NAT activity indicate that both the pre- and the post-transcriptional actions of the β-adrenergic receptor utilize cyclic AMP as a second messenger.

D. <u>Regulation of Sensitivity to β-Adrenergic Stimulation in the Pineal Gland</u>

We have discussed 3 manifestations of the changes in sensitivity which occur during the normal physiologic cycle: the first is an increased response to the same dose of isoproterenol and therefore a decrease in the dose required to produce a given response; the second is an increase in the maximum response attained; and, the third is a progressive lengthening of the lag period for enzyme induction.

The first of these manifestations, a change in the dose response curve to isoproterenol, suggests changes in properties of the receptor, which increase the efficiency of its coupling to intracellular mechanisms for the induction of the enzyme. Second, the changes in the maximum response as a function of prior stimulation, suggest either the activation of inhibitory feedback loops, or the depletion of some essential intermediate for the production of active enzyme.

These phenomena, in addition to the precursor discussed above, indicate the participation of intracellular mechanisms in the regulation of the sensitivity of pineal N-acetyltransferase to induction by catecholamines. This hypothesis was supported by the observation that, in cultured pineal glands obtained at 0600 hrs and at 1800 hrs, the sensitivity of NAT to induction by dibutyryl cyclic AMP also varies with diurnal cycles which parallel the changes which we have found with isoproterenol (28).

This indication that intracellular phenomena participate in the regulation of the sensitivity of the pineal gland to catecholamines does not rule out the possibility that concurrent changes occur at the membrane (receptor-adenylate cyclase complex). The shift to the left in the dose response curve suggests that modifications of receptor properties are also present.

Indeed, the sensitivity of pineal cyclic AMP response to isoproterenol also varies during the diurnal cycle. In the morning, isoproterenol cuases two to three fold increases in the level of cyclic AMP; whereas in the afternoon, the same dose of isoproterenol causes five to ten fold increases in cylic AMP (31).

To summarize, there are diurnal cycles in the sensitivity of NAT to stimulation by catecholamines in the pineal gland. These changes in sensitivity are postsynaptic, occur rapidly, and are in close relationship to the physiologic cycles in sympathetic nerve activity. During the night, when sympathetic nerve activity in the pineal gland is high, a relative subsensitivity develops, which may play an important role in the endogenous cycles of NAT activity. During the day, when nerve activity is low, supersensitivity develops rapidly. The remarkable rate of development of these changes in sensitivity is in sharp contrast to the rate of development of postsynaptic supersensitivity in other systems (19-20).

The β-adrenergic receptor exerts its action intracellularly with cyclic AMP acting as a second messenger. Both pre-transcriptional and post-transcriptional sites are involved in the action of the β-adrenergic receptor in stimulating NAT.

The regulation of the changes in sensitivity also occurs at least at 2 levels. An increase in the sensitivity of cyclic AMP to stimulation by isoproterenol indicates regulation of sensitivity at the receptor-adenylate cyclase complex in the cell membrane. On the basis of our data we cannot distinguish between an increase in the number of receptors, a change in the affinity of the receptor for its agonist, or changes in the efficiency of coupling of the receptor to adenylate cyclase. The second level of regulation of the sensitivity of NAT to induction by isoproterenol is intracellular, probably involving controls in the pathways for synthesis and activation of enzymes.

4. REFERENCES

1. H. Weissbach, B. G. Redfield, Biochem. Biophys. Acta, 43, 352 (1960).

2. J. Axelrod and H. Weissbach, J. Biol. Chem., 236, 211 (1961).

3. D. C. Klein and J. C. Weller, Science, 169, 1093 (1970).

4. J. A. Romero and J. Axelrod, Science, 184, 1091 (1974).

5. J. Axelrod, R. J. Wurtman and S. H. Snyder, J. Biol. Chem., 240, 949 (1965).

6. D. C. Klein and J. L. Weller, Exerpta Med. Int. Cong. Ser. No., 256, 52 (1972).

7. M. J. Brownstein, J. M. Saavedra and J. Axelrod, Molec. Pharmacol., 9 605 (1973).

8. H. J. Lynch, Life Sci., 10, 791 (1971).

9. W. B. Quay, Gen. Comp. Endocrinol., 3, 473 (1963).

10. J. A. Kappers, Z. Zellforsch. Mikrosk. Anat., 52, 163 (1960).

11. J. Axelrod, Science, 184, 1341 (1974).

12. A. N. Taylor and R. W. Wilson, Experientia, 26, 267 (1970).

13. M. J. Brownstein and J. Axelrod, Science, 184, 163 (1974).

14. D. C. Klein, G. R. Berger and J. C. Weller, Science, 168, 979 (1970).

15. T. Deguchi, Molec. Pharmacol., 9, 184 (1973).

16. T. Deguchi and J. Axelrod, Proc. Nat. Acad. Sci., 69, 2547 (1972).

17. D. C. Klein and J. C. Weller, Science, 177, 532 (1972).

18. J. A. Romero, unpublished observations.

19. U. Trendelenburg, Pharmacol. Rev., 15, 225 (1963).

20. W. Fleming, J. J. McPhillips and D. P. Westfall, Rev. Physiol., 68, 55 (1973).

21. T. Deguchi and J. Axelrod, Proc. Nat. Acad. Sci., 69, 2208 (1972).

22. G. Hertting, Biochem. Pharmacol., 13, 1119 (1963).

23. T. Deguchi and J. Axelrod, Molec. Pharmacol., 9, 612 (1973).

24. B. Weiss and S. J. Strada, in Advances in Cyclic Nucleotide Research (Greengard, P., Robison, G. A. and Paoletti, R., eds.), Volume 1, pp. 357-374, Raven Press, N. Y., 1972.

25. T. Deguchi and J. Axelrod, Proc. Nat. Acad. Sci., 70, 2411 (1973).

26. S. A. Brinkley, D. C. Klein and J. L. Weller, Experientia, 29, 1339 (1973).

27. M. J. Brownstein and J. A. Romero, unpublished observations.

28. J. A. Romero and J. A. Axelrod, submitted for publication.

29. J. A. Romero, unpublished observations.

30. J. A. Romero, M. Zatz, and J. Axelrod, Proc. Nat. Acad. Sci., submitted for publication.

31. J. A. Romero and M. Zatz, unpublished observations.

DISCUSSION

Dr. Lovenberg asked if nucleotide incorporation had been studied by Dr. Romero. The speaker replied that he was in the process of doing that.

Dr. Aghajanian wondered if there is a conductive change at the pineal site as the result of beta stimulation, but Dr. Romero indicated that he did not have any data on this.

STRATEGIES FOR THE SYSTEMATIC STUDY OF
NEUROTRANSMITTER RECEPTOR FUNCTION IN MAN

William E. Bunney, Jr., M.D. and Dennis L. Murphy, M.D.

Adult Psychiatry Branch
National Institute of Mental Health
Bethesda, Maryland
and
Section on Clinical Neuropharmacology
Laboratory of Clinical Science
National Institute of Mental Health
Bethesda, Maryland

INTRODUCTION

The systematic study of neurotransmitter receptor function in man remains a neglected area. It is a potentially important issue in understanding disease states and the mechanism of action of pharmacological agents, including drugs affecting behavior.

Although little direct evidence exists, it is clearly possible that changes in neurotransmitter receptor site function may be secondarily or even primarily involved in psychopathological processes, in neurological diseases, and perhaps in other metabolic diseases in man. Disease processes may be reflected in altered or unstable receptor site sensitivity both in chronic illness [1-3] and in a particular phase of recurrent illnesses [4-6]. In the area of behavioral disorders, it has been hypothesized that altered neurotransmitter receptor site sensitivity might exist in the manic and/or depressive phases of bipolar manic-depressive illness [6-8].

It is well known that many of the neuroleptic drugs block post-synaptic dopamine receptors, thus altering the ability of neurotransmitters to bind to these receptors. It has been hypothesized that this action of the neuroleptics may be involved in their therapeutic effects in schizophrenia [9,10]. It is also possible that some of the side effects of chronically administered neuroleptics, for example, tardive dyskinesia, may reflect alterations of receptor site sensitivity [11-13].

It now appears possible to design new therapeutic approaches in the area of psychopharmacology utilizing pharmacologically-induced supersensitivity of a neurotransmitter receptor site prior to a therapeutic agonist in order to increase the potency of the agonist in drug-resistant patients or to accelerate the therapeutic effect.

There are a number of reasons why this area has been relatively neglected in the past. Initial studies of neurotransmitter receptor function in man involved attempts to study it in the periphery, using, for example, blood pressure as a response measure. It is, however, well known that the regulation of blood pressure is a complex phenomenon, only one element of which involves receptor function. A second difficulty in studying receptors in the CNS in man is that only indirect response measures are available. Thirdly, most available agonist drugs have multiple sites of action; for example, amphetamine has often been used as an agonist for testing receptor responsivity. However, it is known that in addition to facilitating the release of norepinephrine and dopamine, amphetamine also has the actions of blocking reuptake and affecting monoamine oxidase activity. Finally, some of the specific drugs which have been particularly useful in animals, such as 6-hydroxydopamine and 5,6-dihydroxytryptamine, are not available for use in man because of apparent irreversible neurotoxicity. Both of these drugs cause degeneration of pre-synaptic neurons.

In the past, there has certainly existed a paucity of basic information concerning pre- and post-synaptic neurotransmitter function and thus the critical data to design human experiments has not been available. Recently, however, there has been an expansion of basic information concerning this area and it is now perhaps possible to develop systematic studies of receptor function in man. In attempting to conceptualize the mode of action of drugs, one site is usually considered. However, it is well known that there are multiple sites for most pharmacological agents. In man, studying receptor function is obviously difficult because one is not able to dissect out the specific sites of drug action as one can in some animal studies. Thus it is necessary to look at final common behavioral reactions such as sleep, activity and neuroendocrine responses.

Figure 1 reviews some of the possible strategies for the study of neurotransmitter receptor function in man. The strategies include pharmacological approaches, the study of lesions, and the utilization of tissue models, all of which are discussed in further detail below.

1. Pharmacological

2. Lesions

   a. traumatic

   b. surgical (sympathectomy)

   c. viral

3. Tissue Models

   a. brain

   b. adipose tissue

   c. platelet

   d. leukocyte

Fig. 1. Strategies for the Study of Neurotransmitter Receptor Function in Man.

With the exception of the tissue models, receptor function studies in man require the use of whole-body responses and some of these are indicated in Figure 2. Blood pressure, pulse, salivation, pupillary changes and temperature are some examples of measurable responses. Sleep parameters provide a possible quantitative and sensitive measure of receptor site changes. Physical activity is a traditional measure utilized in animals, and with the development of sophisticated telemetric monitoring systems it is now possible to accurately measure physical activity throughout a 24-hour period in patients. Neuroendocrine responses deserve special attention. There is an extensive literature suggesting,

1. B.P., Pulse, Salivation, Pupillary Changes, Temperature

2. Sleep Parameters

3. Physical Activity

4. Neuroendocrine Responses

5. Behavior

    examples: psychosis

    mania

    depression

    irritability

6. Neurological Changes

    example: tardive dyskinesia

Fig. 2. Whole Body Indices of Receptor Function Changes.

for example, that dopamine agonists are associated with decreased release of prolactin and luteinizing hormone (LH) [14-17]. In addition, gross behavioral ratings of psychosis, mania, depression and irritability may be shown to reflect alterations in receptor site sensitivity. Finally, neurological changes may also provide indices of receptor function. For example, as mentioned above, it has been hypothesized that tardive dyskinesia following chronic neuroleptic administration may be associated with receptor site changes [11,12].

PHARMACOLOGICAL STRATEGIES

Changes in receptor function are often reflected in changes in super- or sub-sensitivity of the receptor. Pharmacological agents provide a method of assessing or producing such changes. We have selected the dopamine neurotransmitter receptor in order to illustrate pharmacological strategies for studying neurotransmitter receptor site function in man. Figure 3 outlines one possible strategy.

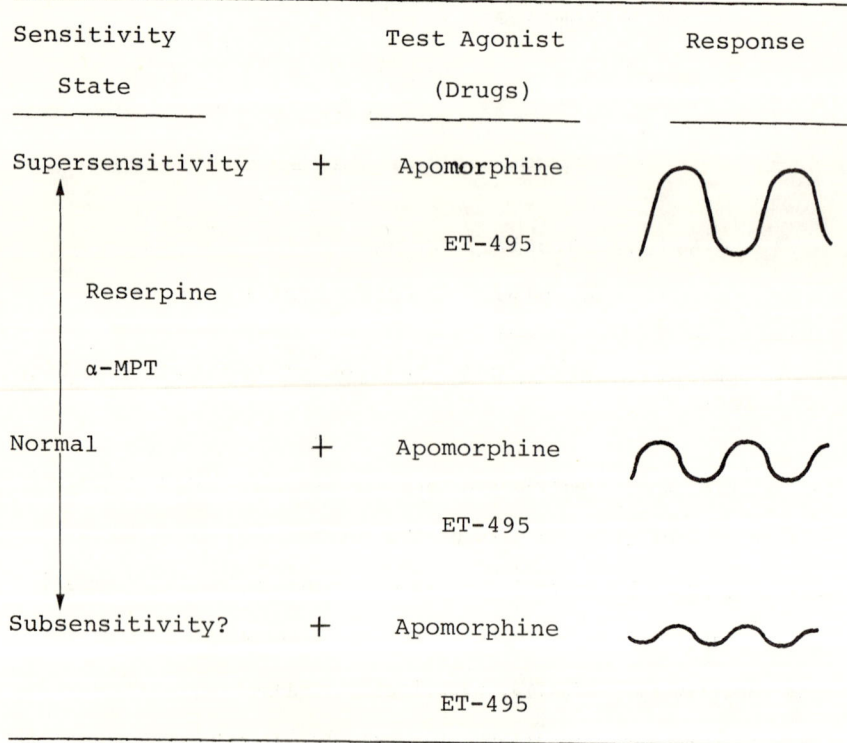

Fig. 3. Evaluation of Directly Produced Receptor Sensitivity Changes in Dopamine Receptor.

RECEPTOR STUDIES IN MAN

Direct Receptor Studies Using Dopamine Agonists

The first strategy would involve the administration of an agonist in the dopamine system. Relatively pure agonist compounds which pass the blood-brain barrier include apomorphine and piribedil (ET-495) [18,19]. We have listed these in the center column as prototypes. Apomorphine, of course, has the disadvantage of producing nausea and vomiting, while ET-495 is associated with less nausea at moderate doses. Other possible drugs include methylphenidate, amantadine, L-DOPA and dopamine. These agonists might be given during disease states or during various phases of illnesses, utilizing some of the whole body indices of receptor site function. These are schematically represented on the right side of the figure.

Receptor Function Studies Following Induced Supersensitivity or Subsensitivity

A second possible strategy for studying receptor site function in disease states might involve perturbing the system with a compound which is thought to specifically increase or decrease neuronal receptor site sensitivity and then to test with a specific agonist. This second approach would allow confirmation of the capacity to develop supersensitivity or subsensitivity states in conditions where previously-identified receptor site abnormalities have been suggested. In the case of the dopamine system, chronic treatment with AMPT or reserpine will produce a state similar to supersensitivity of the receptor which could be tested with an agonist, i.e., apomorphine or ET-495. Many animal studies have documented the supersensitivity associated with these compounds.

Although little animal work and no human studies have been done, it is also possible to consider the investigation of subsensitivity in man, through the strategy of chronic administration of a dopamine agonist.

It is theorized that the bombardment of the neuronal receptor site by the transmitter molecule induces a subsensitivity, while a chronic decrease in the number of neurotransmitter molecules hitting the receptor site results in the development of a supersensitive receptor system. Both of these changes are theoretically followed by adaptive responses, including alterations in uptake of substrates into the neuron, induction or inhibition of synthetic enzymes (particularly those that are rate limiting) [6,20,21], and perhaps changes in degradation enzymes.

In summary, this strategy involves the induction of super- or subsensitivity with specific pharmacological agents. The sensitivity state of the neuronal receptor site is then tested with specific agonists by measuring whole body or tissue changes.

Receptor Function Changes Following Drug Withdrawal

Figure 4 is similar to Fig.3. However, it emphasizes the concept of studying supersensitivity following discontinuation of a compound. The study of physiological and psychological phenomena following the withdrawal of chronically administered pharmacological agents has been neglected. It provides an important research approach and possible therapeutic tool. Supersensitivity associated with phenothiazines and other neuroleptics can probably best be evaluated following withdrawal of the compound.

RECEPTOR STUDIES IN MAN

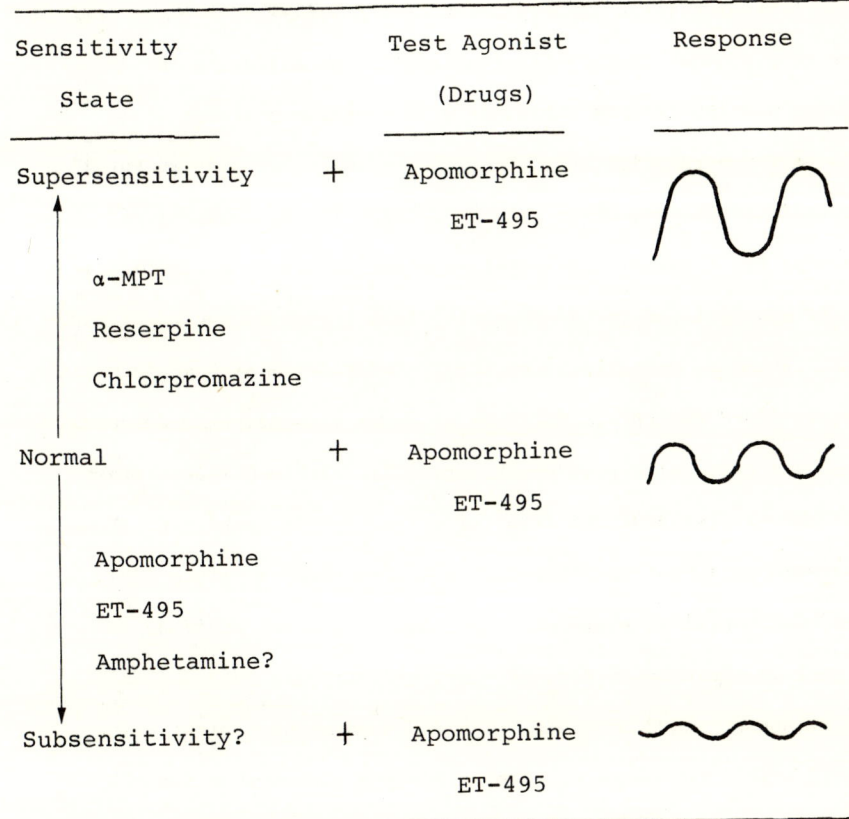

Fig. 4. Evaluation of Receptor Sensitivity Changes in Dopamine Systems Associated with Drug Discontinuation.

In terms of subsensitivity it is also conceivable that the severe crash or depression following the prolonged excessive use of high doses of amphetamine in man may be associated with a subsensitivity of the dopamine system. Again, this could be specifically tested with dopamine agonists.

Two examples of the pharmacological production of supersensitivity in man and its investigation in animal data will be reviewed below. Specifically, the supersensitivity following the discontinuation of alpha-methyl-para-tyrosine (AMPT) and following the discontinuation of phenothiazines will be discussed.

AMPT Supersensitivity. The first example involves the utilization of AMPT in man, which acts as a competitive inhibitor of tyrosine hydroxylase, the enzyme involved in the rate limiting step in the synthesis of the neurotransmitters, dopamine and norepinephrine. Nineteen drug trials of this compound were studied in manic and depressed patients. AMPT was given in an attempt to decrease manic and depressive psychopathology [22]. Table I illustrates that between two and four days following discontinuation of AMPT, depressed patients experienced a marked decrease in sleep [23]. Sleep was monitored every half-hour by the nursing staff on each patient in the drug trials and was systematically recorded on a continuous record of sleep. Table 2 also shows a significant decrease in total hours of sleep following discontinuation of AMPT in seven manic patients on days 3 and 4. It should also be noted that in 15 out of the 19 drug trials, each patient experienced within the first four days following discontinuation of AMPT at least one night in which there was little if any sleep. This decrease is reflected in the mean decreases shown in Tables 1 and 2. In marked contrast to this finding, discontinuation of chronic treatment with large doses of two precursors of biogenic amines, L-DOPA (12 trials) [24] and L-tryptophan (17 trials) [25] produced no change in total hours of sleep during the withdrawal period.

Table 1

Total Sleep Following Discontinuation
of AMPT (Depressed Patients N=7)

	During AMPT Treatment		AMPT Stopped	Post AMPT Treatment		
Days	-6,-5	-4,-3	-2,-1 →	1,2	3,4	5,6
Sleep,	6.85	6.75	6.56	5.24**	4.85*	5.35
Hours	±0.43	±0.42	±0.47	±0.60	±0.65	±0.72

* P < .05, Paired t analysis

** P < .01, Paired t analysis

TABLE 2

Total Sleep Following Discontinuation of AMPT (Manic Patients N=7)

	During AMPT Treatment	AMPT Stopped		Post AMPT Treatment	
Days	-6,-5	-4,-3	-2,-1	1,2	3,4	5,6	7,8
Sleep, Hours	5.56 ±0.32	5.91 ±0.33	6.15 ±0.33	4.81 ±0.51	2.97* ±0.50	4.13 ±0.60	5.01 ±0.79

* $P < .05$, Paired τ analysis

Following AMPT discontinuation, an increased rate of catecholamine synthesis occurs with a hypothetical increase in the concentration of catecholamine molecules available for binding to the receptor site. It is also possible that a continued increase in sensitivity to the catecholamine receptor occurs during this post-AMPT period. Thus, both an increase in synthesis and in receptor sensitivity may be present in man.

Animal studies have clearly documented that an apparent increase in neuronal receptor site sensitivity occurs following AMPT withdrawal [26-29]. All of the studies are consistent in documenting increased motor activity, stereotypic responses and hypothermic responses post-AMPT. These responses have been further augmented by the administration of apomorphine, amphetamine and norepinephrine. One study assessed total stereotypic behavior and demonstrated an increase and shift to the left in a dose response curve one and two weeks following discontinuation of AMPT [29].

Phenothiazine Supersensitivity. A second example of possible supersensitivity produced in the dopamine system involves the discontinuation of chronic neuroleptic agents such as chlorpromazine. Figure 5 lists some of the studies which have documented the existence of tardive dyskinesia following discontinuation of phenothiazines and butyrophenones [30-37]. Eight studies reported a total of 47 patients. Neurological symptoms appeared 3 to 7 days following discontinuation of the neuroleptic. The findings included: spontaneous appearance of tardive dyskinesia (which was not previously manifested), exacerbation of tardive dyskinesia, and appearance of

Studies	Drugs	No. of Patients	Response 3-7 Days (Average) Post Neuroleptic Discontinuation
Uhrbrand and Faurbye, 1960	Phenothiazines and Butyrophenones	47 Patients Reported	1. Appearance of tardive dyskinesia not previously manifested.
Morphew and Barber, 1965			2. Exacerbation of tardive dyskinesia.
Pryce and Edwards, 1966			3. Appearance of other neurological symptoms.
Kennedy, 1969			
Krystof, et al., 1972			
DeMaio, 1973			
Polizos, et al., 1973			
Jacobson, et al., 1974			

Fig. 5. Tardive Dyskinesia Post Neuroleptics.

a variety of other neurological symptoms. It was hypothesized that these neurological symptoms may be the result of a supersensitivity of the dopamine receptor following prolonged receptor blockade.

Preliminary data in our own laboratory has suggested that within four days following discontinuation of the rather specific dopamine receptor neuroleptic blocking agent, pimozide, patients have a marked decrease in sleep for at least one of the four days following the drug [38]. Again, it is possible to interpret these observations as the development of a supersensitivity associated with prolonged administration of a neuroleptic. The observed decrease in sleep is similar to that reported with AMPT.

These findings are compatible with studies in rats and guinea pigs, in which it has been shown that, on an average, 4-14 days following neuroleptic discontinuation, the animals show an increase in spontaneous locomotor behavior, enhanced stereotypic response to apomorphine, and lowered threshold for amphetamine-induced stereotypic responses, as shown in Fig. 6 [29,39-41]. Tarsy and Baldessarini [29] showed an increase in total stereotypic behavior induced by apomorphine one and four weeks following discontinuation of chlorpromazine. There was a shift to the left in the apomorphine dose-response curve following both periods of time, which was more pronounced one week after chlorpromazine.

It is conceivable that one could administer apomorphine or ET-495 to patients following discontinuation of chronic chlorpromazine in patients who did not demonstrate tardive dyskinesia. The appearance of tardive dyskinesia in an individual following

Studies	Drugs	Animals	Response 4-14 Days (Average) Following Neuroleptic Discontinuation
Boyd, 1960	Chlorpromazine and Haloperidol	Rats and Guinea Pigs	1. Increase in spontaneous locomotor activity.
Rubovits, et al., 1973			2. Enhanced stereotypic response to apomorphine.
Gianutsos, et al., 1973			3. Lowered threshold for amphetamine induced stereotypic response.
Tarsy and Baldessarini, 1974			

Fig. 6. Increased Motor Activity Post Neuroleptics in Animal Studies.

RECEPTOR STUDIES IN MAN

administration of a dopamine agonist might then indicate a vulnerability to developing these neurological symptoms.

Studies in man with neurotransmitter agonists utilizing dose response curves provide a powerful tool. This procedure has been almost totally ignored in pharmacological studies in humans.

<u>Norepinephrine Receptor Function</u>. Fig. 7 illustrates a strategy for studying norepinephrine receptor function in man. The pharmacological agent, clonidine, appears to be a norepinephrine agonist. Evidence suggests that in high doses, it may act as a post-synaptic agonist and at low doses, a pre-synaptic agonist.

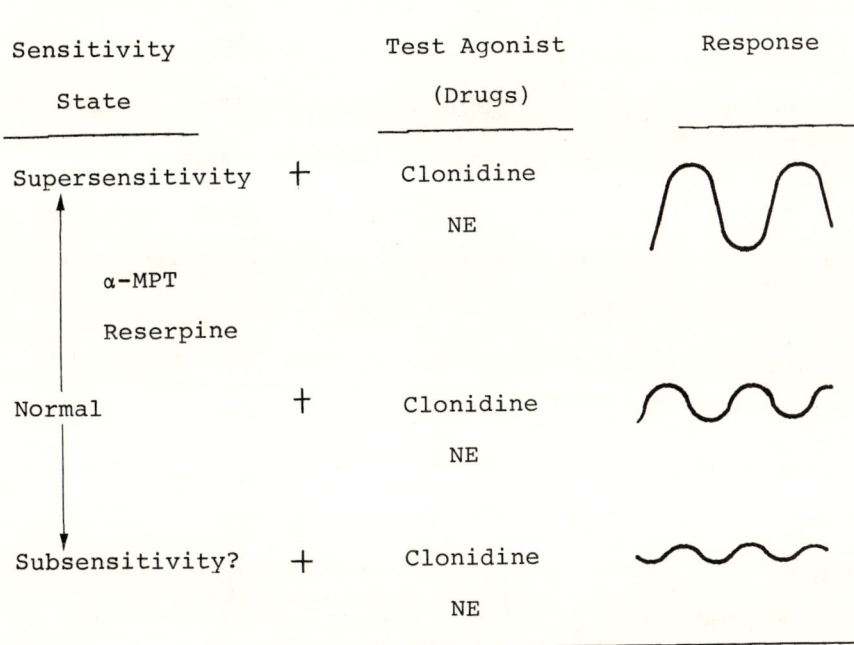

Fig. 7. Possible Evaluation of Directly Produced Receptor Sensitivity Changes in Norepinephrine Receptors.

Its use offers the possibility of dissecting out pre-synaptic from post-synaptic effects in man [42]. Thus, clonidine might be given during illness phases and in different disease states, while monitoring whole body indices of norepinephrine receptor function.

A second strategy would again involve perturbing the system with a compound which is thought to specifically increase or decrease receptor site sensitivity and then to test with an agonist. It would be possible to pharmacologically alter the sensitivity of the norepinephrine receptor utilizing AMPT or reserpine, as previously suggested for dopamine.

In addition, in Fig. 8 the receptor site sensitivity following discontinuation of the beta blocker, propranolol, or following discontinuation of alpha blockers, might be studied with an agonistic compound such as clonidine. This approach is similar to that proposed following discontinuation of the phenothiazines and butyrophenones. It is also suggested in both Figures 7 and 8 that subsensitive states associated with chronic administration of an agonist such as clonidine, or with one of the direct precursors of norepinephrine, threo-dihydroxyphenylserine (threo-DOPS), might be utilized. There is, to our knowledge, no research in man or animals to provide data concerning this approach. There are also conflicts in the literature concerning whether threo-DOPS effectively increases brain ℓ-norepinephrine synthesis [43,44].

Serotonin Receptor Studies. Similarly, one might evaluate directly or indirectly receptor site changes in the serotonin system using serotonergic agonists such as fenfluramine. Super-

RECEPTOR STUDIES IN MAN

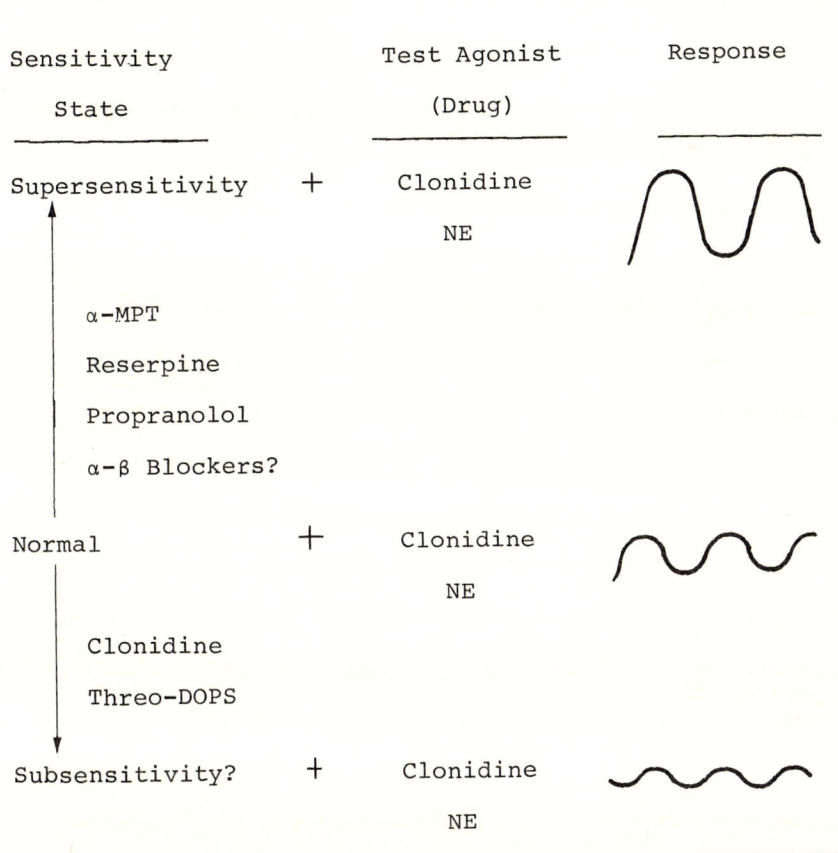

Fig. 8. Possible Evaluation of Receptor Sensitivity Changes in Norepinephrine System Associated with Drug Discontinuation.

sensitivity might be produced with parachlorophenylalanine, a synthesis inhibitor at the rate limiting step, or following discontinuation of serotonergic receptor site blockade with methysergide. Chronic fenfluramine treatment might induce a subsensitivity. All of the compounds mentioned above have been safely administered to man.

Adaptive Mechanisms

To this point we have focused almost entirely on changes in receptor site sensitivity. However, it is well known that this is only part of the complex adaptive neuronal mechanism. Recent studies in animals have demonstrated apparent compensatory changes in brain biogenic amine metabolic pathways in response to pretreatment with psychoactive drugs; for example, the administration of phenothiazines and butyrophenones not only blocks synaptic receptors but is followed by homeostatic increases in striatal tyrosine hydroxylase activity [20]. A similar increase in this rate limiting enzyme in the catecholamine synthetic pathway occurs after 7-9 days of reserpine administration. In contrast, psychoactive drugs which are thought to enhance biogenic amine related synaptic efficacy (imipramine, pargyline, amphetamine) produce a 25-150% increase in the activity of brain tyrosine hydroxylase activity when these drugs are given chronically [6,45]. The finding of these adaptive enzyme responses to chronic drug administration has increased our understanding of the complexity of the metabolic processes involved. It should also be noted that drugs apparently as specific as AMPT or pimozide in affecting the dopamine system may also indirectly affect the norepinephrine, cholinergic, indoleamine and GABA systems. Thus these compounds, which are apparently specific in affecting dopamine systems, may be involved in rather complex interactions with a number of neurotransmitter systems in producing their final behavioral effects.

STRATEGIES UTILIZING LESIONS

Another traditional strategy for the investigation of neuronal receptor site sensitivity alterations in animals is by utilization of surgical and chemical lesions. In man, the traumatic occurrence of lesions following automobile accidents or war wounds provides potential information in this area. In general, however, CNS receptor function has not been systematically evaluated after such lesions. A few isolated studies are provocative. It was found, for example, that a hyperacuity of the phantom limb syndrome in amputees was produced by mescaline [46], which was interpreted as a possible supersensitivity [47]. In another study of an accident case, acetylcholine was applied to both hemispheres of the human brain ten months following a traumatic lesion [48]. The lesion isolated a small segment of the left hemisphere. Acetylcholine had no apparent effect on the intact hemisphere. However, it produced extremely high voltage discharges from the isolated hemisphere. The authors suggested that this might indicate heightened responsivity in cholinergic receptors [48].

The most common type of surgical lesion which may relate to supersensitivity is sympathectomy. Results of a number of studies indicated increased vasoconstriction in response to intravenous epinephrine post-sympathectomy [49-53]. It was suggested that these findings were consistent with a supersensitivity following sympathectomy.

Finally, one of the possible etiologies of Parkinson's Disease may involve degeneration of the pre-synaptic dopamine fibers of the nigrostriatal tract as a result of viral infection. Hypersensitivity of the dopamine system may thus result and explain part of the neuropathology in this illness [54].

Gilles de la Tourette Syndrome has also been studied and it has been proposed that it may involve altered neuronal receptor site sensitivity [55]. Other rare neurological illnesses may also provide uncommon but important clues concerning the role of receptor site sensitivity and the production of neuropathology.

STRATEGIES UTILIZING TISSUE MODELS

This section will review possible tissue models for the study of neurotransmitter-related receptor functions in man, including brain, subcutaneous adipose tissue, platelets and leukocytes. In these examples, α or β catecholamine receptor function changes have been evaluated by measurement of cyclic-AMP or adenyl cyclase changes following catecholamine administration.

Brain

Cyclic-AMP interactions have been studied in human brain biopsy material [56]. Biopsies of cortical grey matter were taken during cancer surgery. Cyclic-AMP elevations were observed following norepinephrine (20-50 times baseline), veratridine (20-50 times), histamine (4-7 times), adenosine (4-7 times) and serotonin (1.5-2 times). Isoproterenol and epinephrine were more effective than norepinephrine in producing cyclic-AMP changes. The effects of all of the catecholamines were blocked by propranolol; thus, it appears as though a dominant beta-receptor adrenergic response is present in human cortex [56]. This study was done in 17 biopsy specimens and at least suggests the possibility of studying receptors in human brain cortex.

Subcutaneous Adipose Tissue

Human subcutaneous adipose tissue taken by biopsy has been utilized to study catecholamine-adenyl cyclase interactions [1,2,57]. Adipose tissue, incubated in buffer, develops increased cyclic-AMP levels and releases glycerol in response to norepinephrine. Propranolol reduces and phentolamine increases the lipolytic effects of norepinephrine, accompanied by corresponding changes in cyclic-AMP. When this system was examined in 84 hypothyroid patients, it was found that adipose tissue from these patients is much less responsive to norepinephrine than the tissue from normals. Studies with combinations of agonists and blocking drugs suggested that increased alpha-adrenergic stimulation is associated with hypothyroidism [1,2,57].

Platelets

The human platelet has been proposed as a model which may be useful for studying alterations in alpha-receptor site sensitivity in man. In platelets separated from blood samples, norepinephrine and epinephrine $\underline{in}$ $\underline{vitro}$ reduce prostaglandin E_1 (PGE_1) stimulated cyclic-AMP elevations [58-60]. Phentolamine but not propranolol prevents the catecholamine effects on cyclic-AMP [60]. Platelets also provide the opportunity to study the marked individual variations in PGE_1, NE and E effects on platelet cyclic-AMP formation.

One of the few instances in which a psychoactive drug interacts with an adrenergic receptor-cyclic-AMP response has been studied in man. Lithium chloride in vitro as well as in vivo was found to have antagonistic effects on PGE_1 stimulated ^{3}H-cyclic-AMP formation and on the norepinephrine inhibition of PGE_1 effects [61, 62].

Platelet cyclic-AMP responses to norepinephrine were also evaluated in two studies of depressed patients. No altered responsiveness to either norepinephrine or PGE_1 was observed in either study [62,63], and hence no evidence in support of a generalized alteration in adrenergic receptor function in depression was obtained. However, as the platelet alpha-adrenergic receptor is not subjected to the same intra-synaptic stimuli as are catecholamine receptors in the CNS, no firm conclusions can be drawn against the hypothesis of CNS receptor function changes in depression.

Leukocytes

The human leukocyte has also been used to study catecholamine cyclic-AMP interactions. Isoproterenol, norepinephrine and epinephrine increase cyclic-AMP levels in human leukocytes studied in vitro [4]. Propranolol blocks the response to catecholamines, indicating that beta-receptors are involved. Some individuals with severe symptomatic bronchial asthma exhibit decreased responses to catecholamines, but normal responses to prostaglandin E_1 [4,5]. Cyclic-AMP responses of mixed leukocytes to various concentrations of propranolol were consistently lower in 52 asthmatic patients studied compared with normal controls. These findings suggest impairment in beta-adrenergic receptor responses in asthmatic patients.

Thus the platelet provides a possible tissue model for studying alpha-adrenergic receptors while the leukocyte offers a model for studying beta-adrenergic receptors in man.

POSSIBLE NEURONAL RECEPTOR SITE SENSITIVITY CHANGES IN BIPOLAR MANIC-DEPRESSIVE ILLNESS

We would like to propose a theoretical model which may be useful in explaining some of the phenomenology observed in this serious mental illness [64]. This model serves as an example of the possible use of our current knowledge of neuronal receptor site metabolism and physiology to construct a heuristic paradigm which may be useful in designing future research in disease states.

Manic-depressive illness is characterized by cyclic alterations in mood and cognition from a depressive phase involving retardation, feelings of worthlessness and hopelessness, to a manic phase involving markedly increased motor and verbal activity, grandiosity, euphoria and, at times, psychotic thoughts.

It is proposed that a supersensitive state of an amine-like receptor exists in the depressive phase of the illness and that environmental stresses or pharmacological agents may result in triggering the release of endogenous amine-like agonists, which then results in the sudden increase in motor and verbal activity and manic behavior. Manic episodes are often two to four weeks in duration and usually terminate spontaneously. This clinical course would be compatible with the gradual development of a tolerance to an amine-like agonist with a shift to a subsensitive state of the receptor molecule. It might be suggested that a defect is present in the normal homeostatic dampening of the ability of the receptor to markedly alter its sensitivity in manic-depressive illness. It is known that in some systems the conformation of the receptor site is affected by sodium levels at an allosteric site [65]. Among several possibilities, it is conceivable that lithium might substitute for sodium in the receptor system, and that this action might be contributory to its clinical efficacy in manic-depressive illness.

SUMMARY

This paper suggests that it may now be possible to initiate systematic studies of neurotransmitter receptor site function in man. Alterations in receptor site function are often manifested by the development of super- and sub-sensitive states. It is suggested that the evaluation of neurotransmitter receptor site function in man may be of particular importance, a) in understanding modes of action and side effects of many acute and chronically administered psychoactive agents; b) that some psychiatric disease states (manic-depressive illness), neurological states (Gilles de la Tourette's Syndrome) and metabolic illnesses (asthma and hypothyroidism) may involve secondary and perhaps even primary defects in dysfunctions of neurotransmitter receptor site activity; c) that it might be possible to develop new pharmacological treatment regimens utilizing the concept of altering and/or stabilizing receptor site sensitivity alone or in conjunction with agonist compounds.

Two general strategies for investigation are suggested: pharmacological and tissue models.

Pharmacologic research strategies involve: a) the measurement of specific behaviors in man which appear to be changed by alterations in receptor site sensitivity; b) the utilization of agonists to test changes in receptor site sensitivity; and, c) the utilization of compounds which in themselves increase or decrease receptor site sensitivity, followed by agonists to test for altered sensitivity states.

Three possible tissue models are suggested: human subcutaneous adipose tissue obtained on biopsy may measure alpha-adrenergic receptors; similarly, platelets offer a system for studying alpha-adrenergic receptors, while human leukocytes provide a model for studying beta-adrenergic receptors in man.

REFERENCES

[1]. U. Rosenqvist, Acta. Med. Scand., 192, 1972A, 353-359.
[2]. U. Rosenqvist, Acta. Med. Scand., 192, 1972B, 361-369.
[3]. H. L. Klawans, C. Goetz, and W. J. Weiner, J. Neural Trans. 34, 1973, 187-193.
[4]. C. W. Parker and J. W. Smith, J. Clin. Invest., 52, 1973, 48-59.
[5]. C. W. Parker, M. L. Baumann, and M. G. Huber, J. Clin. Invest., 52, 1973, 1336-1341.
[6]. D. S. Segal, R. Kuczenski, and A. J. Mandell, Biol. Psychiat., 9(2), 1974, 147-159.
[7]. G. W. Ashcroft, E. Eccleston, L. G. Murray, A. Glen, T. Crawford, I. Pullar, P. Shields, D. Walter, I. Blackburn, J. Connechan, and M. Lonergan, Lancet, 2, 1972, 573-577.
[8]. A. J., Prange, I. Wilson, A. Knox, T. McClane, G. Breese, B. Martin, L. Alltop, and M. Lipton, J. Psychiat. Res., 9, 1972, 187-205.
[9]. S. H. Snyder and S. P. Banerjee, in E. Usdin and S. Snyder (Eds.), Frontiers in Catecholamine Research, Pergamon Press, New York, 1973.
[10]. S. H. Snyder, S. P. Banerjee, H. I. Yamamura, and D. Greenberg, Science 184, 1974, 1243-1253.
[11]. H. L. Klawans, M. M. Ilahi, and D. Shenker, Acta Neurol. Scand. 46, 1970, 409-441.
[12]. H. L. Klawans and R. McKendall, J. Neurol. Sci., 14, 1971, 189-192.

[13]. R. Rubovits and H. Klawans, Arch. Gen. Psychiatry, 27, 1972, 502-507.
[14]. H. Y. Meltzer, E. Sachar, and A. Frantz, "Serum Prolactin Levels in Acutely Psychotic Patients: An Indirect Measurement of Central Dopaminergic Activity" presented at the American College of Neuropsychopharmacology meeting, Palm Springs, California, 1973.
[15]. E. Sachar, "Neuroendocrine Disturbances in the Affective Disorders and Schizophrenia", presented at the American College of Neuropsychopharmacology meeting, Palm Springs, California, 1973.
[16]. A. O. Donoso, W. Bishop, C. P. Fawcett, L. Krulich, and S. M. McCann, Endocrinol., 89, 1971, 774-784.
[17]. I. A. Kamberi, R. Mical, and J. C. Porter, Endocrinol. 88, 1971, 1012-1020.
[18]. N.-E. Anden, A. Rubenson, K. Fuxe, and T. Hökfelt, J. Pharm. Pharmacol. 19, 1967, 627-629.
[19]. H. Corrodi, K. Fuxe, and U. Ungerstedt, J. Pharm. Pharmacol., 23, 1971, 989-991.
[20]. A. J. Mandell, D. S. Segal, R. T. Kuczenski, and S. Knapp, in J. L. McGaugh (Ed.), The Chemistry of Mood, Motivation and Memory, Plenum Press, New York, 1972.
[21]. J. R. Walters and R. H. Roth, J. Pharmacol. Exp. Ther., 191(1), 1974, 82-91.
[22]. H. K. Brodie, D. L. Murphy, F. K. Goodwin, and W. E. Bunney, Jr., Clin. Pharmacol. Ther. 12(2), 1971, 218-224.
[23]. W. E. Bunney, Jr., D. L. Murphy, and R. T. Kopanda, in preparation.
[24]. F. K. Goodwin, D. L. Murphy, H. K. H. Brodie, and W. E. Bunney, Jr., Biol. Psychiatry, 2, 1970, 341-366.
[25]. D. L. Murphy, M. Baker, F. K. Goodwin, H. Miller, J. Kotin, and W. E. Bunney, Jr., Psychopharmacol. 34., 1974, 11-20.
[26]. J. A. Dominic and K. E. Moore, Psychopharmacol., 15, 1969, 96-101.
[27]. F. C. Beuthin, T. S. Miya, D. E. Blake, and W. F. Bousquet, J. Pharmacol. Exp. Ther., 181(3), 1972, 446-456.
[28]. M. A. Geyer and D. S. Segal, Psychopharmacol., 29, 1973, 131-140.
[29]. D. Tarsy and R. J. Baldessarini, Neuropharmacol., 13, 1974, 927-940.
[30]. L. Uhrbrand and A. Faurbye, Psychopharmacol., 1, 1960, 408-418.
[31]. J. A. Morphew and J. E. Barber, Lancet, I, 1965, 650.
[32]. I. G. Pryce and H. Edwards, Brit. J. Psychiatry, 112, 1966, 983-987.
[33]. P. F. Kennedy, Brit. J. Psychiatry, 115, 1969, 103-104.
[34]. J. Krystof, J. Zyg, S. Mitkiewicz, and J. Kaczynski, Polish Med. J., 11(1), 1972, 189-195.
[35]. D. DeMaio, Brit. J. Psychiatry, 123, 1973, 377-378.
[36]. P. Polizos, D. Engelhardt, S. Hoffman, and J. Waizer, J. Autism Child. Schizo., 3(3), 1973, 247-253.
[37]. G. Jacobson, R. J. Baldessarini, and T. Manschreck, Am. J. Psychiat. 131(8), 1974, 910-913.
[38]. D. Van Kammen, R. M. Post, and W. E. Bunney, Jr., in preparation.

[39]. E. M. Boyd, J. Pharmacol. Exp. Ther., $\underline{128}$, 1960, 75-78.
[40]. R. Rubovits, B. C. Patel, and H. L. Klawans, Adv. in Neurol., $\underline{1}$, 1973, 671-679.
[41]. G. Gianutsos, R. B. Drawbaugh, M. D. Hynes, and H. Lal, Life Sci., $\underline{14}$, 1974, 887-898.
[42]. T. H. Svennson, B. S. Bunney, and G. K. Agajanian, in preparation.
[43]. G. Bartholini, J. Constantinidis, R. Tissot, and A. Pletscher, Biochem. Pharmacol., $\underline{20}$, 1971, 1243-1247.
[44]. M. Puig, G. Bartholini, and A. Pletscher, Arch. Pharmacol., $\underline{281}$, 1974, 443-446.
[45]. D. S. Segal, J. L. Sullivan, R. T. Kuczenski, and A. J. Mandell, Science, $\underline{173}$, 1971, 847-849.
[46]. J. Zador, Montasschr. Psychiat. Neurol. $\underline{77}$, 1930, 71-99.
[47]. G. W. Stavraky, "Supersensitivity Following Lesions of the Nervous System", University of Toronto Press, Toronto, Canada, 1961.
[48]. F. A. Echlin, EEG Clin. Neurophysiol., $\underline{11}$, 1959, 697-722.
[49]. N. E. Freeman, R. H. Smithwick, and J. C. White, Am. J. Physiol., $\underline{107}$(3), 1934, 529-534.
[50]. R. H. Smithwick, N. E. Freeman, and J. C. White, Arch. Surg., $\underline{29}$, 1934, 759-767.
[51]. T. J. Fatherree, A. Adson, and E. Allen, Surgery, $\underline{7}$, 1940, 75-94.
[52]. I. D. Stein, K. Harpuder, and J. Byer, Am. J. Physiol., $\underline{158}$, 1949, 319-325.
[53]. F. A. Simeone and D. A. Felder, Surgery, $\underline{30}$(1), 1951, 218-226.
[54]. A. Barbeau and F. McDowell, (Eds.), L-DOPA and Parkinsonism, F. A. Davis, Philadelphia, Pennsylvania, 1970.
[55]. S. H. Snyder, K. M. Taylor, J. T. Coyle, and J. L. Meyerhoff, Am. J. Psychiat., $\underline{127}$(2), 1970, 199-207.
[56]. T. Kodama, Y. Matsukado, and H. Shimizu, Brain Res., $\underline{50}$, 1973, 135-146.
[57]. V. Grill and U. Rosenqvist, Acta Med. Scand., $\underline{194}$, 1973, 129-133.
[58]. S. M. Wolfe and N. R. Shulman, Biochem. Biophys. Res. Commun., $\underline{35}$, 1969, 265-272.
[59]. P. D. Zieve and W. B. Greenough, Biochem. Biophys. Res. Commun. $\underline{35}$, 1969, 462-466.
[60]. J. Moskowitz, J. P. Harwood, W. D. Reid, and G. Krishna, Biochem. Biophys. Acta, $\underline{230}$, 1971, 279-285.
[61]. D. L. Murphy, C. Donnelly, and J. Moskowitz, Clin. Pharm. Ther., $\underline{14}$(5), 1973, 810-814.
[62]. Y. Wang, G. N. Pandey, J. Mendels, and A. Frazer, Psychopharmacol. $\underline{36}$, 1974, 291-300.
[63]. D. L. Murphy, C. Donnelly, and J. Moskowitz, Am. J. Psychiatry, $\underline{131}$, 1974, 1389-1391.
[64]. W. E. Bunney, Jr., A. Andersen, R. M. Post, R. T. Kopanda, and D. L. Murphy, in preparation.
[65]. C. B. Pert and S. H. Snyder, Molec. Pharmacol., $\underline{10}$, 1974, 868-879.

DISCUSSION

Dr. Moore described some of his studies with alpha-methyltyrosine. To prevent the hyperactivity which follows chronic alpha-methyl-tyrosine, the animals were given DOPA together with dopamine hydroxylase blocker; what was found was an enhanced response to apomorphine in these animals. He asked if Dr. Bunney had ever given alpha-methyltyrosine to patients on DOPA to see if this would prevent change in the sleep pattern. Dr. Bunney thought this would be interesting.

Dr. Butcher commented on subsensitivity. He mentioned the work of Dr. Ungerstedt and himself in which a unilateral lesion was placed in the frontal cortex and then rotation behavior was observed following amphetamine and apomorphine. The results were opposite to those observed after B-9 lesions; i. e., the animals rotated in the opposite direction. Thus, the animals rotated contralateral to the lesion side after amphetamine and ipsilateral after apomorphine.

Dr. Lovenberg closed the meeting by pointing out that the meeting had covered a number of aspects of both pre- and postsynaptic receptors, including initial binding of agonists and antagonists to receptors and measurement of such binding. Both primary biochemical events (neurotransmitter and other types of adenyl cyclases) and secondary biochemical events (alterations in tyrosine hydroxylase and messenger RNA) were covered as were cellular electrophysiological events resulting from the biochemical events. The meeting ended with Dr. Bunney's discussion of some of the events occurring in the whole animal and in man.

SUBJECT INDEX

acetylcholine
    and receptors...191
    effect of impulse flow interruption......................21
    generation of nerve impulses.............................69
    receptor..191
    supersensitivity..303
N-acetylserotonin (NAS).....................................265
N-acetyltransferase (NAT)
    control of..267-269
    in formation of N-acetylserotonin.......................265
    light control.......................................272-273
    superinduction..270
ACTH
    and lipolysis.......................................260-261
actinomycin
    and block of N-acetyltransferase induction..............276
action potential..2
adenosine
    increase in cyclic AMP in human brain...................304
adenyl(ate) cyclase.....................2-4, 18, 123-147, 157
    absence from some brain regions.........................208
    activation and receptor occupancy.......................262
    activation by dopamine..................................168
    and N-acetyltransferase.................................268
    and chronic administration of neuroleptics..............242
    as dopamine receptor..........................157, 183-184
    as postsynaptic receptor.................................71
    effect of light...271
    effect of phenothiazines........................76-77, 131
    effect of secretin......................................259
    effect of VIP...259
    lack of relation between blocking potency and neuroleptic
        activity..242
    non-activation by amphetamine.........................75-76
    subcellular distribution in caudate.................131-134
adipose
    cells...227
    tissue and cyclic AMP...................................305
adipsia
    after lesion in substantia nigra........................182
α-adrenergic agonists....................................90, 91
α-adrenergic antagonists............................90, 91, 227

β-adrenergic receptor
 action via adenyl cyclase...............................268
 detection..264
 in adipose cells.......................................227
 in caudate nucleus.....................................143
 in pineal..265-282
β-adrenergic sensitivity....................................146
ADTN
 as stimulator of cyclic AMP................209-210, 212, 214
affinity
 correlation with biological activity...............260-262
 effect of labeling on..................................250
 high vs. low.................................249, 257-259
albumin
 binding of tryptophan..................................249
alcoholism
 effect of apomorphine................................54-55
allopurinol...168
amantadine
 non-stimulator of cyclic AMP......................211, 219
amino acids
 effect on neuronal discharge............................72
AMP..3
amphetamine
 and increase of tyrosine hydroxylase...................302
 and supersensitivity...................................182
 as dopamine releaser.............................94, 98-99
 block of dopamine and dopa.....................32, 98, 120
 effect on neuronal firing..............74-76, 79, 98, 100
 effect on rodent behavior...............................75
 iontophoretic application..........................102-103
 lack of effect on adenyl cyclase..................147, 219
 lack of presynaptic effect on dopamine cells...........111
 local anesthetic effect.............................99-101
 non-stimulator of cyclic AMP...........................209
 stereotypy produced by............................173, 297
 stereotypy reversed by............................174, 175
 vs. apomorphine, effects in lesioned animals...........312
AMPT - cf. α-methyl-p-tyrosine
amygdaloid nucleus...7
anesthetic
 effects of amphetamine at high ejection currents........99
 effects of DMT, lack of................................203
 effects of LSD...203
 use in interruption of impulse flow.....................94
antipsychotic drugs (also cf. individual drugs)
 action on dopamine.........7-8, 94-95, 99, 109, 123, 127-128
aphagia
 after lesion in substantia nigra.......................182
apocodeine
 and production of stereotyped behavior.............212-213

apomorphine
    action on both pre- and postsynaptic receptors...........111
    and stereotyped behavior.......................176, 181, 297
    as dopamine agonist............................74, 93-95, 207
    as test for tendency to tardive dyskinesia...........297-299
    biphasic dose response   57, 64
    block of dopamine and dopa..32, 53-54, 91, 93, 103, 109, 189
    block of dopamine and dopa, overcome by GBL...............33
    block of euphoriant action by α-methyl-p-tyrosine.........55
    block of MAO...189
    block of tyrosine hydroxylase.....46-47, 50-52, 165, 230-232
    effect on mice motility...................................53
    human studies using......................................289
    inhibition of firing of dopaminergic neurons........100, 103
    iontophoretic application............................103, 109
    reversal of ethanol action.............................55-56
    sensitivity to, after dopa and dopamine hydroxylase
        blocker..312
    stimulation of adenyl cyclase................127-128, 212-213
    stimulation of cyclic AMP............................134-135
    stimulation of dopamine receptor.........................127
    supersensitivity due to.........................181-183, 188
    treatment of alcoholism...................................55
    vs. amphetamine, effects in lesioned animals.............312
asthma
    and cyclic AMP response to propranolol...................306
    and response to catecholamines and prostaglandin.........306
ATP..2, 3, 161, 162
ATPase...3
autoreceptors...51-60, 63-84
axotomy...50-53
basal ganglia..123, 207-208
benztropine
    cholinergic inhibitor....................................229
    non-inhibitor of adenyl cyclase..........................219
BH_4
    as cofactor...14-17
bicuculline
    as GABA antagonist..79
binding
    correlation with activity................................264
    nonspecific..247-250
    zones..263
boutons...86
bradykinin
    activation of tyrosine hydroxylase.......................147
8-bromo-cyclic AMP
    as phosphodiesterase inhibitor...........................141
2-bromo-LSD
    action on raphe cells....................................192
    displacement of LSD......................................202

2-bromo-LSD (cont.)
    displacement of serotonin..............................202
bufotenin
    displacement of LSD....................................202
    displacement of serotonin..............................202
bulbocapnine
    as dopamine blocker....................................213
    inhibitor of adenyl cyclase............................219
α-bungarotoxin...184
butaclamol
    inhibitor of adenyl cyclase............................219
    relation to reserpine..................................242
    sterospecificity...................................223-226
butaperazine
    and dystonias......................................120-121
butyrophenones (also cf. individual drugs)..................127
    activation of neuron firing rate........................73
    and cyclic AMP formation...........................220-222
    and tyrosine hydroxylase...............................302
    nullifying dopamine agonist block.......................47
    tardive dyskinesia after withdrawal................295, 296
butyryl cyclic AMP
    increase of dopamine synthesis..........................76
    lack of effect on cyclic AMP level.....................141
calcium
    and adenyl cyclase..................................18, 19
    and cyclic AMP formation...............................26
    and dopamine formation.................................24
    and tyrosine hydroxylase....................23, 38-39, 48
    increase during impulse flow................18, 26, 28, 48
    influx required for transmitter release................70
caudate neurons
    action of phenothiazines............................76-77
    amphetamine action.....................................100
caudate nucleus
    adenyl cyclase.....................................123-147
    and dopamine pathways..................................172
    and LSD binding..193
    blocking in..147
cerebellum
    control of movement.....................................78
    LSD localization.......................................193
cerebrosides...206
cervical ganglia
    formation of cyclic AMP................................207
    transformation of light information to pineal..........266
chloral hydrate
    and trivastal...30
    effect on tyrosine hydroxylase..................12, 14, 16
    increase of impulse flow................................9
    negative effect on firing rate.........................105

chlorimipramine
    inhibitor of adenyl cyclase........................218, 219
chlorpromazine
    and dopa synthesis.....................................55-60
    and stereotyped behavior................................297
    antagonist of dopamine..................................208
    antagonist of glucagon..................................227
    anticholinergic potency............................228, 229
    blockade of dopamine receptors..................53, 111-112
    comparison with butyrophenones.....................220-222
    conformation similarity to dopamine..................93, 214
    effect on catecholamine metabolism..............49, 71, 92
    increase of dopamine turnover...........................155
    increase of firing of dopaminergic neurons..98, 104-106, 109
    inhibition of adenyl cyclase.......................130, 143
    inhibition of cyclic AMP formation.................215-220
    iontophoretically applied...............................110
    nitroxide...220
    sulfoxide(s)......................................219, 220
chlorprothixene
    inhibitor of adenyl cyclase.............................219
choleragen - cf. cholera toxin
cholera toxin
    activation of cyclic AMP...........................233-235
    and neuroleptics..241
cholinergic/dopaminergic potency.......................228-229
cholinergic receptor.............................203, 227-228
circadian rhythm
    in pineal..265-266
clonidine
    as norepinephrine agonist..........................299-300
    decrease of noradrenergic neuron firing............107-109
    decrease of norepinephrine release.........91, 105, 107, 109
    in production of subsensitivity................299, 300, 301
clopenthixol
    inhibitor of adenyl cyclase.............................219
clothiapine
    inhibitor of adenyl cyclase.............................222
clozapine
    and dopa synthesis.....................................56-60
    anticholinergic potency............................228-230
    failure to increase dopamine cell activity.........110-111
    inhibitor of adenyl cyclase....................130, 138-140
    lack of effect in overcoming dopamine inhibition of
        firing rate.......................................104-106
    lack of presynaptic action.............................47-95
    weak blocker of dopamine inhibition of dopaminergic
        neurons...111
cocaine
    increase of sensitivity of norepinephrine..........134-136

conformation
    alteration of serotonin receptor......................201-204
    duality of serotonin receptor............................204
    of dopamine..214
    of dopamine-sensitive adenyl cyclase.................213-214
    of thioxanthenes...317
    of tyrosine hyrdroxylase..................................28
"corollary discharge"...81
cyclic AMP...3, 4
    accumulation during depolarization................18, 19, 26
    activation of protein kinase............15, 18, 19, 124, 125
    and isoproterenol..278
    assay..208-209
    catecholamines vs. propranolol...........................268
    effect on firing rate...............................86, 184
    effect on tyrosine hydroxylase.......14-16, 40, 161-163, 169
    increase after apomorphine...........................134-135
    increase after dopamine....................134-135, 157, 207
    inhibition of formation by phenothiazines............215-220
    in human adipose tissue..................................305
    in human brain...304
    in platelets...305
    mediation of catecholamine action........................208
    mediation of dopamine...............................76, 124
    norepinephrine dependency............................196-197
    stimulation by S584......................................176
cycloheximide
    inhibition of N-acetyltransferase........................268
"dendro-dendritic" synapses...................................70
denervation supersensitivity - cf. supersensitivity
depolarization
    neuronal......................................15, 18-20, 69
depression (also cf. manic-depressive illness)
    lack of response to norepinephrine or prostaglandin......306
desimipramine
    inhibition of adenyl cyclase........................130, 219
    lack of effect on amphetamine supersensitivity...........182
dibenzapines (also cf. dibenzodiazepines and individual drugs)
    and cyclic AMP formation.............................222-224
    block of dopamine effects................................127
dibutyryl cyclic AMP
    induction of N-acetyltransferase.......268, 270-271, 276-277
diethazine
    inhibition of adenyl cyclase........................130, 219
6,7-dihydroxytetrahydroisoquinoline
    stimulation of cyclic AMP............................209-210
N-dimethyldopamine
    stimulator of cyclic AMP.................................211
dimethyltryptamine
    displacement of LSD......................................202
    displacement of serotonin................................202

dimethyltryptamine (cont.)
    lack of anesthetic effects..............................203
    mimic action of serotonin..............................192
diphenhydramine
    non-inhibitor of adenyl cyclase........................219
$DMPH_4$
    as cofactor...13
dopa
    accumulation.............................9-14, 16, 39, 52
    accumulation, after inhibition of dopa decarboxylase......21
    and behavioral supersensitivity....................176, 188
    lack of effect on length of sleep.......................292
    non-stimulator of cyclic AMP.......................209, 211
    use with AMPT to change sleep pattern...................312
dopa decarboxylase
    inhibition..9, 21
    inhibition, block of effects.............................32
    inhibitors delaying dopa behavioral effects.............176
dopamine
    accumulation in neostriatum.....................20, 21, 94
    agonists and antagonists...............................207
    as endproduct inhibitor.......................7, 16, 40
    as neurotransmitter....................................123
    as stimulator of cyclic AMP.134-135, 137, 184, 207, 209, 210
    block by bulbocapnine..................................213
    conformation......................................93, 214
    depletion after 6-hydroxydopamine......................171
    effect on renal artery.................................207
    from labeled tyrosine..........................8, 21, 92
    increased biosynthesis.............................21, 92
    inhibition by phenothiazines of activation of adenyl
        cyclase...76-77
    metabolism.........................49-65, 92, 284
    microiontophoretic application........102, 109-110, 147, 183
    stimulation of adenyl cyclase...................123-147, 168
    stimulation of receptor................................127
    "strategic pool"...26
dopamine(rgic) neurons
    effect of amphetamine...................................98
    fast firing..101
    inhibition of firing.................................37-38
    in substantia nigra zona compacta......................108
    modulation of...97
    regulation of tyrosine hydroxylase....................5-48
    response to impulse flow................................6
dopamine receptors
    action of amphetamine...............................74, 98
    as adenyl cyclase......................................157
    block...1, 38, 91-93, 123
    characterization...............................126-127, 213
    drug interactions with.................................178

dopamine receptors (cont.)
    in transmitter synthesis....................................97
    presence in dopamine neurons..............................102
    requirements for agonists and antagonists................208
    stimulation by apomorphine.................................93
dystonias
    produced by butaperazine.............................120-121
EGTA
    and tyrosine hydroxylase..............................23, 25
electrical stimulation
    chronic..47
    in nigro-neostriatal pathway....................8-15, 95-96
    in nigro-neostriatal pathway with haloperidol..........30-31
    in nigro-neostriatal pathway and trivastal.............30-31
    of adrenergic neurons.......................................6
    of dopaminergic neurons.................................6, 39
emetine
    non-stimulator of cyclic AMP.............................210
end product inhibition
    controlling tyrosine hydroxylase...........5, 53, 95, 149-169
epidermal growth factor
    binding.......................................251, 255-257
epinene
    stimulator of cyclic AMP.......................209, 211,213
epinephrine
    and lipolysis..261
    increase of cyclic AMP in human brain...............304, 305
    increase of cyclic AMP in human leukocytes...............306
    supersensitivity after sympathectomy.....................303
ET 495 – cf. trivastal
ethanol
    reversal of action by apomorphine or trivastal........55, 65
ethopropazine
    cholinergic inhibitor....................................229
    non-inhibitor of adenyl cyclase..........................219
ethoproperazine
    inhibitor of adenyl cyclase..............................130
extrapyramidal side effects (also cf. individual effects).......
    ....112, 127-128, 131
feedback
    deficiency as explanation of action of antipsychotic
        drugs...110
    inhibition..26, 70, 94, 164
    inhibition, receptor-mediated..................156, 157, 159
    in pituitary..80
    loops....2, 37, 50, 60, 80, 91-93, 95, 101, 109-110, 277-278
    mechanisms...97-106
    within synaptic gap.......................................89
fenethazine
    non-inhibitor of adenyl cyclase..........................219

fenfluramine
    and serotonin receptor...................................301
firing rate
    control of..49
    effect of light levels..................................266
    effect of serotonin.....................................191
    generation of spontaneous................................86
    increase after transection of diencephalon..............101
    increase as result of chlorpromazine.....................98
    maximum, after low doses of antipsychotics..............110
    use of GBL to stop.......................................94
fluorescence histochemistry...................................97
flupenthixol
    decrease of apomorphine inhibition......................231
    inhibitor of adenyl cyclase.........................215-221
    lack of stereospecificity in adipocytes.................227
    weak anticholinergic................................228-229
fluphenazine
    inhibitor of adenyl cyclase.......127, 130, 136-137, 215-220
GABA
    and depolarization.......................................69
    in the substantia nigra...............................78-79
    pathway..57, 101
    receptor......................................191, 197, 205
gamma aminobutyric acid - cf. GABA
gamma butyrolactone - cf. GBL
gamma hydroxybutyrate - cf. GHB
GBL
    and dopamine accumulation............................20, 94
    and tyrosine hydroxylase.........................23, 33, 36
    blockade of impulse flow.............................22, 94
GHB
    and tyrosine hydroxylase........................48, 157, 165
    inhibition of firing in substantia nigra.................79
    inhibition of impulse flow...................20, 36-37, 230
Gilles de la Tourette syndrome
    and receptor sensitivity................................304
glia
    in regulation of neurotransmitters.......................71
glucagon
    antagonism by chlorpromazine............................227
    binding...248
glycine
    receptor......................................191, 203, 205
growth hormone
    inhibitor of glucagon binding...........................248
    receptor specificity...............................259, 260
haloperidol
    and behavior..63-64
    and dopa synthesis....................................55-60
    and lesions...182

haloperidol (cont.)
- and tyrosine hydroxylase..............30-32, 36, 95, 98, 105
- antagonist of dopamine...................................208
- block of dopamine receptors.........................111-112
- block of dopamine inhibitory effect......................110
- effect on catecholamine metabolism.............49-50, 71, 92
- increase in dopamine turnover............................153
- increase in dopaminergic neuron activity...98, 105, 111, 121
- inhibitor of adenyl cyclase.........................130, 232
- reversal of apomorphine inhibition of firing....100, 103-104
- reversal of dopamine inhibition of firing............105-106

heparin
- effect on tyrosine hydroxylase.....................160, 162

HF 2046
- inhibitor of adenyl cyclase.............................222

hippocampus
- acetylcholine levels.....................................21
- LSD binding...193
- tyrosine hydroxylase.............................11, 18, 25

histamine
- increase in cyclic AMP in human brain...................304

hormone
- dimerization.......................................252-254
- receptors..245-264

human studies..283-312

HVA
- level reduced by AMPT....................................57

6-hydroxydopamine
- and N-acetyltransferase.................................271
- and cholera toxin..................................234-235
- and dopamine accumulation................................20
- and dopamine neuron degeneration....................171-190
- effect on neuronal discharge.........................74, 86
- lack of behavioral effect.........................171, 173

hydroxyindole-O-methyltransferase (HIOMT)...................265

hyperpolarization
- of postganglionic neuron................................124

hypothalamus
- neurons as targets for noradrenergic synapses............80

hypothermia
- after AMPT withdrawal...................................295

hypothyroidism
- and α-adrenergic stimulation............................305

imipramine
- increase of tyrosine hydroxylase........................302
- inhibition of adenyl cyclase............................130

impulse flow
- alternative explanations.................................90
- in dopamine turnover increase as result of antipsychotic drugs.. 93, 155
- inhibition of..94

impulse flow (cont.)
    in regulation of tyrosine hydroxylase...............5-48, 51
inhibitory potentials...86
insulin
    binding................................247-248, 251-252, 259
    receptor specificity.....................................259
    talc complex..251, 253
intrasynaptic receptors.......................................71
iontophoresis........79, 97-101, 103-106, 109-110, 183, 191, 203
3-isobutyl-1-methylxanthine
    phosphodiesterase inhibitor.....................141-142, 143
isolysergic acid amide
    displacement of LSD.....................................202
    displacement of serotonin...............................202
isomethylxanthine
    phosphodiesterase inhibitor.............................146
isoproterenol
    effect on adenyl cyclase...........................125-126
    increase of cyclic AMP...................134-135, 137, 304
    induction of N-acetyltransferase...................270-276
kinase - cf. protein kinase
lactogen
    receptor specificity.....................................259
lesion (also cf. axotomy)
    and N-acetyltransferase sensitivity................270-271
    differences, with amphetamine and apomorphine............312
    effects...20
    in diencephalon....................................100-102
    in locus coeruleus..21
    in median raphe.....................................21, 192
    in nigro-neostriatal pathway....22, 37, 74, 93, 94, 103-104,
    ....156, 165, 208, 229
    in substantia nigra.............................134, 182
    of superior cervical ganglion...........................266
    studies in man............................285, 286, 303-304
leukocytes
    and cyclic AMP.....................................306-307
light
    effect on N-acetyltransferase..................268, 271-275
    effect on adenyl cyclase.................................271
    effect on melatonin levels...............................266
    effect on metabolism....................................265
    effect on norepinephrine turnover.......................267
    effect on serotonin levels..............................266
limbic area
    adenyl cyclase in..131
    control of behavior.......................................77
    definition..63
    differences from striatal area....................55-56, 60
    involvement in schizophrenia.......................123, 131
lipolysis..260-261, 305

lithium
    inhibition of prostaglandin effect on cyclic AMP.........306
    possible mode of action..................................308
locus coeruleus
    lesion in...21
    neurons......................................72, 86, 105, 108
long-loop receptors..71-72
loxapine
    inhibitor of adenyl cyclase..............................222
LSD
    anesthetic effects.......................................203
    as both agonist and antagonist of serotonin..............192
    binding in brain regions.............................193-204
    effect on raphe neurons..............................73, 192
    iontophoretic application................................203
    lack of effect on noradrenergic cell firing..............107
    mechanism of action......................................192
luteinizing hormone
    and dopamine agonists....................................287
lysergic acid
    displacement of LSD......................................202
    displacement of serotonin................................202
lysine
    binding with vasopressin.................................262
magnesium
    and tyrosine hydroxylase.................................162
manic-depressive illness
    model..307
MAO inhibitors
    and formation of O-methylated catecholamines..............92
    effect on neuronal discharge..............................72
    effect on raphe neurons...................................72
median forebrain bundle
    lesion of...20, 23
median raphe
    lesion in...21
melatonin
    dependence on light level................................266
    synthesis..265
mescaline
    supersensitivity after amputation........................303
methdilazine
    non-inhibitor of adenyl cyclase..........................219
5-methoxytryptamine
    displacement of LSD......................................202
    displacement of serotinin................................202
α-methyldopamine
    stimulator of cyclic AMP............................209, 210
methylenedioxy-apomorphine
    production of stereotyped behavior.......................212
6-methyltetrahydropterin.......................................162

α-methyl-p-tyrosine (AMPT)
 altering sensitivity of norepinephrine receptor..........300
 and receptor supersensitivity.......................289, 292
 and stereotypic responses................................295
 behavioral inhibition.....................................57
 effect on sleep.....................................292-294
 effect on transmitter receptors..........................302
 enhancement of amphetamine action........................182
 enhancement of effect of lesions.........................183
 inhibitor of catecholamine synthesis......................74
 potentiation of phenothiazines........................57, 61
 rapidity of blockade produced by....................121-122
 reversal of amphetamine...................................99
 reversal of apomorphine...................................55
 reversal of hyperactivity from, with dopa................312
 use in manic-depressive illness..........................292
methysergide
 displacement of LSD......................................202
 displacement of serotonin................................202
 supersensitivity after discontinuance....................301
mezapine
 non-inhibitor of adenyl cyclase..........................219
morphine
 non-inhibitor of adenyl cyclase..........................219
 receptor...4
neostriatum............................7, 9-11, 20, 39, 40, 91
 dopamine levels...94
nerve
 growth factor..251
 impulse flow - cf. impulse flow
neurotransmitter
 control..5
 studies in humans....................................283-312
 synthesis..5
nigro-neostriatal dopamine pathway....7-48, 94-96, 97, 156, 171,
 ....174, 176, 208, 230
noradrenergic neurons
 response to impulse flow...................................6
norepinephrine
 and increase after threo-DOPS............................300
 and increase in spontaneous activity................182, 188
 and increase of cyclic AMP...134-135, 137, 209-210, 304, 306
 and induction of N-acetyltransferase.....................270
 and prostaglandin in elevating cyclic AMP................305
 antagonism by phenothiazines..............................77
 depletion after 6-hydroxydopamine........................171
 effect on adenyl cyclase............................125-126
 endproduct inhibitor.......................................7
 increased outflow as result of action of phenoxybenzamine...89, 91
 inhibition by clonidine..................................105

norepinephrine (cont.)
    inhibition of firing of noradrenergic neurons............107
    in locus coeruleus..108
    metabolism..6, 55
    neuronal uptake inhibition................................90
    receptor blockers......................................92-93
    receptor, in man.......................................299-301
    receptor sites..197
    release by α-adrenergic agonists..........................91
    synthesis..6
    turnover...6, 267
NSD 1015...50, 52, 54, 58-59, 60
nucleus accumbens
    amphetamine effect..101
    and adenyl cyclase..131
    and dopamine pathways.....................................184
    and impulse flow...21
    formation of cyclic AMP...................................208
olfactory tubercles
    adenyl cyclase from.................................131, 226
    amphetamine effect..101
    and dopamine pathways.....................................172
    and impulse flow...21
    formation of cyclic AMP...............................207-208
    in control of behavior.....................................77
opiate receptor...203, 206
"osmo-receptors"..80
oxymetazoline
    decrease of norepinephrine release.........................91
oxytocin
    receptor specificity......................................259
pallido-nigral pathway..101
pargyline
    increase of tyrosine hydroxylase..........................302
Parkinsonism
    and supersensitivity..................................303-304
    as result of block of adenyl cyclase......................143
    dopaminergic degeneration or blockade.....................123
    mechanism of therapeutic action of trivastal..............177
    prevention by anticholinergic activity....................228
PCPA
    and supersensitivity......................................300
pentolamine
    non-inhibitor of adenyl cyclase...........................219
perlapine
    inhibitor of adenyl cyclase...............................222
permeability
    in regulation of tyrosine hydroxylase activity..........38-39
phenothiazines (also cf. individual drugs)
    and tyrosine hydroxylase..................................302
    antagonism of action of adenyl cyclase.77, 127, 130, 215-220

phenothiazines (cont.)
    antagonism of action of norepinephrine....................77
    effect on neuron firing rate..............................73
    nullify dopamine agonist block............................47
    relation between potency and inhibition of adenyl
        cyclase..215-220
    site of action...76-79
    supersensitivity.....................................295-297
    tardive dyskinesia after withdrawal.................295, 296
phenoxybenzamine
    increase of norepinephrine outflow....................89, 91
phentolamine
    and lipolysis..305
    increase of norepinephrine outflow........................91
    inhibitor of catecholamine effect on cyclic AMP..........305
phosphatidyl serine
    effect on tyrosine hydroxylase...........................160
phosphodiesterase...............................3, 165, 184
    inhibition.......................................141-142, 146
phosphorylation
    in activation of tyrosine hydroxylase...18-20, 158, 161-162,
    ....164-165, 168-169
    in dopaminergic transmission........................228, 229
picrotoxin
    as GABA antagonist..79
pimozide
    and dopa synthesis...............................56, 58, 60
    decrease in sleep..297
    inhibitor of adenyl cyclase...............130, 219, 220, 222
    lack of presynaptic action................................47
    weak anticholinergic................................228, 229
pineal
    β-adrenergic receptor.........................4, 265-282
    stimulator of cyclic AMP.................................184
pinocytosis
    effect on binding..250
piribedil - cf. trivastal
platelets
    in study of α-receptor sensitivity..................305-306
presynaptic receptor
    in regulation of tyrosine hydroxylase...................5-48
prochlorperazine
    inhibitor of adenyl cyclase.....................130, 215-220
prolactin
    and dopamine agonists...............................286-287
    receptor specificity.....................................259
promazine
    inhibitor of adenyl cyclase.....................139, 215-220
promethazine
    ineffective in reversing inhibitory effects of dopamine
        receptor stimulants...................................37

promethazine (cont.)
    inhibitor of adenyl cyclase......................130, 215-220
propranolol
    and lipolysis...305
    block of N-acetyltransferase.........................267-268
    block of catecholamine increase of cyclic AMP........304-306
    effect on cyclic AMP levels...............136, 137, 143, 268
    non-inhibitor of adenyl cyclase.....................219, 305
propyl-norapomorphine
    stimulator of adenyl cyclase.............................212
prostaglandins
    and cyclic AMP elevation............................305, 306
    differentiation from short-loop receptors..............70-71
    inhibitory effect on adrenergic terminals.................90
    non-inhibitor of adenyl cyclase..........................219
protein kinase.....2, 15-19, 124-125, 139, 158, 161-162, 164, 169
pterin
    requirement as cofactor..............................152-153
Purkinje cells
    inhibition of...74, 86
pyrathiazine
    non-inhibitor of adenyl cyclase..........................303
raphe nuclei
    discharge..72-73
    effect of serotonin......................................191
receptor(s)
    blockers..90
    characteristics..2
    identification.......................................245-264
receptor-ligand complex...2
receptor site
    saturation...2
renal artery
    effect of dopaminergic drugs........................207, 213
reserpine
    alteration of norepinephrine receptor sensitivity........300
    and N-acetyltransferase..................................271
    and blockade of vesicular stroage.........................74
    and butaclamol...242
    and depletion of dopamine.................................53
    and receptor supersensitivity............................289
    and sensitivity to apomorphine....................51-52, 182
    and tyrosine hydroxylase.................................302
    time effect on receptors.................................121
retina
    dopamine responses..................................76, 207
    handling of information...................................78
reuptake..189
RO 4-4602
    as dopa decarboxylase inhibitor.................9, 178, 179

S 584
    and behavioral supersensitivity..........................176
    and stereotypy..180
    stimulator of cyclic AMP....................176, 184, 211-212
schizophrenia
    action of drugs..........................1, 57, 61, 123, 284
secretin..259
septohippocampal cholinergic pathway...........................21
serotonin
    acetylation...245
    cerebral...53
    circadian rhythms...246
    displacement of LSD.......................................202
    effect on firing rate.....................................191
    neurons...72-73
    receptor..................................191-206, 300 -301
    uptake..195-196
serotonin N-acetyltransferase - cf. N-acetyltransferase
short-loop receptors....................................... 70-71
sleep
    effect of AMPT..............................292, 293, 294
    effect of AMPT plus dopa..................................312
    lack of effect on length by dopa..........................292
    lack of effect on length by tryptophan....................292
snail neurons...213
"spare receptors"...261-262
spiroperidol
    inhibitor of adenyl cyclase..................219, 220, 232
    weak anticholinergic..................................228-229
stereospecificity
    of apomorphine..212
    of butaclamol................................219, 223-226
    of flupenthixol.......................215-217, 221, 232
    of LSD binding.............................192, 201, 202
    of norepinephrine...209
    of tryptophan binding.....................................249
    lack, in adipocytes.......................................227
stereotyped behavior...53
    after amphetamine.....................................173-174
    after AMPT withdrawal...............................295, 297
    after apocodeine......................................212-213
    after chlorpromazine..................................... 177
    after methylenedioxy-apomorphine......................212-213
    after S 584...178
    reversal by 6-hydroxydopamine.............................174
striato-nigral pathway...79
striatum
    adenyl cyclase in............................157, 208, 210
    differences from limbic area............................13-14
    formation of dopamine......................................24
    tyrosine hydroxylase in..7, 11-14, 23, 25, 152-154, 159, 231

structure-activity relationships..........................207-243
subcellular localization
    of GABA..193
    of LSD binding..193
    of muscarinic binding...................................193
subsensitivity
    after chronic fenfluramine..............................301
    induced...289-290
    in pineal gland.....................................269-280
    of receptors..288
substantia nigra
    and GABA...79
    effects in, resulting from peripheral dopamine agonists
        and antagonists.....................................155
    lack of effect of clonidine.........................105-107
    lesion of..20
    zona compacta....................7, 72-73, 100, 108, 171-172
    zona compacta, dopamine applied to.......................38
supersensitivity
    induced..289, 300-301
    in manic-depressive illness.............................307
    in pineal gland.....................................269-280
    in therapy..284
    of receptors..287
    postsynaptic..171-190
    presynaptic...178
    to mescaline after amputation...........................303
snyaptic cleft
    and LSD binding....................................197, 200
    diffusion of dopamine across............................124
    dominance of postsynaptic receptor.......................54
    increase of dopamine via stimulation of presynaptic
        receptors..96
tardive dyskinesia
    and receptor site sensitivity.....................284, 287
    after withdrawal of butyrophenones................295, 296
    after withdrawal of phenothiazines................295, 296
    presynaptic blocking in production of.............112, 182
telencephalon
    catecholamine pathways...................................81
tetrahydrobiopterin
    requirement for, by tyrosine hydroxylase................153
tetrahydropapaveroline
    non-stimulator of cyclic AMP............................210
threo-DOPS
    increase of brain norepinephrine........................300
    in production of subsensitivity.....................299-301
theophylline
    as phosphodiesterase inhibitor..........................146
    effect on lipolysis.................................260-261

thioridazine
    and dopa synthesis.....................................56-50
    anticholinergic potency..............................228-230
    failure to increase dopamine cell activity...............110
    inhibitor of adenyl cyclase.........................130, 219
    potentiation by AMPT......................................61
thioxanthenes
    antagonism of dopamine action on adenyl cyclase......215-221
transmitter -cf. neurotransmitter
TRH
    binding sites..197
trifluoperazine
    inhibitor of adenyl cyclase.....................130, 215-220
    weak anticholinergic.................................228-229
triflupromazine
    inhibitor of adenyl cyclase..............................130
N-trimethyldopamine
    stimulator of cyclic AMP.................................211
trivastal..29-31
    and behavioral supersensitivity..........................177
    and stereotypy...180
    as dopamine agonist...............................53, 94-95
    as test for vulnerability to tardive dyskinesia......297-299
    block of dopamine and dopa................................32
    block of dopamine and dopa, overcome by GBL...........33, 36
    human studies using......................................289
    mechanism of therapeutic action in Parkinson's disease...177
    metabolite as stimulator of adenyl cyclase...............127
    non-stimulator of cyclic AMP.............................212
    reversal of ethanol action................................55
    stimulator of dopamine receptor..........................127
tryptamine
    displacement of LSD......................................202
    displacement of serotonin................................202
tryptophan
    effect on raphe neurons...................................73
    lack of effect on length of sleep........................292
    stereospecificity of binding to albumin..................249
tyramine
    non-stimulator of cyclic AMP........................209, 211
tyrosine
    as substrate..................................14, 16, 21
    conversion of labeled, by antipsychotic drugs.............92
    conversion of labeled, by apomorphine................230-231
    conversion of labeled, by electrical stimulation...........8
tyrosine hydroxylase
    activation.......................15, 18, 94-95, 106, 147
    affinity for cofactors.....................6, 13, 22, 24, 26
    affinity for dopamine.....................13, 14-17, 22, 24
    affinity for substrate....................6, 12-14, 22, 26
    allosteric activation.................................15, 20

tyrosine hydroxylase (cont.)
    and lialoperidol..96
    and trivastal.....................................29-31, 94
    assay...11
    association with membrane...............................159
    as substrate for protein kinase.........................161
    block by apomorphine................................230-232
    brain region activity..............................150, 151
    conformation..28
    cytoplasmic origin vs. synaptomes.......................158
    differential effects of calcium.......................24-25
    effect of amphetamine...................................302
    effect of butyrophenones................................302
    effect of imipramine....................................302
    effect of pargyline.....................................302
    effect of phenothiazines................................302
    effect of reserpine.....................................302
    endproduct inhibition...........................22, 149-169
    regulation of.................................5-48, 149-169
    release from feedback inhibition........................156
vas deferens
    tyrosine hydroxylase from.............................11, 25
vasoactive intestinal polypeptide (VIP).......................259
vasopressin
    binding with lysine.....................................262
    inhibitor of glucagon binding...........................248
    receptor specificity....................................259
ventral tegmental area
    block of dopamine neurons................................20
veratridine
    increase in cyclic AMP in human brain...................304
withdrawal effects.......................................290-292
zona compacta - cf. substantia nigra

AUTHOR INDEX

Adler, M.W. 190
Aghajanian, G.K. 5, 20, 21, 38, 41, 42, 49, 51, 62, 64, 68, 73, 74, 83, 84; cf. Bunney and Aghajanian 89-122; 155, 166, 191, 192, 201, 204, 282
Agid, Y. 20, 42, 171, 176, 185
Ahlenius, S. 55, 56, 57, 63
Alousi, A. 5, 42
Anden, N.-E. 8, 20, 42, 49, 53, 56, 62, 63, 68, 72, 83, 84, 91, 92, 93, 94, 97, 103, 113, 123, 127, 144, 145, 171, 176, 185, 228, 240, 289, 310
Angst, J. 228, 240
Arbuthnott, G.W. 5, 42
Ashcroft, G.W. 284, 309
Axelrod, J. cf. Romero and Axelrod 265-282
Azzaro, A.J. 98, 113
Barbeau, A. 304
Barker, J.L. 69, 83
Bartholini, G. 300, 311
Bedard, P. 53, 62
Bell, L.J. 20, 42
Ben-Ari, Y. 80, 86
Bennett, J.L. 192, 193, 200, 204
Bennett, J.P., Jr. cf. Snyder and Bennett 191-206
Bernheimer, H. 92, 113
Besson, M.J. 98, 107, 114
Beuthin, F.C. 295, 310
Binkley, S.A. 272, 281
Birnbaumer, L. 227, 240
Bloom, F.E. 67-87, 110, 114, 121, 143, 146
Boakes, R.J. 203, 205
Bockaert, J. 259, 262, 263
Boyd, E.M. 297, 298, 311
Brodie, B.B. 150, 166

Brodie, H.K. 292, 310
Bromer, W.W. 250, 263
Brown, B.L. 209, 237
Brown, G.L. 89, 114
Brown, J.H. 76, 85, 207, 208, 214, 219, 236
Brownstein, M.J. 266, 267, 280, 281
Bruckwick, E.A. cf. Lovenberg and Bruckwick 149-169
Bunney, B.S. 9, 37, 42, 73, 74, 84, 89-122, 123, 127, 145, 155, 166
Bunney, W.E., Jr. 1-4, 283-312
Burgen, A.S.V. 228, 240
Burkard, W.P. 92, 114
Burt, D.R. 197, 205
Butcher, L.L. 312
Campbell, B.A. 183, 187
Campbell, D.B. 212, 237
Cannon, J.G. 214, 238
Carlsson, A. 9, 20, 21, 42, 49-65, 68, 71, 72, 78, 79, 83, 92, 94, 95, 98, 110, 115, 121, 123, 127, 144, 150, 151, 155, 156, 158, 164, 165, 166, 167
Changeux, J.-P. 203, 205
Chasin, M. 197, 205
Cheramy, A. 91, 93, 109, 115
Christiansen, J. 230, 232, 241
Cicero, T.J. 151, 168
Clark, W.G. 264
Clement-Cormier, Y.C. 76, 85, 128, 129, 130, 131, 133, 141, 145, 157, 167, 208, 214, 219, 236
Cole, J.O. 228, 240
Connor, J.D. 110, 115, 143, 146
Cooper, B.R. 183, 187
Cooper, J.R. 21, 22, 42

Corrodi, H.   72, 84, 92, 98, 115, 123, 127, 144, 177, 186, 289, 310
Costa, E.   47, 95, 115, 150, 157, 159, 166, 169
Costall, B.   177, 186, 213, 238
Coyle, J.T.   11, 43, 98, 115
Creese, I.   171-190
Cross, B.A.   80, 85
Crow, T.J.   230, 240
Cuatrecasas, P.   227, 233, 240, 241, 245-264
Dahlström, A.   7, 43, 97, 115
DaPrada, M.   92, 115
Davidoff, R.A.   69, 83
Davis, J.   120-121
Deguchi, T.   184, 187, 267, 268, 270, 271, 272, 275, 281
DeMaio, D.   295, 296, 310
De Meyts, P.   250, 263
De Robertis, E.   131, 133, 140, 145
Desbuquois, B.   259, 263
Dixon, M.   17, 43
Dominic, J.A.   182, 186, 295, 310
Donoso, A.O.   287, 310
Dunitz, J.D.   217, 238
Eccles, J.C.   68-69, 83
Echlin, F.A.   303, 311
Ehringer, H.   123, 145
Enero, M.A.   90, 115
Ernst, A.M.   93, 103, 115, 176, 186
Evarts, E.   80, 81, 86
Everett, G.   46, 120, 147, 242
Evetts, K.D.   171, 185
Fairbanks, G.   139, 146
Farnebo, L.-O.   50, 62, 74, 75, 77, 84, 89, 90, 91, 98, 109, 115, 116
Farrow, J.T.   192, 204
Fatherree, T.J.   303, 311
Faull, R.L.   20, 43
Feltz, P.   74, 84, 99, 101, 116, 183, 187
Fibiger, H.C.   183, 187
Finkelstein, R.A.   233, 241
Fjalland, B.   112, 116
Fleming, W.   269, 279, 281
Forn, J.   cf. Krueger et al. 123-147

Frank, K.   69, 83
Frazier, W.A.   251, 263
Free, C.A.   227, 239
Freedman, R.   76-77, 85
Freeman, N.E.   303, 311
Fuxe, K.   68, 83, 97, 116, 121
German, D.C.   75, 85
Gessa, G.L.   20, 43, 47, 63, 189
Gey, K.F.   92, 116
Geyer, M.A.   295, 310
Gianutsos, G.   112, 116, 297, 298, 311
Glick, S.D.   183, 187
Glowinski, J.   98, 116, 208, 237
Goldberg, L.I.   207, 213, 236
Goldstein, A.   255, 263
Goldstein, M.   24, 43, 177, 186
Goodwin, F.K.   292, 310
Greengard, P.   cf. Krueger et al. 123-147; 207, 208, 236
Grill, V.   305, 311
Guroff, G.   154, 166
Häggendal, J.   89, 116
Haigler, H.J.   106, 107, 116, 192, 203, 204
Harris, J.C.   76, 85
Harris, J.E.   14, 24, 43, 163, 167, 235, 241
Hartzell, H.C.   184, 187
Hattori, T.   101, 116
Hedqvist, P.   70, 71, 83, 90, 116
Herr, B.E.   21, 43
Herting, G.   134, 146
Hertting, G.   270, 281
Herz, A.   110, 116
Hess, S.M.   146
Hoffer, B.J.   67, 74, 75, 76, 82, 84, 208, 237
Hökfelt, T.   171, 185
Horn, A.S.   93, 116, 131, 141, 145; cf. Iversen et al. 207-243
Hornykiewicz, O.   65, 122, 123, 144, 145, 188, 242, 243
Huang, M.   184, 187
Humber, L.G.   223, 239
Hynes, M.D.   183, 187

Iversen, L.L. 64, 78-79, 85, 168, 207-243
Iversen, S.D. cf. Creese and Iversen 171-190
Jacobson, G. 295, 296, 310
Javoy, F. 95, 116
Jenner, P. 212, 237
Joh, T.H. 153, 159, 167
Johnson, E.M. 125, 145
Kaiser, C. 217, 239
Kakiuchi, S. 15, 43
Kalisker, A. 184, 187
Kamberi, I.A. 287, 310
Kappers, A.N. 266, 280
Karlin, A. 203, 205
Karobath, M. 131, 141, 145, 157, 167, 214, 219, 230, 238, 241
Kaufman, S. 153, 166
Kebabian, J.W. 76, 85, 124, 126, 128, 141, 145, 157, 167, 177, 183, 186, 208, 212, 236
Kehr, W. 10, 29, 32, 43, 49, 50, 53, 62, 94, 95, 103, 109, 117, 155, 156, 167, 230, 241
Kennedy, P.F. 295, 296, 310
Kettler, R. 153, 154, 166
Kim, J.S. 78, 85
Kirpekar, S.M. 90, 117
Klawans, H.L., Jr. 182, 187, 283, 284, 287, 309
Klein, D.C. 265, 266, 267, 268, 280, 281
Kodama, T. 304, 311
König, J.F.R. 101, 117
Korf, J. 5, 21, 43
Krueger, B.K. 123-147
Krystof, J. 295, 296, 310
Kuczenski, R.T. 159, 160, 162, 167
Kuhar, M.J. 195, 196, 205
Kuo, J.F. 124, 145, 161, 167
Lal, S. 212, 238
Langer, S.Z. 29, 44, 70, 83, 90, 117, 178, 186
Langlais, P.J. 64, 146-147
Langley, J.W. 69, 83
Laverty, R. 92, 117, 171, 185
Lindvall, O. 78, 80, 85

Lineweaver, H. 35, 44
Lippman, W. 223, 226, 239
Lloyd, T. 152, 159, 160, 162, 166, 167
Loh, H.H. 249, 263
Lovenberg, W. 149-169, 241, 282, 312
Lynch, H.J. 266, 280
Maeno, H. 124, 145
Malkinson, A.M. 139, 146
Mandel, L.R. 146, 242
Mandell, A.J. 290, 302, 310
Masland, R.L. 69, 83
Matthysse, S. 123, 145, 207, 235
McAfee, D.A. 123, 145
McGeer, E.G. 230, 241
McGeer, P.L. 101, 117
McKenzie, G.M. 98, 117
McLean, J.R. 98, 117
McLennan, H. 110, 117
Meltzer, H.Y. 47, 287, 310
Miledi, R. 184, 187
Miller, J.P. 141, 146
Miller, R.J. 76, 85, 127, 131, 141, 145, 157, 167, 177, 183, 186; cf. Iversen et al. 207-243
Mishra, R.K. 134, 141, 145, 177, 183, 184, 186, 187, 208, 236
Miyamoto, E. 124, 145
Moller-Nielsen, I. 216, 238
Moore, K.E. 63, 98, 117, 189, 312
Morgenroth, V.H., III cf. Roth et al. 5-48
Morphew, J.A. 295, 296, 310
Moskowitz, J. 305, 311
Mujec, M. 91, 117
Murphy, D.L. cf. Bunney and Murphy 283-312
Murrin, L.C. cf. Roth et al. 5-48
Musacchio, J.M. 153, 158-159, 167
Muscholl, E. 70, 83, 134, 146
Nagatsu, T. 164, 168
Nauta, H.J.W. 79, 85
Neff, N.H. 92, 118

Nybäck, H. 8, 20, 44, 92, 93, 118, 123, 127, 144, 145
Olson, L. 74-75, 84
Palkovits, M. 195, 196, 205
Palmer, G.C. 184, 187
Pappas, G.D. 69, 83
Parker, A.H. 251, 263
Parker, C.W. 283, 306, 309
Patrick, R.L. 230, 241
Persson, T. 92, 93, 103, 118
Pert, C.B. 200, 203, 205, 308, 311
Petersen, P.V. 217, 239
Phillips, A.G. 75, 85
Pijnenburg, A.J.J. 233, 241
Pohl, S.L. 227, 240
Polizos, P. 295, 296, 310
Post, M.L. 217, 238
Prange, A.J. 284, 309
Precht, W. 79, 85
Pryce, I.G. 295, 296, 310
Puig, M. 300, 311
Quay, W.B. 266, 280
Randrup, A. 123, 145
Recker, R.F. 214, 238
Ritter, S. 75, 85
Rodbell, M. 4
Romero, J.A. 265-282
Rosenqvist, U. 283, 305, 309
Roth, R.H. 5-48, 72, 74, 79, 84, 94, 96, 103, 109, 118, 157, 164, 165, 167, 168-169
Rubovits, R. 112, 118, 284, 297, 298, 310, 311
Sachar, E. 287, 310
Sahakian, B.J. 183, 187
Sayers, A.C. 230, 240
Schaefer, J.P. 217, 238
Schanberg, S. 168
Scheel-Kruger, J. 183, 187
Schelkunov, E.L. 228, 240
Schlatter, E.K.E. 55, 62
Schoenfeld, R. 176, 186
Sedvall, G.C. 5, 45, 207, 215, 230, 236
Seeman, P. 77, 85, 222, 232, 239
Segal, D.S. 182, 186, 283, 284, 290, 302, 309, 311
Segal, M. 67, 73, 82, 84, 203, 205
Sethy, V.H. 21, 45

Shader, R.I. 228, 240
Sheppard, H. 76, 85, 212, 213, 214, 238
Shiman, R. 11, 45
Shimizu, H. 15, 45
Shiu, R.P.C. 259, 263
Siggins, G.R. 67, 74, 76, 82, 84, 143, 146, 183, 184, 187
Simeone, F.A. 303, 311
Skolnick, P. 77, 85
Smith, R.C. 188
Smithwick, R.H. 303, 311
Snyder, S.H. 86, 123, 145, 188, 191-206, 207, 228, 235, 240, 249, 262, 263, 284, 304, 309, 311
Soloff, M. 259, 263
Sotelo, C. 171, 185
Soudijn, W. 222, 239
Spector, S. 205
Starke, K. 70, 83, 90, 91, 109, 118, 119
Stavraky, G.W. 303, 311
Stein, I.D. 303, 311
Stein, L. 98, 119
Stevens, J. 123, 145
Stewart, K.K. 249, 262
Stille, G. 223, 230, 239
Stjärne, L. 90, 119
Stock, G. 20, 46
Stricker, E.M. 181, 186
Strömberg, U. 53, 62
Strömbom, U. 53, 54, 63
Studier, F.W. 138, 139, 140, 142, 146
Svensson, T.H. 105, 108, 119, 299, 311
Symchowicz, S. 180, 186
Szentagothai, J. 70, 78, 81, 83
Tarsy, D. 112, 119, 182, 186, 295, 297, 298, 310
Taylor, A.N. 266, 281
Taylor, K.M. 171, 185
Tebecis, A. 78, 85
Teuber, H.L. 80-81, 86
Thoenen, H. 89, 119
Tilson, H.A. 98, 119
Trendelenburg, U. 178, 186, 269, 279, 281
Tseng, F. 213, 238
Ueda, T. 125, 139, 140, 142, 145

Uhrbrand, L. 295, 296, 310
Ungerstedt, U. 7, 46, 78, 80, 85, 123, 127, 144, 171, 172, 176, 180, 182, 185, 186, 187
Uretsky, N.J. 171, 176, 185, 186
Usdin, E. iii
Van Kammen, D. 297, 310
Volle, R.L. 69, 83
Von Voigtlander, P.F. 98, 119, 184, 187, 208, 236
Walinder, J. 61, 63
Walters, J.R. cf. Roth et al. 5-48; 72, 79, 84, 94, 95, 103, 105, 109, 119, 120, 155, 156, 167, 230, 241, 290, 310
Wang, Y. 306, 311
Weiner, N. 5, 46, 147, 168, 206
Weiss, B. 165, 168, 184, 187, 197, 205, 208, 236, 271, 281
Weissbach, H. 265, 280
Werner, U. 91, 120
Wolfe, S.M. 305, 311
Wolff, J. 227, 239
Woodruff, G.N. 213, 238
Yamabe, H. 150, 151, 166
Yamamura, H.I. 191, 196, 200, 204, 205
York, D.H. 104, 110, 120
Young, A.B. 191, 200, 203, 204, 205
Zador, J. 303, 311
Zieve, P.D. 305, 311
Zigmond, M.J. 182, 187
Zirkle, C.L. 217, 239
Zivkovic, B. 153, 157, 159, 162, 164, 167
Zukin, S.R. 191, 197, 200, 204